Essential Abnormal & Clinical Psychology

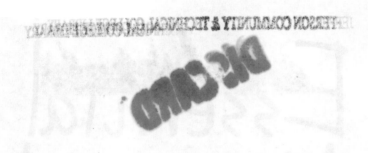

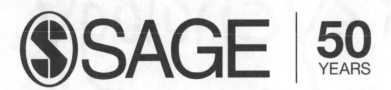

SAGE was founded in 1965 by Sara Miller McCune to support the dissemination of usable knowledge by publishing innovative and high-quality research and teaching content. Today, we publish more than 850 journals, including those of more than 300 learned societies, more than 800 new books per year, and a growing range of library products including archives, data, case studies, reports, and video. SAGE remains majority-owned by our founder, and after Sara's lifetime will become owned by a charitable trust that secures our continued independence.

Los Angeles | London | New Delhi | Singapore | Washington DC

Essential Abnormal & Clinical Psychology

Matt Field & Sam Cartwright-Hatton

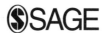

Los Angeles | London | New Delhi
Singapore | Washington DC

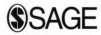

Los Angeles | London | New Delhi
Singapore | Washington DC

SAGE Publications Ltd
1 Oliver's Yard
55 City Road
London EC1Y 1SP

SAGE Publications Inc.
2455 Teller Road
Thousand Oaks, California 91320

SAGE Publications India Pvt Ltd
B 1/I 1 Mohan Cooperative Industrial Area
Mathura Road
New Delhi 110 044

SAGE Publications Asia-Pacific Pte Ltd
3 Church Street
#10-04 Samsung Hub
Singapore 049483

Editor: Luke Block
Production editor: Imogen Roome
Copyeditor: Audrey Scriven
Proofreader: Leigh C. Timmins
Marketing manager: Alison Borg
Cover design: Wendy Scott
Typeset by: C&M Digitals (P) Ltd, Chennai, India
Printed in India at Replika Press Pvt Ltd

Library of Congress Control Number: 2014951829

British Library Cataloguing in Publication data

A catalogue record for this book is available from the British Library

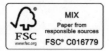

ISBN 978-0-7619-4188-0
ISBN 978-0-7619-4189-7 (pbk)

At SAGE we take sustainability seriously. Most of our products are printed in the UK using FSC papers and boards. When we print overseas we ensure sustainable papers are used as measured by the Egmont grading system. We undertake an annual audit to monitor our sustainability.

Contents

List of Figures and Tables

Figures

Table

About the Authors

Matt Field is a Professor of Psychology at the University of Liverpool. While an undergraduate student at Swansea University, his experience of research investigating depressed mood and alcohol craving motivated him to pursue a career in research. He went on to study conditioning processes in tobacco addiction for his PhD, which he received from the University of Sussex in 2001. Following a three-year spell at the University of Southampton, he moved to the University of Liverpool in 2004. He leads the addiction research group, teaches abnormal and clinical psychology to undergraduate and postgraduate students, and does far too much university administration. He is on the editorial boards of the journals *Addiction*, *Drug and Alcohol Dependence* and *Psychopharmacology*, has published more than 100 articles in peer-reviewed journals (some of them are even quite good!), and this is his first book. He lives with his wife and three cats in Formby.

Sam Cartwright-Hatton is a Professor of Clinical Child Psychology who specialises in anxiety disorders and parenting processes. She started out with an undergraduate degree at the University of Liverpool, and then a PhD at the University of Oxford. This PhD was on anxiety disorders in adults, and despite having almost no existing knowledge of or interest in clinical psychology, by the end of it, she was hooked. At the end of the PhD, to the exasperation of her parents, who thought she might never leave university, she moved to Manchester to train as a clinical psychologist. Since then she has specialised in researching and treating anxiety in young children. She has produced around 50 publications, and this is her fourth book. In 2011 she left rainy Manchester for sunny Brighton, where she continues her research at the University of Sussex and lives with her husband and little girl.

Acknowledgements

Writing this book has been an enjoyable and stimulating experience, but like all big projects it took up *much* more of our time than we anticipated. We are very grateful to the following people who helped to shape it into the finished product: the team at SAGE, particularly Michael Carmichael, Keri Dickens and Chris Kingston, who made some really helpful suggestions to improve the first draft and generally tighten things up; the anonymous reviewers of the first draft, for their thoughtful and detailed comments; Noreen O'Sullivan for sending us *lots* of important articles for the Schizophrenia chapter; Helen Startup for feedback on the Personality Disorders chapter; Andy Jones for his constructive comments on the first drafts of many of the chapters; and Andy Field and Learning Matters for allowing us to adapt some of the material from *Crucial Clinical Psychology*.

Matt Field and Sam Cartwright-Hatton, September 2014

Foreword

This is a timely book, coming in an era when even the most ardent student will find it challenging to navigate through the shifting paradigms that generate waves of often conflicting research findings in the psychological sciences. The authors, with complementary backgrounds in experimental and clinical psychology, make light work of integrating a burgeoning body of research into a clear, comprehensive and engaging volume. I particularly welcome this book because it enables the reader to grasp the fact that they are embarking on a journey of exploration of what is in truth an interdisciplinary, multi-faceted subject: Understanding the mechanisms that govern normal and abnormal psychological processes requires both a wide angle lens and a sharp focus. The authors accomplish this with a lightness of touch that belies the complexity of the subject matter.

The opening chapters equip the reader with the necessary methodological and conceptual tools in areas such as the metrics of normality and abnormality. These and successive chapters begin with a clear set of learning objectives and then offer lucid descriptions of key features, core mechanisms, theoretical models and treatment approaches. This encourages the reader to embrace both the research findings and the 'real world' applications that evolve from them. This also creates an ideal platform on which the student can develop the 'scientist–practitioner' perspective that defines applied psychology, especially in clinical settings. Addressing core processes such as cognitive biases or trans-generational influences such as coercive behaviour in developmental contexts, and much else besides, will provide the reader with plenty of scope for more intensive study or in time the pursuit of definitive career pathways.

Common mental health problems including childhood disorders, depression, anxiety disorders, psychoses, substance misuse problems, eating disorders and personality disorders are thus addressed. In the process the reader is able to gauge and to appreciate the complex interplay of factors that are involved and the sometimes gentle, and often controversial, gradient between what is deemed normal or abnormal and thus needing remediation. In relation to the latter, the book introduces the reader to the key evidence-based treatments for these frequently occurring mental health problems.

I wholeheartedly recommend this book as a comprehensive introduction to the student at undergraduate or postgraduate level.

Dr Frank Ryan

Preface

Many students choose to study psychology because they are interested in psychological disorders. Some want to pursue a career in clinical psychology, counselling or cognitive behaviour therapy so that they can help people who suffer from them. Because abnormal and clinical psychology are so intensively researched, there is a lot of information out there and a correspondingly huge choice of abnormal and clinical psychology textbooks on the market.

We decided to write this book because we felt that many textbooks provide a good overview of everything, but most don't 'drill down' into the details, controversies or debates in research or treatment, and this is because they are trying to give equal coverage to such a huge amount of material. We want this book to be different: we don't pretend to cover everything, but we do introduce the topics and encourage you to think critically about the details of research and the way that research findings are interpreted. If you can develop these critical skills now, you will be able to apply them to other pieces of research that you read in addition to this book.

Who is this book for?

This book is intended to introduce you to the *essentials* of abnormal and clinical psychology. It is an accessible resource for students from a range of disciplines and at different levels. For high school (e.g. A level) and level 1 university courses, it contains everything you need to get a broad understanding of the topics and some idea of the current debates and controversies. At higher levels (e.g. final year undergraduate, and postgraduate) the book should be used as a framework on which to build your own independent reading. Our intention is that all students will benefit from reading the first two chapters, and then you can pick and choose from the other chapters depending on which topics are being covered in your particular course.

Overview of the structure and features of this book

The first two chapters are an introduction to some fundamental issues and you should read these before you dip into any of the subsequent chapters. The first chapter explains some of the current controversies in the way that psychological disorders are categorised and diagnosed, and then introduces you to some important issues regarding research, including how to evaluate research findings in a critical way. The second chapter provides an overview of how psychological disorders are treated, and covers key topics such as the practical problems involved in deciding the best way to treat a distressed patient, and the many ways that we can test whether treatments actually work.

Subsequent chapters (3–11) focus on specific disorders or classes of disorders and you may not need to read all of these, depending on the syllabus of the module you are studying. However, we would hope that you will be sufficiently interested in these topics to want to read the whole book anyway, even if you don't have to! Most of the chapters have the following structure:

- *What is the disorder?* In this section we introduce the classic symptoms and features of the disorder(s), explain how it is diagnosed, and discuss the controversies that surround diagnosis.
- *How does the disorder develop?* In this section we discuss risk factors for the disorder. These usually include heritability, environmental risk factors, and interactions between the two.
- *What is going on in the mind and brain of the sufferer?* In this section, which is usually the longest in the chapter, we introduce theories from psychology and neuroscience that try to make sense of the disorder. In most cases, these theories attempt to explain how risk factors for the disorder lead to changes in psychological function that ultimately lead to the symptoms of the disorder. So, the material in these sections is linked back to the things that were discussed in the previous section.
- *How is the disorder treated?* Here we provide an overview of the most common treatments and we discuss studies that have evaluated how effective those treatments are. Again, we link these treatments back to theories of the disorder(s) and we discuss options for the development of new treatments in the future, based on those theories. To give you a feel for how the theory is actually put into practice, some of the chapters focus on the nuts and bolts of what happens during treatment.

Each chapter includes a number of specific features and text boxes that highlight important issues and will help you to think critically about the material. These are:

- *Assessment targets*: Bear these in mind before you start to read the chapter, and then go back to them when you have finished the chapter. If you cannot answer 'yes' to these questions then look over the chapter again. If you still cannot answer these questions, you should return the book to the shop and demand a refund!
- *Essential diagnosis* boxes: These contain essential criteria for diagnosis of the disorder(s) and are taken straight from the main diagnostic manuals (the *Diagnostic and Statistical Manual of Mental Disorders* and/or the *International Classification of Diseases*). These boxes are important because people tend to have different opinions about what, for example, 'depression' is, so it is necessary to be clear about what clinicians and researchers mean when they talk about any particular disorder
- *Essential experience*: These are usually case studies of people who suffer from a psychological disorder in which they describe their symptoms, how the disorder has affected their life, or how treatment has affected them. You should think about how

these relate to the diagnostic criteria (which can be a bit 'dry' and formal) and also about how they fit, or do not fit, with the theories and evidence described elsewhere in the chapter.

- *Essential debate*: Here we discuss some of the current controversies in a given topic, sometimes based around a published article in a scientific journal. We want you to think about these issues carefully, and also search for other papers that have been published more recently that relate to this debate. For broader issues, these debate boxes have a 'pros versus cons' format, or similar, and in these cases you should think carefully about the issues and make sure that you understand both sides of the argument.

- *Essential research*: Towards the front of the book, these boxes tend to introduce specific research methods that crop up throughout the book, and later on, highlight particular studies that have been influential, or controversial, or both. We want you to think carefully and critically about the research and, as above, conduct your own literature searches to see what has changed since this work was published. Sometimes we discuss fairly old studies that nicely illustrate a particular methodology or robust finding, and have become 'classics'. Other times we focus on more recent studies that could fundamentally change the way we understand a particular disorder, and in other cases we show you why some studies are a bit rubbish and should not be trusted!

- *Essential treatment*: These boxes might describe how a treatment actually works in practice (the 'nuts and bolts'), they might summarise important studies that have evaluated the effectiveness of treatments, or they might highlight recent research that has investigated new types of treatment. Again, we want you to think critically about the material that is presented in these boxes, and ask yourself: Am I convinced by this treatment? Does it follow from the evidence about the disorder, and would I recommend it to a close friend or family member that suffers from this disorder?

- *Essential questions*: These are some examples of coursework or exam questions that test your understanding of the material in the chapter. You could write short essay plans for each question, or if you are really keen you could have a go at writing the essay itself.

Companion Website

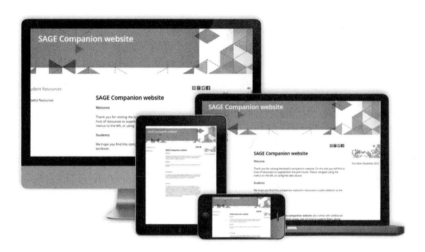

Essential Abnormal and Clinical Psychology is supported by a wealth of online resources for both students and lecturers to aid study and support teaching, which are available at: **study.sagepub.com/fieldcartwrighthatton**

For Students

- **Watch author-selected videos** to give you insight into how an understanding of abnormal and clinical psychology is applied in practice.
- **Interactive quizzes** allow you to test your knowledge and give you feedback to help you prepare for assignments and exams.
- **Weblinks** direct you to relevant resources to deepen your understanding of chapter topics and expand your knowledge of abnormal and clinical psychology.
- **Selected journal articles** give you free access to scholarly articles chosen for each chapter to reinforce your learning of key topics.

For Lecturers

- **PowerPoint slides** featuring figures and tables from the book which can be downloaded and customised for use in your own presentations.
- **Test banks** that provide a diverse range of pre-written options as well as the opportunity to edit any question and/or insert personalised questions to effectively assess students' progress and understanding.

THE BIG ISSUES IN CLASSIFICATION, DIAGNOSIS AND RESEARCH INTO PSYCHOLOGICAL DISORDERS

General introduction

In this chapter, we consider whether it is possible to define what makes some psychological characteristics and behaviours 'abnormal'. We then introduce the *Diagnostic and Statistical Manual of Mental Disorders* and the *International Classification of Diseases*, the two most important classification and diagnostic manuals for psychological disorders. We explain how psychological disorders are diagnosed, and think critically about the problems that arise when applying a 'medical model' of diseases to psychological disorders. In the second part of the chapter we describe and evaluate research methods that are used to study psychological disorders, before considering how very diverse approaches to psychological disorders actually complement rather than compete with each other.

Assessment targets

At the end of the chapter, you should ask yourself the following questions:

- What distinguishes abnormal from healthy psychological functioning?
- Should we categorise and diagnose psychological disorders in the same way as other medical conditions?
- What types of research methods are used to study psychological disorders, and what are the limitations of those methods?
- What are the main approaches to the understanding of psychological disorders, and can they be integrated?

Section 1: What is abnormal?

Defining abnormality

No two people are the same; we all differ in psychological characteristics such as intelligence, sociability, and our general outlook on life ('glass half full or glass half empty'). Because people are so different from each other, this makes it difficult to decide what makes someone 'abnormal' rather than just 'different from me'. To start thinking about what makes behaviour abnormal, it is helpful to think of the 'four Ds' (Bennett, 2005):

- *Deviance* (from the norm) This assumes that there is a normal range for specific aspects of psychological function, and that anyone who falls outside that range might be classed as abnormal. For example, let's imagine that the majority of the population score between 25 and 75 on a 100-point measure of depressed mood. If this was the case, anyone who scored below 25 or above 75 would be considered 'abnormal', and the more extreme their score was, the more abnormal they would be.
- *Distress* This means that a person might be considered abnormal if they feel distressed in some way. This requires us to define 'distress', which isn't too difficult, but what level of distress makes a person abnormal?
- *Dysfunctional* This means that a person is thinking and/or behaving in a way that is hindering their daily life, for example their relationships or their performance at work or school. Again, we need to set a threshold to determine at what point psychological dysfunction is abnormal: nobody is perfectly functional all of the time!
- *Dangerous* This means that a person can be considered abnormal if their psychological condition puts them or other people at risk of harm – for example, someone who feels suicidal, or a person with paranoid delusions that drive them to physically hurt other people.

The 'four Ds' are not intended to be a prescriptive checklist, but they are a useful way of thinking about which kinds of human behaviour are normal, and which kinds are abnormal. Most psychological disorders fit some but not all of the four Ds. For example, a person with generalised anxiety disorder (GAD; see Chapter 6) is in distress, and this is dysfunctional (it prevents them from engaging in many activities). However, it is difficult to say how 'deviant' this is: we all feel anxious from time to time, and GAD is a very common disorder, so is it fair to say that people with GAD are actually any different from 'normal' people? Furthermore, most people with GAD are not a danger to themselves or others.

With regard to the notion of deviance, on what types of individual differences can somebody be 'deviant', in order to be considered abnormal? Perhaps we can start with an extreme depressed mood, but what about intelligence? Is someone abnormal if they are extremely intelligent? As for distress, we need to decide how to define this. It is relatively uncontroversial to say that someone who feels very depressed or anxious is in a state of distress. But we all feel these emotions from time to time, and at certain periods of our lives we may experience them more intensely than others (e.g. when starting a new job, or after a relationship break-up). At what point does distress become a sign of abnormality? Or maybe we shouldn't talk about the severity of distress, but instead focus on how long people have been distressed?

Dysfunctional behaviour is also tricky. If someone is so paralysed by anxiety or depression that they cannot go to work or talk to their friends, then that is dysfunctional. But many other behaviours are dysfunctional in some sense, and we don't consider that people who engage in them are abnormal. For example, young people who use fake ID to buy alcohol and then drink it in the park on a school night are doing something dysfunctional (it is illegal, not good for them and won't help their performance at school). But even though we might not approve of this type of behaviour, many people would not see it as 'abnormal'.

Finally, defining abnormality based on a person being a danger to themself or others is fraught with difficulty. The vast majority of people with psychological disorders do not intend to harm themselves and they pose no risk to others. On the other hand, some people are just bad tempered and physically aggressive – which makes them a risk to others – but this wouldn't necessarily make them candidates for a psychiatric evaluation.

The overarching point is that each of these things is very difficult to define because there are no objective measures for them, and that is because our personal network dictates how we view these things. The example of teenage drinking is a case in point here: this might be viewed as dysfunctional by most members of society, particularly schoolteachers (!), but other groups, such as teenagers, may see it as completely normal and even something to aspire to! There are also cross-cultural differences. For example, in some cultures a person who has 'visions' and speaks to themself is considered to have magical powers, whereas the same behaviour in many European countries would be considered 'abnormal' and cause for psychiatric investigation. Finally, these things have changed over time within cultures. For example, homosexuality was categorised as a psychological disorder until as recently as 1973, but today most people (extreme fringe groups aside) are quite shocked by that historical fact! To give another example, the distinction between someone who suffers from major depressive disorder and someone who is just a bit miserable and pessimistic (but basically 'healthy') is always going to be a difficult call to make. Successive revisions of psychiatric diagnostic manuals have generally reduced their thresholds for making this distinction, such that some-one who would have been considered miserable but healthy in the 1950s might be diagnosed with a major depressive disorder from 2013 onwards (see Chapter 5). We revisit this issue throughout the book.

Section summary

It is impossible to agree on a universal definition of what makes a person 'abnormal'. This is because definitions of abnormality are heavily influenced by broad social and cultural factors, and these are constantly shifting. However, it can be useful to think of the 'four Ds' (deviance, distress, dysfunctional and dangerous) as a starting point.

Section 2: How are psychological disorders classified?

In this section we describe the two main diagnostic systems for psychological disorders: the *Diagnostic and Statistical Manual of Mental Disorders* (or *DSM* for short) and the *International Classification of Diseases* (*ICD*) which includes psychological disorders and is published by the World Health Organisation (WHO) (see www.who.int/classifications/icd/en/). We will show

how these diagnostic systems have changed over time and explain why they are structured in the way that they are. We will also talk about *why* we diagnose psychological disorders, and the advantages that diagnosis offers for their management and treatment.

The *Diagnostic and Statistical Manual of Mental Disorders*

The American Psychiatric Association published the fifth edition of the *Diagnostic and Statistical Manual of Mental Disorders* in 2013 (*DSM*-5; American Psychiatric Association, 2013a) after more than 10 years of development and consultation. The previous version of the *DSM* had separate 'axes' for personality disorders and mental retardation (axis 2) and for all other disorders (axis 1), but this distinction was abolished for *DSM*-5. Disorders are grouped together under the following categories:

- Neurodevelopmental disorders.
- Schizophrenia spectrum and other psychotic disorders (includes Schizophrenia; see Chapter 4).
- Bipolar and related disorders (see Chapter 5).
- Depressive disorders (includes major depressive disorder; see Chapter 5).
- Anxiety disorders (includes Generalised Anxiety Disorder; see Chapter 6), phobias (Chapter 7), panic disorder and social anxiety disorder (Chapter 8).
- Obsessive-compulsive and related disorders.
- Trauma and stressor-related disorders.
- Dissociative disorders.
- Somatic symptoms and related disorders.
- Feeding and eating disorders (includes binge-eating disorder, bulimia nervosa and anorexia nervosa; see Chapter 10).
- Elimination disorders.
- Sleep-Wake disorders.
- Sexual dysfunctions.
- Gender dysphoria.
- Disruptive, impulse-control and conduct disorders.
- Substance-related and addictive disorders (see Chapter 9).
- Neurocognitive disorders.
- Personality disorders (see Chapter 11).
- Paraphilic disorders.

Most categories contain a number of specific disorders that are related to each other. For example, the 'Anxiety Disorders' category contains 12 different disorders including Generalised Anxiety Disorder (GAD). The distinctive features of each disorder are then listed, together with any exclusion criteria. When we talk about 'features' we can distinguish between 'symptoms' (which the patient can report on, and is often distressed by) and 'signs' (which are directly observed, usually by a clinician). The diagnostic criteria for GAD are shown in Box 1.1.

Box 1.1   Example of *DSM* diagnostic criteria

The *DSM*-5 (American Psychiatric Association, 2013a) characterises generalised anxiety disorder as follows:

A. Excessive anxiety and worry (apprehensive expectation), occurring more days than not for at least 6 months, about a number of events or activities (such as work or school performance).
B. The individual finds it difficult to control the worry.
C. The anxiety and worry are associated with three (or more) of the following six symptoms (with at least some symptoms present for more days than not for the past six months):

   * restlessness or feeling keyed up or on edge;
   * being easily fatigued;
   * difficulty concentrating or mind going blank;
   * irritability;
   * muscle tension;
   * sleep disturbance (difficulty falling or staying asleep, or restless, unsatisfying sleep).

D. The anxiety, worry or physical symptoms cause clinically significant distress or impairment in social, occupational, or other important areas of functioning
E. The disturbance is not attributable to the physiological effects of a substance, or another medical condition.
F. The disturbance is not better explained by another psychological disorder

When we look at these features it is helpful to think back to how these relate to our conceptions of 'abnormality' which we discussed in the previous section. In particular, some of the 'four Ds' are evident in the criteria for GAD: sufferers feel *distress*, and the anxiety is *dysfunctional*. However, it is difficult to get an idea of how *deviant* these features are: Would you say that someone who had these symptoms is different from another person who is 'normal'? Do you think different people would agree on this?

The *International Classification of Diseases*

The tenth version of the International Classification of Diseases was published by the World Health Organisation in 1992 (World Health Organisation, 1992). Another revision is now underway and is likely to be published in 2017. Unlike the *DSM*, which is published by a psychiatric association and is limited to mental disorders, the *ICD* is a broad diagnostic bible for every kind of medical condition imaginable. A subsection is devoted to 'Mental and Behavioural Disorders', and within this are different categories of disorders (e.g. 'Mood Disorders'; 'Neurotic, Stress-Related and Somatoform Disorders'), and within these categories sit the specific disorders. As with *DSM*-5, specific disorders are described in terms of their characteristic signs and symptoms, and any exclusion criteria that they might have. The *ICD*-10 criteria for Generalized Anxiety Disorder are shown in Box 1.2, and you can compare them with the *DSM*-5 criteria for the same disorder in Box 1.1.

Box 1.2   Essential diagnosis

Generalised Anxiety Disorder

The *ICD*-10 (World Health Organisation, 1992) criteria for Generalised Anxiety Disorder are:

A. A period of at least six months with prominent tension, worry, and feelings of apprehension, about every-day events and problems.
B. At least four of the following symptoms are present, one of which must be from (1):

1. Palpitations or pounding heart; sweating; trembling or shaking; dry mouth.
2. Difficulty breathing; feeling of choking; chest pain or discomfort; nausea or abdominal distress; feeling dizzy, faint or light-headed; feeling that objects are unreal ('derealisation') or that one's self is distant or 'not really here' (depersonalization); fear of losing control, going crazy, or passing out.

We can see that both classification systems highlight the importance of 'worry' and physical indicators of anxiety, and both specify that symptoms need to be present for at least six months in order for a diagnosis to be made. Both *DSM*-5 and *ICD*-10 require symptoms to cause impairment or distress, and they specify the requirement to rule out other medical conditions or psychological disorders as causes of the symptoms (these criteria are explicit in *ICD*-10, but they are listed elsewhere in the manual rather than alongside the criteria for individual disorders). There are some differences too: the *DSM*-5 criteria are explicit that worry should be 'uncontrollable', whereas the *ICD*-10 criteria attach more weight to the physical signs of increased arousal. These points of divergence may be important, because different people may meet the criteria for GAD depending on which diagnostic system is used (Nilsson et al., 2012).

There are also some differences in the way that *DSM*-5 and *ICD*-10 are organised. For example, *ICD*-10 puts the Somatoform disorders in with other Anxiety Disorders, whereas *DSM*-5 treats them as distinct categories. However, overall there are more similarities than differences between the two classification systems. In most chapters of this book we list the *ICD*-10 criteria, but we point out notable differences between *ICD*-10 and *DSM*-5 where they occur.

Most significantly, both classification systems treat psychological disorders as distinct from each other: they specify that each disorder has characteristic clusters of symptoms, and disorders are qualitatively different from 'normal' human experience.

Why do we classify psychological disorders in this way?

In other branches of medicine, disease classification systems are incredibly useful because the signs and symptoms of medical conditions are (relatively) easy to detect and measure. This enables doctors to quickly and efficiently check that a patient has the symptoms of a given disorder (e.g. influenza or tonsillitis), and then make a diagnosis that determines the most appropriate treatment. The same logic has been applied to the classification of psychological disorders, resulting in the *DSM* and *ICD*. Looking beyond the individual patient, the idea is that classification and diagnosis help us to understand psychological disorders and devise better treatments for them. It would be impossible for us to diagnose, understand, conduct research into and treat schizophrenia if we could not agree on what schizophrenia was, and what its defining features were. This is discussed in Box 1.3.

Box 1.3   Essential experience

What if we didn't categorise psychological disorders?

Imagine a parallel universe in which psychological disorders are not categorised, everyone is treated as an individual and similarities between people are ignored. A patient, Bob, goes to see his doctor, complaining of hearing voices that tell him what to do. Bob is also paranoid that the government are following him. While talking to Bob the doctor notices that his mood seems 'flat' (he doesn't react to things that would make other people happy or sad), and he doesn't seem to have washed or changed his clothes for several weeks.

The doctor has no idea what to do, so he just tries different treatments at random. He refers Bob for some counselling, but this doesn't help. Neither do antidepressant drugs.

If only somebody had recorded the details of previous patients who had similar symptoms and signs to Bob! With enough patients, we might have seen that certain symptoms and signs seem to cluster together (in this case hallucinations, delusions, affective flattening and social dysfunction). Eventually we might conclude that these symptoms point towards the diagnosis of a particular disorder (schizophrenia, in this case). Once we get this far, we can conduct some research into its causes, how it progresses, and what is the best way to treat it. Over time we can build up a lot of useful information about this 'disorder'. And once we reach this stage, the next time a patient like Bob presents to his doctor with these symptoms, the doctor can make a diagnosis and quickly work out which types of treatments are likely to be effective.

Both the *DSM* and the *ICD* are constantly being refined. As new research is published we gain a better idea of the key features of different disorders: we learn about which disorders are distinct from each other and which share sufficient overlap with other disorders to suggest that they should be categorised together. In the next section, we consider the general limitations of this approach to describing and categorising psychological disorders.

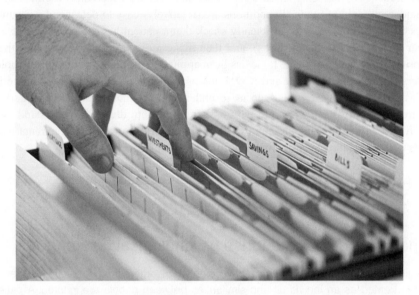

Figure 1.1   Is it appropriate to categorise psychological disorders in the way that we do?

Section summary

We have shown how the *DSM* and *ICD* organise their categorisation of psychological disorders, and have given some examples of how the 'four Ds' are applied in practice. We have also offered a broad defence of this general approach to psychological disorders. In the next section we consider some of the problems that are caused by this approach to psychological disorders, and we consider the alternatives.

Section 3: What are the problems with the diagnostic approach?

In this section we take a critical look at the diagnostic approach. In particular, we consider whether a diagnosis helps patients, and whether it is a good way to progress our understanding of psychological disorders. We discuss the assumptions that psychological disorders fit into neat categories that can be reliably discriminated from each other, and that people with psychological disorders are qualitatively different from 'normal', psychologically healthy people. We then evaluate alternatives to diagnosis including case formulation and the symptom-based approach. We will focus on the *DSM* here, but this discussion applies equally to the *ICD*.

Are the *DSM* and *ICD* reliable and valid?

A good classification system needs to be both reliable and valid. Reliability refers to the fact that if different clinicians were to diagnose the same person, that person should always be classified with the same disorder. A diagnostic system would not be reliable if, for example, one clinician used it to diagnose someone as having obsessive-compulsive disorder whereas another clinician interviewed the same person and diagnosed them with schizophrenia. Generally, *DSM* diagnoses have acceptable reliability (Regier et al., 2013), although reliability may be higher for common disorders such as the anxiety and mood disorders (Brown et al., 2001) compared to disorders with more diverse symptoms (Bentall, 2003; Hyman, 2010). According to the APA, the use of standardised interview techniques and more explicit criteria in successive versions of *DSM* have improved its reliability.

Reliability is necessary for validity, but it is not sufficient. The validity of a classification can be assessed in many ways. We could ask whether the diagnostic criteria have intuitive validity: Do they describe the disorders in an intuitively accurate way? In some cases this is arguably not the case (see 'Homogeneity of sufferers', below). Other issues are whether we can isolate causal factors for particular disorders (*etiological validity*), and many critics of the *DSM* and *ICD* would argue that this is not the case: there are shared causes for many different psychological disorders (e.g. experiencing a stressful life event during childhood), as you will see throughout this book. We can also ask whether a diagnosis can be used to predict how someone with a particular disorder will respond to treatment. Arguably the *DSM* and *ICD* fail this test, because many clinicians who diagnose their patients with a psychological disorder will try several different medications and/or psychological treatments before they find one that 'works'. These criteria for assessing validity may seem harsh, but classification systems used in other branches of medicine tend to fare much better than the *DSM* does.

Are disorders distinct from each other?

A good classification system should produce mutually exclusive disorders, yet there is considerable co-occurrence between disorders (known as *co-morbidity*). For example, the lifetime co-morbidity between major depressive disorder and generalised anxiety disorder may be as high as 73% (Lewinsohn et al., 1997) and there is considerable overlap between the symptoms of schizophrenia and those of bipolar disorder (particularly manic episodes): some treatments seem to be equally effective for both conditions. But this overlap in symptoms is not really acknowledged in the *DSM*, which treats them as totally distinct entities. Substance use disorders (see Chapter 9) are also highly comorbid with most other psychological disorders, including mood disorders (see Chapter 5), anxiety disorders (see Chapters 6, 7 and 8), schizophrenia (see Chapter 4) and personality disorders (see Chapter 11). If there is so much overlap between (supposedly distinct) disorders, this undermines a core assumption of the diagnostic approach.

Homogeneity of sufferers: Are all patients the same?

Classification imposes homogeneity within disorders and encourages clinicians to ignore the individual characteristics of a particular patient. One criticism that has been levelled at the *DSM* is that the diagnostic criteria for schizophrenia (for example) are so broad that, in principle, two patients could present with totally different symptoms – with no overlap between them at all – yet they may both receive a diagnosis of schizophrenia (we discuss this in more detail in Chapter 4). This is not an ideal situation for the patient, because a clinician may make the diagnosis and then use that to prescribe medication or a psychological treatment which may not help that particular patient.

It is worth pointing out, however, that some clinicians would argue that this issue has been exaggerated, and would also counter-argue that, for example, 'I know a schizophrenic patient when I see one'. The point here is that although disorders can present in many different ways, there are sufficient similarities between most patients with (for example) schizophrenia that a diagnosis can be made quite quickly and without difficulty in the majority of cases.

Lowering the thresholds

A big criticism of *DSM*-5 in particular is that the thresholds for diagnosing some disorders have been lowered from those used in *DSM-IV*, which continues a historical trend. For example, a person who might have been classed as healthy but 'a bit of a worrier' 50 years ago might receive a diagnosis of generalized anxiety disorder if they were to be assessed today (see Chapter 6). Someone who is in the depths of despair after a bereavement might receive a diagnosis of major depressive disorder now, whereas the 'bereavement exclusion' in *DSM-IV* meant that they would probably not have received that diagnosis before 2013 (see Chapter 5). We give other examples of this throughout the book.

The consequence of this slippage of diagnostic criteria is that the boundaries between 'normal' and 'abnormal' are becoming blurred, to the extent that we may soon reach a point where there will be more people in the world with a psychological disorder than without one (if we haven't already reached this point). A fundamental feature of classification approaches to psychological disorders (and indeed any illness) is that there must be a clear distinction between people who are healthy and those who are unwell: a dichotomy between 'normal' and 'abnormal' psychological functioning. This dichotomy looks increasingly implausible as the thresholds are adjusted downwards.

What are the alternatives to diagnosis?

The symptom-based approach

Some psychologists favour abolishing the diagnostic approach to psychological disorders altogether, and would prefer to treat *patients* according to their individual symptoms. For example, patient A might have moderate depressive rumination, moderate problems controlling their drinking and occasionally experience auditory hallucinations, but have no other symptoms. On the other hand, patient B might have serious problems getting to sleep, and severe depressive rumination and uncontrollable worry, but no other symptoms. A radical alternative to the diagnostic approach would be to conduct research into the causes and optimal treatment for these different symptoms (rather than disorders), such that patients A and B here would receive treatment that is tailored to their own individual symptoms. In principle, this might even stretch to prescribing drugs for one symptom (e.g. antidepressant drugs for depressed mood) and psychological treatment for another (e.g. CBT to help someone reduce their alcohol consumption). There have been some notable successes of this approach when applied to our understanding of the development of different symptoms of schizophrenia (see Chapter 4), and in many ways this approach is similar to what happens during psychological case formulation (see below). Another advantage here is that it does not require clinicians to set a threshold for determining whether a person's levels of a psychological construct (e.g. depressed mood) are 'normal' or 'abnormal'. Instead, a symptom only requires treatment if a patient is bothered by it!

If we go back to the original rationale for diagnosing and classifying psychological disorders (discussed in Section 2), however, we arrive at a criticism of this type of approach. Clinicians will readily acknowledge that many of their patients do not neatly 'fit' the diagnostic criteria for one particular disorder to the exclusion of all other disorders. For example, patient A, above, seems to have some (but not all) of the symptoms of major depressive disorder, alcohol use disorder and schizophrenia. But this is just one individual: when we study large numbers of people, we see that certain symptoms do tend to cluster together, which implies that there is some kind of underlying 'disorder' that is characterised by a cluster of symptoms. If we were to focus on individual symptoms, this might be less useful than trying to treat the disorder as a whole.

Psychological formulation (or case formulation)

Psychological formulation is employed by clinical psychologists and psychotherapists, particularly those who are sceptical of the medical model and diagnostic approach to psychological disorders. The aim of psychological formulation is to identify the nature and causes of patients' symptoms and then devise the most appropriate treatment on an *individual basis*. For example, patient A may experience auditory hallucinations and delusions along with other symptoms of schizophrenia (see Chapter 4). An overworked clinician following the diagnostic approach and medical model might make a diagnosis of schizophrenia and recommend a standard course of antipsychotic medication, without giving this much thought. On the other hand, a clinician who has the time might work up a case formulation to identify the root causes of *that particular patient*'s hallucinations and delusions (which might, for example, be related to sexual abuse experienced during childhood), and then develop a psychological intervention that is tailored to the specific symptoms of that patient.

After reading this chapter you may be encouraged to learn that if you ever have psychological problems and you are seen by a psychologist or psychiatrist, they may diagnose you with a psychological disorder (so, they will follow the diagnostic approach). However, any treatment that you receive will probably be heavily influenced by their psychological formulation of you as an individual. The weaknesses of a case formulation approach are similar to those for the symptom-specific approach. You could also go back to Box 1.3 and think about the risks of this approach if completed instead of (rather than in addition to) a diagnosis. However, the case formulation approach is often used alongside the diagnostic approach, so any benefits from following the diagnostic approach are not lost. We will come back to this issue in Chapter 2.

Section summary

In this section we have highlighted the limitations of a diagnostic approach to psychological disorders. While classification systems such as the *DSM* and *ICD* are generally reliable, their validity is questionable. Different disorders are supposed to be distinct from each other, which makes it difficult to explain high rates of comorbidity between these. On the other hand, two people could be diagnosed with the same disorder even if they have no symptoms in common at all. Finally, the gradual lowering of thresholds for diagnosis of psychological disorders means that the boundaries between 'normal' and 'abnormal' psychological function are becoming less distinct over time. Alternatives to diagnosis such as the symptom-specific approach and case formulation offer some advantages, but they have their own problems.

Section 4: How do we conduct research into psychological disorders?

Developments in research mean that we are constantly expanding our knowledge of psychological disorders, and coming up with new ways to treat them. In this section we will take a critical look at some of the research methods that are used in the field and highlight some controversies that have arisen because of poor research methods, statistics or an inappropriate interpretation of results. This will help you evaluate the research presented in this book, as well as any scientific papers you read alongside it. Research methods used to evaluate treatments for psychological disorders are covered in Chapter 2.

What do researchers measure?

Many psychological disorders are characterised by 'abnormal' subjective experience, and therefore it is important to record subjective states accurately. A clinician may get an initial idea of how an individual is feeling and what they are thinking during an informal consultation or a more formal and structured clinical interview. However, the most widely used measures of subjective states in research are self-report measures, such as single item visual analogue scale (VAS) measures of mood, and standardised questionnaires of depressed mood such as the Beck Depression Inventory (BDI; see Beck et al., 1988), that contain many different items.

Measurements of physiological activity can also provide a good indicator of a person's emotional state. For example, heart rate, blood pressure and skin conductance (which measures sweat gland activity) are used to measure the degree of physiological arousal, which can be particularly useful if you are interested in the strength of a spider phobic's reaction to a picture of a spider and how this reactivity changes over the course of therapy, for example (see Chapter 7).

Cognitive processes play a key role in many psychological disorders. In some cases these cognitions are best measured by simply asking participants what they are thinking about (e.g. in the case of delusions in schizophrenic patients). However, in other cases more indirect measures might be used. For example, many disorders are characterised by an *attentional bias* for disorder-relevant stimuli (e.g. an anxious patient may find their attention drawn to sources of threat in their environment; see Chapter 6). While people may know that their attention tends to be captured by certain types of things in their environment, they will rarely have good insight into the magnitude of their attentional biases (which can be very subtle), and for this reason it can be useful to measure their attention directly. To overcome this, we can measure attentional biases directly by monitoring participants' eye movements, or we can use reaction time tests that allow us to make inferences about what people are attending to (see Box 6.4, Chapter 6).

Other reaction time measures can be useful for measuring subtle cognitive distortions that people may not be aware of. For example, the implicit association test (IAT) requires people to quickly categorise different types of words in order to calculate the strength of their automatic associations between different categories of objects, for example associations between the concepts of 'spider' and 'bad' as opposed to 'spider' and 'good'. The strength of their automatic associations can be a better predictor of their actual response to spiders than their self-reported attitudes to spiders (Teachman & Woody, 2003; see Chapter 7). Moving beyond reaction time tests, researchers have developed thousands of cognitive tests that are used to obtain direct measures of psychological constructs (e.g. working memory, risk taking), which is particularly useful when people don't have a very good insight into a particular construct.

Finally, activity in the brain can be directly measured using techniques such as electroencephalography (EEG) and functional magnetic resonance imaging (fMRI). These methods work in different ways: EEG involves placing electrodes on the scalp to measure tiny fluctuations in electrical activity, which can then be used to make inferences about activation in areas of the brain close to the position of the electrodes. With fMRI, changes in blood flow in the brain are used to make inferences about which parts of the brain are most active (and which areas are relatively less active) in research participants. These techniques have led to rapid advances in our understanding of the patterns of brain activation that correspond to different psychological states (e.g. feeling afraid, or craving a drug), and they have helped us to characterise abnormalities of brain structure and function in psychological disorders.

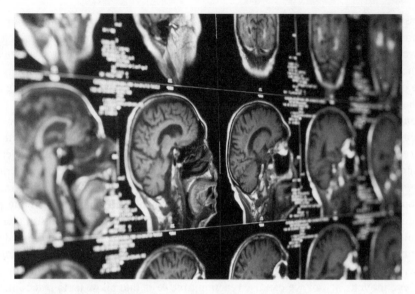

Figure 1.2 Different instruments can be used to measure brain structure and activity in the brain while people perform tasks or look at different types of stimuli

Each of these research methods plays a crucial role in our understanding of psychological disorders, and the best types of research will use a combination of these methods to answer a research question.

What types of research methods are used?

Qualitative versus quantitative methods

Most of the methods we will discuss are *quantitative*: you take a group of people, measure something or other (e.g. their blood pressure, or how anxious they feel), and then you report the *average* value for that measurement for all of your participants. You might test two different groups (e.g. one group that have been diagnosed with a spider phobia and a control group who have not), or you might do something to your participants (e.g. show them a picture of a spider) before you take your measurement, or perhaps take your measurements twice (e.g. once before a course of exposure therapy and once afterwards). The important point here is that you are not just testing one person; you are testing a group of people, measuring something or other, and you are interested in how these measurements vary *on average*.

Qualitative research methods are used less frequently but you will come across them. Their aim is to gather an in-depth understanding of human experience by talking to only a few people, asking them some broad questions and then letting them talk while you record what they say. The discussion is transcribed and the researcher looks for recurring themes that crop up across different people. To give an example, Cutting and Dunne (1989) administered an open-ended interview to patients with schizophrenia in order to understand the subjective experience of being in a psychotic state. They then conducted some additional studies in which they refined the questions that they asked, which enabled them to 'hone in' on the most important aspects of the experiences of schizophrenic patients.

Qualitative research has a long history in psychology. Wilhelm Wundt, who is often seen as the founder of scientific psychology, viewed it as a vital bridge between philosophy and rigorous experimental research. For the majority of the twentieth century (when behaviourism and then cognitive psychology were the dominant paradigms in psychology) qualitative research was viewed as subjective, prone to bias from the experimenter, and therefore something to be avoided. It is important to note that modern qualitative methods go to great lengths to minimise bias from the experimenter and make things as objective as possible. Furthermore, as we will see later in this chapter, there are many biases in quantitative methods that manifest themselves in more subtle ways. Many researchers would agree that qualitative research continues to occupy the important niche that was advocated by Wundt: a way to gain rich insights into human experience in order to generate new measures and theoretical models, which in turn lead to hypotheses that can be tested in quantitative research.

Box 1.4   Advantages and disadvantages of qualitative research

Advantages

- It allows for a rich and deep understanding of human experience.
- It can form the basis for the development of theories and hypotheses that can be tested in quantitative research.

Disadvantages:

- It is prone to bias from the researcher, because whatever a person says can be interpreted to fit the existing beliefs of that researcher (although modern qualitative methods take steps to avoid this).
- One must be cautious when generalising findings beyond the individuals who were studied, although this problem also affects most quantitative research too.

We now move on to discuss the various types of quantitative methods.

Cross-sectional research

Cross-sectional studies are probably the easiest type to do and for that reason there are a lot of them! Here, you take a group of participants with a psychological disorder, and a control group of participants who don't have that disorder. You measure various things and look for differences between the two groups. For example, one of your authors was involved in a study (Mogg et al., 2003) which recruited a group of dependent tobacco smokers and a control group of non-smokers. All participants completed a computerised measure of attentional bias for smoking cues whilst their eye movements were recorded. Their results showed that the tobacco smokers had an attentional bias for smoking pictures: they looked at those pictures for longer than neutral pictures. However, the non-smoker control group did not show this bias.

Cross-sectional research is a very powerful tool for describing and characterising psychological disorders, and along with clinical observations such studies are often the starting point for the development of theories. Theories then make novel hypotheses that need to be tested with different types of research designs (often prospective and experimental studies, to be discussed next).

Another way that cross-sectional studies are used is to look at the relationships between different psychological constructs within groups of people. For example, in the Mogg et al. (2003) study, a secondary finding was that in smokers attentional biases for smoking cues were positively correlated with the strength of the self-reported craving for tobacco.

The main limitation of cross-sectional studies is that we cannot make any *causal inferences* from this type of research. To return to the study from Mogg et al., this study tells us that smokers have an attentional bias for smoking pictures and non-smokers do not, but we cannot work out from this whether regular smoking causes an attentional bias to develop, or whether attentional bias is what makes people start smoking. It is possible that both explanations are true, and a third possibility is that neither variable causes the other, but both are linked by a hidden third variable that was not measured in that particular study. In this example, it could be that favourable attitudes to smoking develop in some people (perhaps because they hang around with others who smoke), and this increases both their attentional bias for smoking pictures and the likelihood that they will start smoking.

Box 1.5   Advantages and disadvantages of cross-sectional research

Advantages

- It enables us to characterise psychological disorders accurately (e.g. 'cigarette smokers have an attentional bias for smoking pictures, but non-smokers do not').
- It enables us to characterise the relationships between different psychological constructs.

Disadvantages

- It cannot be used to infer causal relationships between variables, or to infer that psychological process X is what causes psychological disorder Y to develop.

Prospective (or longitudinal) research designs

With prospective studies we measure one or more things in our participants at one point in time (as we would in a cross-sectional study), but then we arrange to see our participants again at a later point in time in order to take some more measurements. The two main uses of prospective designs in clinical psychology are to predict the *onset* of psychological disorders in people who do not have the disorder at the beginning of your study, and to predict general psychological functioning or the *recurrence* (or *relapse*) of symptoms in people who have been diagnosed with a disorder but have recovered after treatment. One example of the first type of prospective study is the Cognitive Vulnerability to Depression Project (Alloy et al., 1999), which showed that young people who had a pessimistic thinking style (but were not actually depressed at the time) were much more likely to be diagnosed with major depressive disorder five years later compared to people who were not so pessimistic (this study is discussed in detail in Chapter 5). Examples of the second type of prospective study are those which show that general cognitive impairments in schizophrenic patients are very good predictors of how well individuals will function (e.g. live independently, maintain friendships) after they have received treatment (Green, 2006; see also Chapter 4).

Prospective studies are very useful for several reasons. From a theoretical perspective most psychological disorders have several distinctive symptoms (e.g. depressed mood, anhedonia and sleep disturbance in major depressive disorder), and it can be difficult to know which (if any) of these symptoms plays the most important role in maintaining the disorder, or in causing it to develop in the first place. Prospective studies go beyond cross-sectional studies (which can only ever be descriptive) because they move us closer to an understanding of the psychological characteristics that cause the disorder to develop, or maintain it once it has initially appeared.

Prospective studies are also useful from a clinical perspective. It can be very helpful to know which psychological characteristics in a schizophrenic patient are related to their future recovery, because the clinician can track changes in these characteristics in order to gauge when the patient is sufficiently well recovered. Even more useful, in many cases it is possible to directly target those characteristics during therapy, for example targeting depressogenic cognitions during CBT for major depressive disorder (see Chapter 5).

However, despite going beyond cross-sectional studies and hinting at causal relationships, prospective studies still don't tell us about causality because they don't enable us to rule out hidden 'third variables', as discussed in the previous section about cross-sectional research. To expand on the example that we discussed there, it could be that attentional bias predicts a relapse to smoking in the future among people who have been successfully treated and have managed to quit. But that wouldn't mean that attentional bias is the *cause* of a relapse to smoking. Instead, attentional bias might just serve as a cognitive marker of an underlying social or biological process that is what really determines whether someone will relapse or not. If this is true, then we wouldn't expect attentional bias modification (see Chapter 6) to be a useful treatment for nicotine addiction (Field et al., 2014; see also Chapter 9).

> # Box 1.6 Advantages and disadvantages of prospective research designs
>
> *Advantages*
>
> - They enable us to move beyond characterising psychological disorders and investigate the specific psychological processes that are related to the development of disorders, their maintenance, or a recurrence of symptoms after treatment.
> - They can help clinicians to identify (and target) the most important symptoms.
>
> *Disadvantages*
>
> - Although they hint at causal relationships, prospective studies cannot definitively show cause and effect because there is always the possibility of results being influenced by a hidden variable.

Experimental research designs

With experimental research designs, we experimentally manipulate one or more variables (the *independent variable(s)*) in order to examine its influence on one or more *dependent variables*. For example, Broeren and colleagues (2011) were interested in the influence of peer modelling on fear beliefs in children. They conducted an experimental study in which children watched a short video that showed a child of their own age interacting either fearfully or confidently with a novel animal (a rare type of guinea pig). Before and after watching the video, the children reported how fearful they felt about that animal. They found that children who had seen the 'fearful' video reported being more fearful of the animal after seeing the video, but the children who had seen the 'confident' video were less fearful of the animal after seeing the video.

Studies such as this are very useful because they establish a clear cause-and-effect relationship between two variables. In this case, the variables were the peer modelling of fear (the independent variable) and fear beliefs (the dependent variable). The aim of the study was to test theoretical models which predict that children acquire fear beliefs (e.g. 'spiders are dangerous') because they see other people behaving fearfully in response to spiders. The best way to test this theoretical prediction was to experimentally manipulate the peer modelling of fearful behaviours, and to do this using a novel animal which people didn't have any pre-existing fear beliefs about (so, not spiders then!). And that is exactly what the researchers did.

One criticism of experimental studies is that they often seem very artificial and far removed from the 'real world'. In the example above, you might say that a staged video of a child acting fearfully in the presence of an odd-looking rodent, followed immediately by questions about how scary that rodent is, is *not* how peer modelling works in real life. That might well be true, but researchers designing an experimental study will (usually) go to great lengths to remove or control for any 'confounding' variables that could obscure or exaggerate the influence of the independent variable on the dependent variable. Often, the resulting experiment can seem a bit 'silly' and artificial, detached from the real world, but you have to keep sight of the goal of experimental studies (which is to observe the influence of variable X on variable Y). It's also worth pointing out that many experimental studies are more complex than this: they might, for example, investigate how two independent variables interact to influence a dependent variable. In addition, there are lots of good examples of experimental research being conducted in more naturalistic settings outside of the laboratory.

Box 1.7   Advantages and disadvantages of experimental research designs

Advantages

- They allow us to study the causal relationships between two variables, which goes beyond showing that these variables are related (cross-sectional studies) and that one predicts the other over a period of time (prospective studies).

Disadvantages

- A well-controlled experiment can seem very artificial, and far removed from how psychological disorders work in the real world.

The combination of experimental, prospective and cross-sectional research designs has great explanatory power. Cross-sectional designs can tell us about the psychological variables that characterise psychological disorders, prospective studies can tell us which of those variables is actually an important determinant of the onset of the disorder or a recurrence of symptoms after treatment, whereas experimental studies complement this by telling us that variable X does (or does not) have a causal influence on variable Y. A nice example comes from research on the role of depressogenic cognitions in major depressive disorder. The first step was to establish that depressed people think in a more pessimistic way than non-depressed controls, which they do (Haaga et al., 1991). Subsequent years saw a combination of prospective and experimental studies that established cause and effect. Prospective studies revealed that depressogenic cognitions preceded the onset of major depressive episodes several years later, and experimental studies showed that the induction of negative mood led to the reactivation of pessimistic cognitions in formerly depressed patients, and the degree of reactivation predicted the recurrence of symptoms several months later (Scher et al., 2005; see also Chapter 5).

How to think critically about research

When we read about a piece of research we would like to think that it is describing some fundamental 'truth'. For example, if we read about a research study which shows that people who possess a certain gene variant are more likely to develop depression if they also experience traumatic life events (Caspi et al., 2003) we would like to file this away as a proven 'fact'. Unfortunately, with this example (and many others in psychology, and science in general), other studies will try to replicate this research study, but they will get different results from those reported in the original study (see Box 5.4 in Chapter 5) which is called a *failure to replicate*. This state of affairs can be very confusing for students and researchers, because we need to know about what is 'true' and what isn't. In this section we will think about why a published research finding does not necessarily represent the 'truth'.

Sampling

Firstly, we have to remember that any research project can only take a *sample* of people with a given characteristic (e.g. a diagnosis of schizophrenia). Imagine that you were given the task of coming up with an answer to the question of 'How much salt is there in seawater on planet Earth?'. You could just pop down to your nearest beach (let's say this is Brighton), take a litre of seawater, give it to someone who can analyse the salinity of that water, and wait for the results. You might then use those results to make a generalisation about the salinity of all of the seawater on Earth. But why should we assume that the salinity of seawater near Brighton is the same as that in the sea somewhere else (e.g. off the coast of Indonesia)? What about sea water that is at the bottom of a 12-mile deep trench in the Pacific Ocean; does our generalisation apply here? The answer to this question – which is 3.5%, on average – can only come from taking multiple different samples, from as many sites as possible, as far apart as possible, at different depths, and by making sure that each sample is based on an *accurate measurement* of salinity.

Unfortunately, a lot of psychology research is based on a fairly specific sample, and the things that psychologists are interested in are not easy to measure. This has big implications for the generalisability of findings from one study to another. For example, let's say we work in Liverpool and we want to recruit some patients with eating disorders for our research project. If we were to do the project properly, we would do our best to recruit from different cities (e.g. Liverpool and Manchester), as well as rural areas (e.g. Cheshire and Lancashire) nearby, and we would try to recruit people with different socio-economic backgrounds and levels of education. Good quality research projects will achieve this. In an ideal world, researchers would work with other researchers in other countries in order to make sure that the final sample of participants is as diverse as possible. Sometimes this happens, but for practical and financial reasons it usually doesn't. Even when it does, and research participants come from different countries, the recruiting countries tend to be quite similar, for example the UK and the USA rather than the UK and China.

What this means is that the vast majority of research findings are based on fairly restricted samples of people (in the aforementioned example, this would be people from the north west of England), but those findings are used to make generalisations about the psychological processes involved in psychological disorders for all human beings. It is of course possible that the psychology of eating disorders will be similar in people recruited from Liverpool and Beijing, but it is also very possible that there will be important differences: when people look for cross-cultural differences, they tend to find them. To make matters worse, the participants who are tested in a lot of psychology research (particularly research involving 'healthy' participants) are drawn from an even more restricted population: well-educated and relatively affluent people aged between 18 and 21 (i.e. university undergraduates)!

Publication bias

One pessimistic view is that many, perhaps the majority, of published research findings may be 'false' (Ioannidis, 2005) in the sense that they do not describe reality accurately. This is because results that are novel and which support the researchers' hypotheses are likely to be published in scientific journals, whereas studies that don't find what the researchers expected to find, or fail to replicate earlier findings, are less likely to be published. Unfortunately, scientific progress is heavily dependent on such negative findings, because the biggest advances come from *disproving* hypotheses (forcing us to think of better theories) rather than confirming hypotheses. However, 'false positive' findings are more likely to be published in scientific journals than 'true negative' findings, for several reasons:

1. Most published studies do not test enough participants and therefore they do not have adequate statistical power, which means that they are more likely to reveal statistically significant findings by chance, or fail to detect 'real' effects if these exist (Button et al., 2013).
2. The way in which we test for statistically significant relationships or differences (called Null Hypothesis Significance Testing) is applied incorrectly most of the time (Dienes, 2011).
3. The 'incentive structures' in place for researchers tend to encourage this whole state of affairs. In essence, scientific journals prefer to publish novel and statistically significant findings, and researchers – including your lecturers, and the authors of this book – progress up the career ladder by publishing lots of research papers. To make matters worse, it is common for researchers to engage in 'Questionable Research Practices' (QRPs) which basically involve 'bending the rules' in order to nudge their research findings over the threshold of statistical significance (Simmons et al., 2011). Some people argue that QRPs are so widespread in psychology and some other sciences that we need a complete overhaul of the way in which scientific journals select papers for publication, and the ways in which researchers are promoted up the ranks by their employers.

4. Finally, much research is conducted by commercial organisations that have a clear financial interest in the outcomes of that research. The most obvious example here is pharmaceutical companies, who are frequently accused of painting an overly-optimistic picture of the effectiveness of their own drugs (Goldacre, 2012). But they aren't the only ones. For example, a researcher may have invested a lot of time and effort in developing and evaluating a particular psychological therapy, and they would be only human if they really wanted to demonstrate their therapy worked! Everyone who works in research has some kind of vested interest in the outcome of their research.

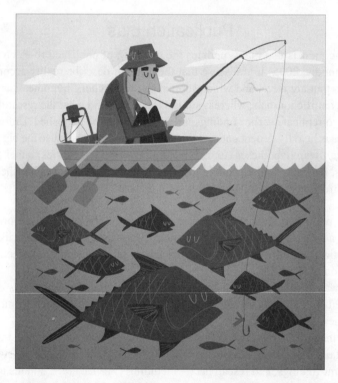

Figure 1.3 Some published findings may arise from researchers 'fishing' for the results that they expected to find

You shouldn't be thinking here that all of psychology research is an unregulated and immoral mess: most researchers are honest, and many systems are in place to ensure that research is done properly and that results are interpreted and reported in an unbiased way. However, the combined impact of all of the things discussed above is that there are lots of subtle ways in which research can be biased. Furthermore, researchers who engage in QRPs aren't necessarily 'evil' (although some probably are), they are just conducting their research according to established norms and trying to progress their career (and the careers of the people who work with them) as best they can.

What can be done?

Fortunately, there are many things that you can look out for when you are reading scientific papers in order to make a decision about how much you can believe that a piece of research is 'true'. With regard to sampling, you should read the descriptions of study participants, and how they were recruited, very carefully. This will enable you to make a judgment on the extent to which you can generalise the research findings to different groups of people. Findings from a research project conducted in London can probably be generalised to similar groups of people elsewhere in the UK, but you might need to think carefully before generalising those findings to other countries. You should also pay attention to the ethnicity and demographic characteristics of the sample: findings from a white middle-class sample should be treated more cautiously than those from a more mixed sample of study participants. With regard to identifying dodgy research methods and statistics, this requires an eye for detail, although we would highly recommend reading Simmons et al. (2011) who highlight some of the more commonly used tricks.

Perhaps a more practical solution than carefully evaluating the information about study participants, methods and statistics for every single study that you read – as this would take you absolutely ages – is to rely on evidence syntheses that are written by others. There are two main types. *Narrative reviews* are a written summary of all of the available evidence on a given topic (e.g. the influence of heritable factors on schizophrenia) and can prove very useful for gaining an overview of a topic. Furthermore, narrative reviews are generally written by specialists in a research area who are usually quite good at pointing out many of the methodological weaknesses of individual studies – things that can be difficult to spot – and this is an important detail that meta-analyses (see below) often miss. Unfortunately, narrative reviews can be subject to subtle biases from the people who write them, and the absence of any quantitative information means that it can be difficult to grasp the magnitude or practical relevance of the influence of X on Y, or the relationship between X and Y.

For this reason *systematic reviews* – and in particular a subset of these, called *meta-analyses* – are incredibly useful, and ideally these should be the first thing you read when you are researching a new topic for the first time. When writing a meta-analysis, the author will find *every published study* on a given topic (good authors will also try hard to find results that have not been published), and they will then extract a numerical value from each study to indicate the size of the effect for example the magnitude of the correlation between the number of life stressors and major depressive episodes that a person experiences, or the size of the effect of antidepressants on depressed mood. These values are then combined before being analysed together, in order to calculate the average effect size across all of the studies. This approach is very powerful because larger studies (with more statistical power) have a bigger influence on the overall estimate of effect size than smaller studies. Furthermore, it is possible to estimate 'publication bias' for a given research question – the likelihood that negative findings exist, but haven't been published – using some clever statistical techniques, and to correct for this estimated publication bias before arriving at a calculation of the average effect size. In summary, meta-analysis is a very powerful tool for getting an estimate of the true state of affairs for a given topic in psychology. A meta-analysis is much more useful than any individual study could ever be, and it is less prone (although not completely immune) to many of the biases that afflict individual studies.

It's fair to say that the volume of psychology research has proliferated to such an extent in recent years that it is impossible to keep track of it, even if you limit yourself to a very narrow field. However, the mass of published data means that meta-analyses are viable for even the most specialist and 'niche' topics (the authors of this book have written a few between them!) and they are becoming more and more common. When you evaluate the evidence for a given topic, remember that a meta-analysis can be really useful.

Section summary

In this section, we have discussed the advantages and disadvantages of the different research methods that are used to study psychological disorders. We showed how a combination of different methods can have great explanatory power. We then discussed some of the problems that affect scientific research, and why you have to be careful before concluding that a piece of published research represents 'the truth'. Paying close attention to the characteristics of the sample, the methods used and the statistical analyses, and making use of systematic reviews and meta-analyses when possible, are the best ways to get an accurate and unbiased idea of what is real and what is probably rubbish!

Section 5: What are the main approaches to understanding psychological disorders?

Heritability and genetics

Most characteristics of individuals, including their psychological characteristics (e.g. their IQ), are at least partly heritable, which means that these are passed from parents to their offspring. A *heritability estimate* refers to the percentage of variability in a *phenotype* within a population that can be attributed to genetic variability, as opposed to environmental variability or random factors. For example, the heritability estimate for the phenotype of being dependent on nicotine is estimated at about 50% (see Chapter 9). At first glance, you might assume that this means that YOUR risk of becoming a smoker is half determined by your genes, and half determined by your environment. This is not the case, because the heritability estimate refers to variability in a *population*, not variation within *individuals*. A better example of this is to think about the heritability of body height, which stands at about 90% for men. This does *not* mean that if we take a 200cm male, 180cm of his height (90%) were determined by his genes and the other 20cm (10%) were determined by his environment. Research methods used to assess heritability are discussed in Box 1.8.

Box 1.8   Essential research

Running in the family: Making sense of heritable and environmental influences on psychological disorders

Do psychological disorders run in families? If so, how much, and how does it happen? The debate around these questions has been going on for decades and shows no sign of being resolved any time soon. If techniques for unpicking the human genome progress at the rate they are currently progressing, then we *may* one day have an answer. But until now this field has depended on good old-fashioned detective work, using three main research designs: family studies, twin studies and adoption studies.

Family studies

These studies are used to estimate the risk to other family members if one member of that family has a particular disorder. For instance, if Fred suffers from depression, what is the likelihood that his siblings, parents and children will also become depressed? These studies are usually run using a 'case control' design. That is, a person with the condition is identified, and then matched with a very similar person (in terms of age, gender, background, and whatever other variables the researchers deem important) who does not have that condition. Once a large group of pairs has been identified in this way, their family members will be assessed to determine whether any of them has the condition. If the disorder turns out to be more common in the families where one person is already known to have the condition, this suggests that the disorder is not a random thing, and researchers will want to try to understand what causes it, and perhaps try to prevent it in family members who are at risk. However, this type of study cannot give a clear indication of whether a disease 'runs in families' because of genetic processes, or as a result of environmental ones: two members of the same family could have the same condition because they share genes, or because they share a similar environment. That is why twin studies and adoption studies are needed.

Twin studies

Twin studies rely on the fact that twins come in two types: identical (or monozygotic, meaning that they came from the same egg and the same sperm) and fraternal/non-identical (or dizygotic, meaning that they each came from a separate egg and sperm). Monozygotic (MZ) twins share 100% (or nearly 100% . . . it's complicated) of their genes. Dizygotic (DZ) twins share *on average* 50% of their genes. So, imagine you manage to find 100 people with a diagnosis of an anxiety disorder (they are called the 'proband') who also just happen

(Continued)

(Continued)

to have an MZ twin. If anxiety disorders were an entirely heritable condition, you would expect to find that almost all of the MZ probands with anxiety disorders would have a twin with the same condition (i.e. a 'concordance rate' of almost 100%). Now let's imagine that as well as probands with MZ twins, you find 100 probands with anxiety disorders and a *DZ* twin. If heritability is the whole cause, you would expect to find much lower rates of anxiety disorders in the twins of the DZ probands (i.e. a much lower concordance rate), because they share only 50% (on average) of their genetic material.

On the other hand, if anxiety disorders were purely environmental in origin, what would you expect to find? Well, MZ twins will share a lot of their environment – they will have shared a uterus, parents, home, most probably a school, many friends … but then, so will DZ twins. The two twin types will not differ a great deal in how much environment they have shared. So, if anxiety is just down to environment you would expect twins of anxious probands to be effected equally, in other words to have a similar concordance rate, regardless of whether they were MZ or DZ.

No psychological disorder is entirely caused by heritable factors, and no psychological disorder can be purely attributed to environmental factors, so all disorders fall between the two examples that are described above. And, by looking at the difference in concordance rates for a disorder in MZ and DZ twins, you get an indication of the relative importance of genes and environment. If the two concordance rates are very similar, you would conclude that a shared environment is the key factor. However, if the concordance rates are very different (with MZ twins having the higher concordance rate) then you would conclude that the heritable, genetic influence was stronger.

Adoption studies

Adoption studies make use of the fact that in families where a child has been adopted at an early age, that child will share a common environment with their adoptive family, but will not share their genetic make-up. On the other hand, the child will share their genes, but not their environment, with their biological parents. This allows researchers to tease apart the relative contributions of genes and environment. So, a typical adoption study design would measure a trait of interest (e.g. shyness) in children, and also in their biological parents and in their adoptive parents. If the children's levels of shyness are more closely related to the adoptive parents' levels of shyness (or related behaviours) than the biological parents' level of shyness, then the researchers will conclude that this trait is most heavily influenced by environmental factors. However, if the children's levels of shyness are more closely related to their biological parents' shyness, then the conclusion would be that genetic factors are more important. In a study employing this design, Daniels and Plomin (1984) showed that shyness in young children was related both to shyness levels in their biological mothers, indicating a genetic contribution to the trait, *and* to low sociability in their adoptive mothers, indicating an environmental contribution as well.

The other thing to be aware of is that heritability estimates assume that there is at least *some* variability in genetic and environmental factors within a given population. If there is no variability in either genetic or environmental factors, a heritability estimate is meaningless. For example, we know that cigarette smoking causes lung cancer. Try to imagine a parallel universe in which the entire population smoke 20 cigarettes per day, that is, there is no variability in smoking behaviour within this population. In this population the heritability estimate for lung cancer would approach 100% – in other words, it would appear to be almost entirely heritable – whereas we *know* that lung cancer is strongly influenced by environmental factors, cigarette smoking in particular (thanks to Richard Bentall for this example).

We now have a pretty good idea about how heritable different disorders are, and heritability estimates will be discussed throughout this book. Arguably more interesting developments in heritability research are attempts to identify specific gene variants that are associated with psychological traits or disorders, and the study of gene × environment interactions (discussed in Box 1.9). We will look at these things throughout the book.

Box 1.9   Essential research

Gene–environment interactions

It used to be thought, basically, that our genes contributed a bit to our mental health, and our environment contributed another bit, and together they dictated whether we would develop a psychological disorder. We are now starting to realise that it's a lot more complicated than that …

We now understand that genes and environments both influence how the other works. Therefore, the genes that we are born with can affect the type of environment we end up with. Also, the environment that we are in can change the way our genes express themselves, and while a particular environment might be really toxic for someone with genotype A, it might be no problem at all for someone with genotype B. All of this is known as gene–environment interaction.

Our genes effect our environment. The environment that children develop in is not random. People with certain genes are more likely to end up in certain environments. So, for example, we know that people with a particular genetic profile are more likely to seek out friendships with people who have a relaxed attitude to illegal drug use. In other words, their genes encourage them to place themselves in a 'risky' environment. Unsurprisingly, they are then much more likely to end up using drugs themselves (Agrawal et al., 2010). In this situation, was it their genes or their environment that caused them to use drugs?

Our environment affects our genes. This finding has come as a bit of a shock. Until a few years ago we thought that all of us had the genes we were conceived with, and

(Continued)

(Continued)

that was that. However, in recent years a new field called *epigenetics* has emerged. Epigenetics is based on the discovery that the activation of our genes can be dramatically altered by our environment. One major way in which genes are regulated is called methylation, and involves groups of a chemical called Methyl attaching to the gene and then deactivating it. For example, researchers interested in a number of different psychological disorders have looked at the methylation of a group of genes that influence the behaviour of glucocorticoid receptors, which are important in dictating how the brain responds to stress hormones. Those who have lots of methylation to these genes are known to be particularly sensitive to stress hormones, and, perhaps as a result, tend to be at significant risk of psychological disorders characterised by impulsivity and aggression. So how do these genes become methylated? The answer is that there are probably various ways, but it is becoming clear that mothers who are very stressed when they are pregnant (e.g. because they are experiencing domestic violence) give birth to children with high levels of methylation to glucocorticoid genes (e.g. Radtke et al., 2011). And we know that this group of children goes on to have higher than normal levels of emotional and behavioural problems. Again, ask yourself what has caused the difficulties that these children experience? Is it their genes, or their environment … ?

Environment affects different genotypes in different ways. Some people can have a seemingly awful childhood, but emerge basically unscathed. Others can have a pretty good childhood, but still experience significant psychological difficulties. So what's going on? It may be that we need a particular genotype to experience the worst effects of a problematic childhood. For instance, we know that experiencing childhood abuse increases the risk of developing behaviour problems. However, it may be that this is only the case for people with a certain genotype.

Conversely, some genes only cause problems if the environment is right. Fox et al. (2005) studied a serotonin transporter gene, known as the 5-HTT allele. They found that having a short version of this allele was associated with behavioural inhibition (a combination of shyness and fear of new situations, which is thought to put children at risk of anxiety disorders). However, this association was only present for children where the parent reported low levels of social support. For children whose families experienced high levels of social support, having the short version of this allele did not put them at increased risk of behavioural inhibition.

Examples of gene x environment interactions are discussed throughout this book.

Biological and psychological models of psychological disorders

Most abnormal and clinical psychology textbooks will outline the main approaches to the understanding of psychological disorders. These will usually include the psychodynamic approach (heavily influenced by famous psychologists including Freud and Jung), the behavioural approach (which usually means classical and operant conditioning so Pavlov and Skinner will get a mention), the cognitive approach (Beck usually makes an appearance here), and finally the biological approach (where Kraepelin's name tends to pop up). These various approaches are important to historians of psychology, because each emerged at a different period in history and each was the dominant view for a period of time. Furthermore, they have all had a lasting influence on how we view psychological disorders.

When we were writing this book, we decided that it would not be helpful to present these different approaches as distinct 'camps' that compete with each other to explain psychological disorders. Unfortunately many textbooks are structured in this way, and many introductory undergraduate psychology courses are taught in this way too. This approach is used because it demonstrates how these ideas have developed over time, and also because it helps to simplify and pigeonhole the material in order to structure lectures and textbooks, and to aid students' understanding of it. Therefore, the material is often taught a bit like this:

Theory A predicts that chicken nuggets cause schizophrenia; evidence X supports this theory whereas evidence Y is inconsistent with this theory. On the other hand, theory B predicts that chocolate ice cream causes schizophrenia; evidence Y supports this theory but evidence X is inconsistent with the theory.

Does this sound familiar? We have opted for another route in this book. While we would acknowledge the different types of processes in psychological disorders (e.g. biological and cognitive processes), we have not organised the material into different approaches that are forced to compete with each other, in a kind of theoretical fight to the death until only one theory remains. Instead, we have tried to demonstrate how, for example, cognitive and biological explanations can explain the same psychological phenomena in slightly different ways, and how the cognitive and biological accounts are *not* necessarily inconsistent with each other. Of course, where there are conflicts between different theories we have explained these and presented the evidence so that you can evaluate the theories yourself. In addition, we have limited our discussion of many well-known theories that are of historical importance but do not add anything to our current understanding of psychological disorders. A good example of this is the Freudian approach, from which many of the more strange ideas (e.g. the idea that young boys desire sexual relations with their mothers) have been disproved by research. On the other hand, some of Freud's ideas (motivational and emotional states that operate below the threshold of conscious awareness, traumatic events during childhood as determinants of psychological disorders during adulthood) have been influential, and these continue to echo through contemporary theories of psychological disorders. We have also tried to describe and evaluate modern theories without getting bogged down in the history or evolution of those theories.

Box 1.10 gives an example of how these different approaches can all contribute to our understanding of psychological disorders. Although the box is focused on explaining how disorders develop, you can also use it to think of different approaches to the treatment of psychological disorders, something that we discuss in more detail in Chapter 2. For example, we could target a brain dysfunction directly with surgery or with medication, which might then alter cognitive distortions and *that* might then alleviate symptoms. Another approach would be to try to rectify the cognitive distortions directly, which might have the same effect on symptoms (and may also change the underlying biology; see Chapter 5 for a discussion of how this works for depression). Finally, there might be ways we can help people to 'un-learn' any unhealthy associations they have formed, which may affect the symptoms of the disorder and perhaps also affect the cognitive distortions (see Chapter 7 for a of how this works for specific phobias).

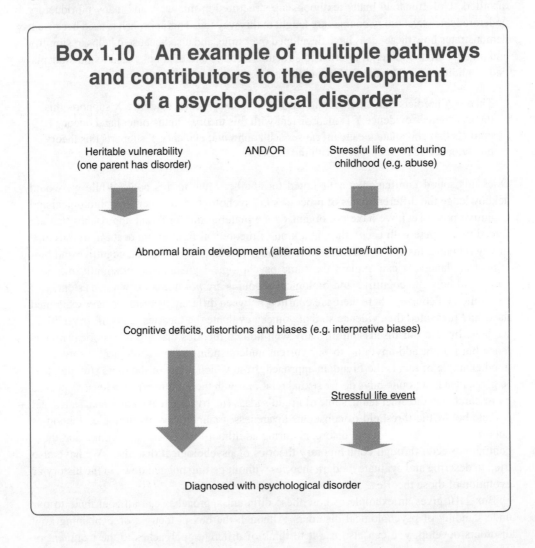

Box 1.10 An example of multiple pathways and contributors to the development of a psychological disorder

Heritable vulnerability (one parent has disorder)

AND/OR

Stressful life event during childhood (e.g. abuse)

Abnormal brain development (alterations structure/function)

Cognitive deficits, distortions and biases (e.g. interpretive biases)

Stressful life event

Diagnosed with psychological disorder

Stressful life events and broader social factors

As you will see throughout this book (and in Box 1.10), stressful life events can trigger the development of many different psychological disorders. Such events might not be sufficient to produce a psychological disorder (most people who experience a bereavement do not become depressed, for example), but they may interact with some other vulnerability, such as a heritable risk for the disorder.

Broader social factors also play a role in the development of psychological disorders and in the likelihood that people will make a recovery. For example, it is obvious when you think about it but people who live in Muslim countries are less likely to develop an alcohol problem than people who live in Western countries in which alcohol is readily available and drinking is part of the culture. Within such countries, there may be a culture of heavy drinking within some social groups, but a culture of abstention (or infrequent, 'social' drinking) in others. If someone is a member of such a social group then they are more likely to drink heavily and develop an alcohol problem, and less likely to recover, compared to a person in a different social group (see Chapter 9). To give another example, schizophrenia is more common in immigrants and in people who live in dense urban environments. Furthermore, recovery from schizophrenia is more unlikely in people who have high levels of expressed emotion in their immediate family environment (see Chapter 4). Throughout this book we have given an overview of the influence of these broad social factors on specific psychological disorders, and we cover these things in more detail where their interactions with psychological processes are well established. You should also be able to think about how social factors might fit into the multiple pathways model shown in Box 1.9.

Section summary

In this section we have introduced the notion that many psychological disorders are partially heritable and are influenced by broad social factors. Biological and psychological explanations for psychological disorders have evolved considerably over time, and the most influential modern theories and models manage to integrate biological, cognitive and learning processes to explain how disorders develop (and can be treated). We have also demonstrated how it can be useful to think of biological, cognitive and learning processes as complementary processes that can explain different aspects of psychological disorders, rather than as independent viewpoints that must conflict with each other.

Essential questions

Some possible exam questions that stem from this chapter are:

- Are people with psychological disorders qualitatively different from 'normal' people?
- What are the problems with a diagnostic approach to psychological disorders, and are the alternatives any more useful?

- What methods do we use to study psychological disorders? Give examples of what we can learn from different types of methods, and the limits of what we can infer from the different types of methods.
- How can we decide whether the research that we read about is 'true'?

Further reading

Simmons, J. P., Nelson, L. D., & Simonsohn, U. (2011). False-positive psychology: Undisclosed flexibility in data collection and analysis allows presenting anything as significant. *Psychological Science*, *22*(11): 1359–1366. (A very entertaining read that illustrates how easy it is to produce flawed research that appears to be 'true', and some of the things you should look out for in order to judge the quality of research.)

www.theguardian.com/commentisfree/2012/feb/10/diagnostic-manual-mental-illness (Richard Bentall and Nick Craddock debate the value of a diagnostic approach to psychological disorders, with a focus on *DSM*-5.)

www.thementalelf.net/ (This website provides very useful summaries of mental health research, including studies of treatments for psychological disorders. The summaries are brief and appropriately critical, and are a good way to 'dip into' a topic before you turn to look at articles published in scientific journals.)

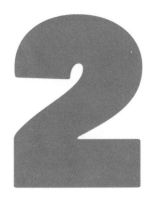

HOW ARE PSYCHOLOGICAL DISORDERS TREATED?

General introduction

Mental health professionals treat the symptoms of psychological disorders in a multitude of ways. This chapter will outline some of the most common ways in which they work. We will begin with a look at the debate surrounding the use of medication versus psychological techniques. After this cursory overview of the medical approach, we will then focus on approaches that are taken by psychologists (well this *is* a psychology book, after all). We will discuss preventative approaches, which have become an increasing focus in recent years (although still not nearly enough), and also discuss treatment approaches that are used when symptoms are already present. Within both prevention and treatment work there are many ways of working. Psychologists may work with individual clients or with groups. They may use a manual-based 'package', which is applied to the client with a minimum of tailoring, or they may use the gold-standard, formulation-based approach which is custom-built for each client. Psychologists also work from a number of theoretical perspectives, including cognitive-behavioural and psychodynamic. They may specialise in the treatment not just of adults, but also of children and adolescents, people with learning disabilities, older adults, and other specialist groups.

This chapter will give a brief introduction to all of these approaches, but thenceforth both this chapter and the rest of the book will give most attention to what typically happens in clinics (as opposed to research trials). This is the individual treatment of one individual, using a selection of techniques that are hand-picked for that client, based on a thorough assessment of their needs. Because the bulk of the scientific evidence base is devoted to cognitive-behavioural theories and treatments, it is these that we will focus on in the rest of the book. Although there is now a growing literature on the treatment of children, families, couples, people with learning disabilities and older adults (amongst others), this chapter, and most of those that follow, will focus largely on the treatment of individual, non-disabled adults. We will also give some thought as to how researchers evaluate the usefulness of psychological therapies. Finally, we will examine the ethical framework within which all psychologists are expected to work.

Assessment targets

At the end of the chapter, you should ask yourself the following questions:

- Can I explain the pros and cons of medication and psychological interventions for psychological disorders?
- Can I explain how researchers evaluate the usefulness of treatments for psychological disorders?
- Do I know the basic components of a simple CBT treatment programme?
- Do I understand the principles of ethics and conduct that psychologists should adhere to when delivering psychological therapies?

Section 1: Medication versus psychological approaches

Most people who seek treatment for a mental health condition will, if they are offered any help at all, be offered medication. Only a minority will be offered psychological therapy. Although in the UK psychologists are not licenced to prescribe medication (as they are in some other countries), they work closely with others who are, and many of their clients will take medication or have the option to. Therefore it is important that psychologists understand a little about the role of medication in the treatment of mental health conditions. A detailed

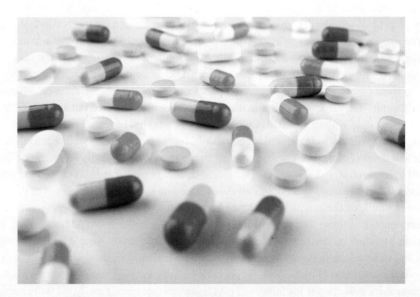

Figure 2.1 Most people who get any treatment for their condition will receive medication ... but would they be better off with a psychological therapy?

description of medications that are used to treat mental health conditions is beyond the scope of this book. Instead this section will look at situations when medications might be used, and the pros and cons of doing so.

Pros and cons of medications for mental health problems

Psychologists often tend to be quite negative about medications. Why is this, and are there times when it might be preferable to prescribe a medication? See Box 2.1 for some answers.

Box 2.1   Essential debate

The pros and cons of prescribing medications for psychological disorders

Pros	Cons
It is usually cheaper to medicate than to offer therapy.	Medication does not usually work in the long term (unless you keep taking this long term). Good psychological therapies have been shown to have long-lasting effects that are maintained after they are terminated.
There are nowhere near enough therapists qualified to give therapy to all who would benefit. Giving medication means that people do at least get some help.	Medications often have unpleasant side-effects. This means that quality of life is impaired. It also means that some people will stop taking the medication, and end up relapsing.
Some patients prefer medication to therapy. Taking medication requires less time and effort, and it can be less stressful and difficult.	Some medications are dangerous if an overdose is taken.
Sometimes therapy fails, and medication is the only approach left. Sometimes, in these situations, the medications work quite well.	Medications have been linked to fatalities. Although these are rare, they can occur through an overdose or side effects, or interactions with food or other drugs.
	Some drugs (particularly the older ones) require lifestyle changes that can cause problems. For instance, if someone is taking Monoamine Oxidase Inhibitor (MAOI) drugs (usually prescribed for depression), they will have to stay away from a wide range of foods, including most cheeses, pickled things, red wine and chocolate.

What do you think? Should medications be prescribed to patients in some circumstances? Although most psychologists would rather see people getting therapy as a first-line approach, we can recognise that there are situations in which medications will be the only or the best option.

Combination treatment

Nowadays psychologists do not usually work in isolation and typically they will work as part of a 'multi-disciplinary team'. This team will have a whole range of professionals who are contributing to each client's care. Depending on the setting, there may be psychologists, psychiatrists, social workers, cognitive-behaviour therapists, nurses, speech and language therapists, occupational therapists, primary wellbeing practitioners and a whole host of others. This means that as well as the psychological therapy (which is probably directed by the psychologist, but delivered by a number of members of the team) the client may also have medication. This is a very typical scenario, and on the face of it sounds as if that person will be getting the best of both worlds. In many cases they will be. However, we are now starting to realise that sometimes giving both medication and therapy at the same time might not be as sensible as it sounds. There is intriguing evidence available that taking medication at the same time as the therapy might, in some cases, mean worse results for the client. Foa et al. (2002) reported that in three studies of cognitive behaviour therapy (CBT) plus medication for panic disorder, only one study showed more improvement for those receiving medication plus CBT, compared to those getting CBT alone. Moreover when the patients were followed up much later, in two of the studies, those receiving both medication and CBT were doing *worse* than those who had received CBT alone. It was not entirely clear why this might be. Some people have suggested that medication dampens down the emotions and cognitive processes that therapy attempts to work on. If these emotions and cognitive processes are not fully activated during CBT, then a patient cannot learn fully to deal with them, and in the end, the therapy does not work as well as it could have done.

However, the research into combining medications and therapy is in its early days, and the interactions between the two are not yet fully understood.

What works best: Medication or therapy?

At this point you might well be thinking 'Yeah, but are the meds as good as the therapy?'. Good question. But the answer is not a simple one, and it depends on who you ask. There are now a fair few trials comparing medications to psychological therapies. These have been run for quite a few of the major psychological disorders, and will be discussed in the relevant chapters. However, in summary, the jury is still out. It seems that when a researcher who favours medications runs a trial, medications do better. And when a researcher who favours psychological treatments runs the trial … Well, can you guess the outcome? Yep, psychological treatments tend to do better. This is not usually due to any kind of fraud on the part of the researchers, but because of the difficulties inherent in running treatment outcomes research, which leads nicely on to our next section.

Section summary

In this section we have learnt that many people with psychological disorders will use medication to treat their symptoms, either by choice or because that was all that was available to them. We have also learnt that there are some advantages to using medication, either alone or in combination with psychological therapy, but that these need to be balanced against a number of significant drawbacks.

Section 2: Researching and evaluating treatments for psychological disorders

New therapies (or, more usually, variants of old therapies) are constantly being invented by us creative psychologists. It is *very* important, however, that new therapies are tested to find out whether they do actually work (and that they are as wonderful as their inventors imagine). It is also vital that the professionals using those therapies are able to read the treatment outcome research and understand its limitations. In this chapter we will look at the stages that researchers go through as they evaluate the usefulness of psychological therapies. We will then discuss some of the main difficulties that researchers face in carrying out this type of research and the limits that this puts on the conclusions that can be drawn. Finally, we will briefly look at how successful psychological therapies are.

What are the difficulties in treatment research?

Randomised Controlled Trials (RCTs) are often seen as the gold standard of treatment outcome research. In a typical RCT, half of the participants will be randomly assigned to get the new intervention, whilst the remainder will receive no treatment, a placebo treatment, or a different treatment. They will then be followed up to see which group has the best outcomes. However, this design is not without its flaws and RCTs are very difficult to conduct. Therefore the results of any single trial should be examined very carefully, and it is not until a number of different trials have been conducted that the efficacy of a new intervention can be accepted with some degree of confidence. So what are the main difficulties with running an RCT of a psychological intervention?

- As mentioned at the end of the last section, it is well known that when researchers carry out a trial of an intervention that they are personally excited about, that intervention will do better than other treatments the researcher is comparing it to but is less excited about. In most cases this is not fraud, although we must accept, as a profession, that fraud probably does sometimes happen. Instead, most of the time a researcher who is passionate about their new therapy will be more enthusiastic about treating people with this, and little unconscious messages about this are likely to leak out to those taking part, and to the research assistants who are measuring the outcomes. Although researchers running treatment trials always aim for outcomes to be measured 'blind' (i.e. by someone who doesn't know which treatment the patient received), it is very difficult to stop them sometimes finding out by accident, and to also stop this from unconsciously influencing their ratings. For example, a patient might accidentally mention how nice that Prof Cartwright-Hatton is, thus letting the research assistant know that they *must* have received the psychological therapy, and so it can then be difficult for the research assistant to be objective about assigning an outcome rating to that client.

- In trials of drug treatments the control group are often given a 'placebo' treatment', such as a sugar-pill, so that neither the patient nor the doctor knows who is getting the new treatment and who is in the control group. This is known as a 'double-blind' trial, and it means that neither the patient nor the doctor can influence the results of the study. However, this is nearly impossible to do in psychological outcomes research. Can you think of how you would make a placebo psychological treatment? (If you can think of a way of doing this that no patient or psychologist would rumble, please can you contact the authors.) Because of this problem, both the psychologist doing the treatment and the client receiving it know who is getting the new treatment and who is not. Although most researchers will be at pains to make sure that this knowledge does not influence the result of their trial, it would be highly unlikely that well-meaning patients and/or passionate researchers wouldn't sometimes inadvertently bias the results just a little bit.

- In trials of treatments for other medical conditions the outcome can usually be objectively measured. For instance, is the patient still alive? Have they still got four limbs? Has their haemoglobin increased? These are all things that can be measured objectively. There is very little room for personal opinion in judging whether someone is dead. However, when measuring whether someone's psychological symptoms have improved there is huge room for subjective opinion. Ask 10 different psychologists and you will get 10 different opinions. Although psychologists have worked very hard to generate objective ways of measuring symptoms (structured interviews, standardised questionnaires) there is still room for disagreement, and this causes big problems in trials of psychological interventions. The way that this is usually (partially) resolved is to have two separate psychologists assess patients' outcomes (maybe not all patients, but a good proportion). These psychologists will have been trained in the outcome measurement in the same way, so that they will be looking for the same things, but when they come to assess the clients they will do this separately, and then they will compare their results. The 'inter-rater reliability' of these outcome assessors should be reported along with the main results from the trial.

- Drop-out rates from treatment trials are often very high. Taking part in an RCT is an arduous task. Participants (who, let's remember, are struggling with a psychological disorder) not only have to come for their treatment (or sit getting nothing or a placebo, if they are in a control group), they also have to come for assessments before, after, and sometimes during treatment, and sometimes again months or years later.

These assessments can be tiring, distressing, long, boring and inconvenient. As a result, the drop-out for RCTs can be very high, meaning that we can't be sure whether the results of the study can really be generalised to the entire population of people with the disorder in question. There are statistical methods for dealing with missing data caused by participant drop-out, but none of these are completely satisfactory.

- Sometimes, even when the RCT has gone very well, it can be difficult to generalise its results to real-world settings. The fact is that most RCTs are run in very carefully controlled university-based settings. The clients are very carefully selected to make sure that everyone is able to benefit maximally from therapy. People with weak English (or whatever the local language is) will be excluded, as will those with learning disabilities. The study may also only include people with very pure conditions. So in a study of a treatment for social anxiety disorder, the researchers may exclude patients who have comorbid depression or personality disorders. This can result in a very rarefied (i.e. unusual) pool of participants. The participants are then treated by very carefully selected therapists (jobs on trials are sometimes seen as cushy numbers, so they get lots of applicants!) who spend their time focusing just on this one condition, perhaps just seeing a couple of clients a day, to allow careful thought about each client. They will receive tons of training, and careful supervision, often from a world-leading expert in the area. Unsurprisingly, the results of the trial will be very good. Treatment manuals will be published, to great fanfares, and announced at big conferences, where on-the-ground therapists will flock to a two-hour workshop to learn How To Do It. They will then take this back to their clinic. Here, they will try to apply what they have learnt with their client, one of the six that they are seeing that day. Their client has social anxiety disorder, but is also very depressed. He doesn't speak great English, is recently bereaved, in horrible debt and about to lose his job. How well do you think the therapy works in these rather different circumstances … ? Unsurprisingly, studies of new treatments that are applied in the real world usually produce substantially less shiny results.

Box 2.2   Essential research

Stages in treatment outcome research

There are lots of methods that researchers employ in order to test whether interventions are effective. In approximate order of how powerful the evidence is, and the order that they are used in when developing a new therapy, these are as follows.

(Continued)

(Continued)

Case studies

When trying out a new technique, a researcher will probably start with just one or two clients. Clearly this only produces very preliminary evidence, and sweeping generalisations cannot be made on the basis of case studies. However, a well-conducted case study, with careful measurement of the symptoms of interest, and of the mechanisms that the treatment seeks to change, before, during and after the intervention, can provide early evidence that a new technique is worthy of further research.

Pilot/feasibility studies

The next stage is usually to carry out a pilot study. The aim here is to try out the new technique with a slightly larger selection of clients, and to test whether it would be feasible to carry out a full-scale trial.

Randomised Controlled Trials

RCTs are considered to be the gold-standard of treatment outcome research. In an RCT a large sample of clients with a particular condition will be recruited to take part. They will then be 'randomised' so that some of them get the new treatment and some do not. Those who do not receive the new intervention will either receive no intervention at all, or better still some type of placebo treatment, or best of all an alternative type of therapy. The outcomes for these groups of clients are then compared. If the clients who received the new intervention do better than those who did not, then the intervention will start to be taken seriously. However, several more successful trials will be required (preferably run by different researchers) before the new treatment can be considered 'well-established'.

Meta-analyses

When a number of trials of a new intervention have been carried out, it can be useful to pool the results from these to get a bigger picture of how effective the intervention really is. When results are pooled in this way it is known as a 'meta-analysis'. RCTs of interventions for mental health problems are usually rather small. Pooling the results from various trials gives a much more powerful insight into an intervention's effectiveness. In addition, pooling the results of lots of trials 'irons out' any random results that do sometimes occur. Clever statistics can also be utilised to find out whether there is any publication bias. It is a sad but well-recognised fact that studies that don't find an effect for an intervention are difficult to publish in scientific journals, because the editors of those journals want to publish exciting new findings, not articles stating 'it didn't work' (see Chapter 1). Also, if a treatment didn't work, it will sometimes not be clear whether this was because it was no good or because there was something wrong with the study, for example, perhaps not enough people to have the power to detect a significant effect. Because of this, negative trials often don't get published and this is a real problem. A well-conducted meta-analysis will be able to estimate how many of these unpublished 'file-drawer' studies are in existence, and therefore will give a clearer idea of whether the intervention in question really is effective or not.

Meta-meta-analysis

An enterprising team from Germany (Huhn et al., 2014) have taken things a step further ... and have done a meta-analysis of meta-analyses! They searched for all existing meta-analyses of psychological or drug treatments for psychological disorders, only including meta-analyses that had compared two active treatments or had compared an active treatment to a placebo treatment (i.e. they didn't include studies that compared people getting treatment to people getting nothing). In the end they included 61 meta analyses on 21 disorders, incorporating 852 trials and over 137,000 participants. They reported that the average intervention showed a medium effect size, which was slightly higher for psychological interventions than for drug treatments, although in head-to-head comparisons these types of intervention did not come out as being significantly different. Interestingly, they also reported a slight indication that combining psychological and drug interventions was a little better than having either individually. However, they noted as well that most of the meta-analyses in this meta-meta-analysis only included data on patients up until the end of treatment, so the study could tell us nothing about the long-term usefulness of the interventions.

How successful is therapy?

The success of therapy varies hugely from client to client. Some disorders are more 'treatable' than others. For instance, some trials of a treatment for panic disorder have claimed success rates of over 80%. This is despite the fact that, until about 30 years ago, panic disorder was considered 'untreatable' by psychological therapy. For other disorders, particularly the more severe and enduring ones such as personality disorders (see Chapter 11), the figure is much lower. The success rates for each disorder that we cover in this book will be discussed in the relevant chapters.

It is worth pausing here, however, to think about what we mean by success in therapy. See Box 2.3 for a discussion of this.

Box 2.3   Essential debate

What do we mean by 'successful therapy'?

What do we mean by 'successful therapy'? Do we mean a complete remission of all symptoms? Of course not. It would be an unusual human being who never had the occasional symptom of unhappiness or anxiety. Most people even have the occasional 'psychotic' symptom, such as hearing a voice that was not really there (see Chapter 4). So what do we mean by this? Well the definitions of illness and health have been subject to substantial philosophical debate, going back over many centuries, so you are not going to get an easy answer here. In the research literature success is often defined as being free of a diagnosable disorder, as described by the *DSM* or *ICD* (see Chapter 1). However, many psychologists have their own opinions on this. A psychologist treating relatively mild cases of anxiety and depression may be unhappy with anything less than return to completely normal functioning for their clients. A psychologist working with clients diagnosed with psychosis, on the other hand, would quickly burn out if they set this as their goal. So, as with many things in life … it depends. We think that this is something that, generally speaking, should be between the client and their psychologist to decide.

Section summary

In this section we have seen how necessary it is that psychologists properly evaluate the therapies they develop. We have also seen that there are various ways and stages of doing this, and that even in randomised controlled trials, which are considered the gold-standard of treatment outcome research, there are hazards that can compromise the validity of the conclusions.

Section 3: The range and scope of a psychologist's work

In this section we provide an overview of the various ways in which psychologists work with their clients. We will explore treatment versus prevention, working with manuals versus formulation-based approaches, and working with groups versus individuals. We will also touch on the psychodynamic approach, before focusing on the cognitive-behavioural approach in more detail. Finally, we will briefly look at the different client groups with whom cognitive-behaviour therapy has been used.

Treatment versus prevention

In the past, the predominant approach in psychology has been to treat symptoms once they are full-blown and causing problems. However, in recent years, we have become aware that we might be able to stop symptoms before they are fully developed, and before they are causing difficulties. There are a few different types of prevention.

Primary versus secondary prevention

Primary prevention   When a psychologist wants to prevent symptoms before they have ever become full blown and have caused problems, this is known as 'primary prevention'. An example of primary prevention would be a psychologist going into schools and teaching children the skills for coping with stress, with the intention of preventing emotional disorders from arising later on, even though there was no indication that any of those children were going to have problems with this.

Secondary prevention   Secondary prevention is when a psychologist takes a population who have already suffered from psychological disorders and tries to prevent them from suffering again. An example here might be a psychologist who runs a coping skills group for people who have had an episode of depression but are fine at the moment. These clients might be taught skills for spotting changes in their mood, and ways of avoiding triggering low mood, such as getting enough sleep and exercise, eating properly, watching out for negative thinking and so on. In this case the clients have already suffered from depression, and the goal of this approach is to prevent them from suffering relapses (or to reduce the number that they experience).

Universal versus targeted prevention

Universal prevention   Sometimes a psychologist will take the view that the problems they are attempting to prevent are so common, or it is so difficult to predict who is and is not at risk, that the best approach is to offer the prevention to everyone. This is known as universal prevention, that is, everyone is offered the prevention, whether they are likely to need it or not. Almost everyone reading this book will have been the recipient of some universal prevention – albeit of the medical kind, rather than the psychological kind. Most developed countries now aim to vaccinate most of their populace against a whole variety of ills. It may be that you were never going to get diphtheria, or measles, or mumps, or tetanus, or any of the multitude of other diseases that you were probably vaccinated against. But you were vaccinated anyway, and this is a good example of universal prevention. In the past, psychological prevention programmes have not usually been offered universally. They were simply too expensive and too unproven to do this. However, in some parts of the world there are now psychological treatment programmes that are so widely offered as to be considered 'universal prevention'. A great example of this is a parenting programme called 'Triple P', which is designed to prevent behavioural and emotional problems in children. In some areas of the world (mostly in parts of Australia) all parents, whether they are fantastic parents or terrible ones, and whether their kids are little angels or little horrors, are offered a free short course in parenting (Sanders, 2012). This is discussed in more detail in Chapter 3.

Targeted prevention   Offering a psychological prevention treatment to everyone, regard-less of whether they are at risk of developing problems, is very expensive (see Box 2.4). Because of this, most psychologists who want to prevent a problem from arising will target people that they know are at a high risk of developing symptoms and impairment. This is known as 'targeted prevention'. An example of targeted prevention is a study by Ron Rapee and colleagues (Rapee and colleagues, 2005), where children who scored high on a measure of 'behavioural inhibition' were identified. Behavioural inhibition is not a disorder in itself. Instead, it is better described as a childhood temperament style, typified by being shy and withdrawn. We know that children who are behaviourally inhibited are at increased risk of developing anxiety disorders further down the line. So having identified a group of children who were behaviourally inhibited, Rapee and colleagues set about training the children's parents in techniques to prevent anxiety from developing. Although only a small study, the results were very promising, with those who received the intervention having fewer diagnosa-ble anxiety disorders 12 months after treatment, when compared to those who did not receive the intervention.

Box 2.4   Essential debate

Pros and cons of universal prevention and targeted prevention

	Universal prevention	Targeted prevention
Pros	No-one is stigmatised or labelled by being invited to take part.	It is cheaper, as fewer people are treated.
	Less effort is needed to identify who needs what.	Efforts can be focused on engaging those who really need the treatment (and who, typically, may be more difficult to engage).
	You catch everyone, including some low-risk people who would have gone on to develop difficulties, and would have been missed by a targeted approach.	
	Psychological disorder is not black and white. Most people exist in the grey areas, and universal treatment may still be beneficial to those who run the risk of very minor problems.	

	Universal prevention	Targeted prevention
Cons	It is very expensive. Typically you have to treat very many healthy people to prevent one person from becoming symptomatic.	Those who are identified as at risk may be stigmatised or labelled.
	Typically, it is the people who need it least who are most likely to take up the offer.	Identifying someone as at risk who was not actually going to develop any problems may be damaging for that person.
	There may be a risk to the intervention, which for those with very low risk might outweigh the benefits. The concept of risk from psychological therapies is fairly new and under-researched.	It is almost impossible to accurately predict who is and is not at risk of developing a psychological disorder. With targeted prevention, some people who are at risk will always be missed. Likewise, you will always end up treating some people who didn't need to be treated.

Formulation versus treatment manual

This book will focus on the individual 'formulation-based' approach. This is where a psychologist meets a client, works out exactly what the goals are for that specific person, also works out exactly what is causing their particular difficulties, and then designs a tailor-made intervention just for them. This is often seen as the 'gold-standard' approach. However, there is another approach which is also widely used. This is often called a 'manual-based' approach. This is where a psychologist takes a ready-made treatment off the shelf and gives this to their client. Usually the psychologist will have done some sort of assessment with the client to work out which 'package' might be best for them, and then monitors the client to make sure all is going well. Also, a good psychologist will adapt the package manual a little bit to fit it more closely to a client's particular needs. Although most clinic-based psychologists would say that they use a 'formulation-based' approach, once they have worked out their formulation they will usually address their client's difficulties using bits and pieces of manualised approaches, carefully selected to fit their formulation. However, research psychologists usually work tightly to manuals with little room for manoeuvre with individual clients, and it is these manual-based treatments that we see reported in treatment trials.

As usual there are a number of advantages and disadvantages to the 'manual-based' approach. These are presented in Box 2.5.

Box 2.5   Essential debate

Advantages and disadvantages to using the 'manual-based' approach to treatment

Advantages

- Manualised treatments can be used by less experienced and less highly-trained therapists. Therefore, they are cheaper and can be offered to more needy people.
- Manual-based treatments have usually undergone years of rigorous research. They will have been developed by experts in the field, and shown to work well in research trials. Therefore, we know that they are reasonably theory based and likely to work. This cannot always be said for 'formulation-based' approaches, which are often built on an individual therapist's ideas, and are never tested in a rigorous scientific environment.

Disadvantages

- A manual-based approach is always designed to cover as many areas as possible, and lots of these may not be relevant to your client. Most psychologists who have ever used a manual will tell you of clients they lost because the first few bits of the manual just didn't feel useful to them.
- You very rarely get clients with nice clean-cut disorders. A client might have been referred with Generalised Anxiety Disorder, but when you dig a bit deeper you will nearly always find some comorbidity ... perhaps a little depression, a sub-clinical social anxiety ... So which manual should you go for? An experienced therapist will have the skill to deal with this, and to pick and choose bits from different manuals. However, opting for this route does wipe out some of the advantages of using a manual.

Working with individuals versus working with groups

This book mostly focuses on treatments for individuals. However, psychologists are increasingly attempting to provide therapy for groups of clients together, and there are a number of advantages to this approach:

- It can be more cost-effective than just seeing one person at a time. However, it is rarely as cost-effective as it would first seem, because groups usually need to be run by two therapists, and all of the after-care (between-session phone calls to clients, their carers, other professionals involved in their care; catch-up sessions for those who couldn't come this week, etc.) still has to be done individually.

- For some problems, it can be helpful for clients to come together in a group. For instance, for mildly to moderately depressed people, coming to a group can provide a social setting that actively helps their condition. One of us (Sam) runs groups for parents who are learning to deal with an excessively anxious child. This seems to work best as a group – the parents swap ideas, they get support and empathy from other people who have faced the same problems as them, and finally, coming together as a group means that you can have a bit of fun and laughter. There is nothing like a little bit of appropriate humour to diffuse tension and to get across a difficult therapeutic message.

However, there are also a number of disadvantages to working with groups:

- You cannot give a tailor-made approach to each person in a group. Everyone has to get what is on offer. This brings the same problems as using a 'manual-based' therapeutic approach (see Box 2.5 above).
- Group dynamics can be difficult, and groups are most definitely not for the novice therapist. Just one difficult client in a group can make the whole thing very difficult to run. For this reason, groups are nearly always run by two psychologists, at least one of whom will be very experienced in running groups.

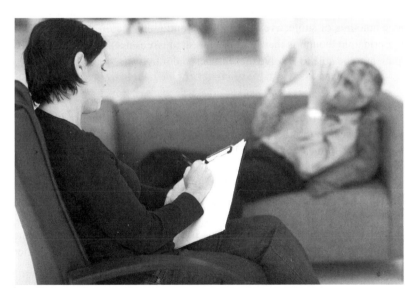

Figure 2.2 You are unlikely to have a couch in your office if you work in the NHS (as most UK psychologists do). You might get a couple of nice plastic chairs, with not *too* many mystery stains, if you're lucky

Different theoretical approaches to treatment

The psychodynamic approach: Freud's theory and psychoanalysis

Summing up the wealth of Freud's ideas is no easy task, but essentially his entire theoretical framework revolved around the simple idea that people are influenced by 'unconscious' desires. Freud's early conceptions of neurotic behaviour were that it stemmed from some kind of traumatic early experience that a patient had buried deep in their unconscious.

Therapeutically, Freud initially used hypnosis (regression to a childhood state) as a means to unlock early traumatic experiences, but eventually he moved away to use other techniques such as dream analysis and the 'talking cure' (free association) to unearth the cause of trauma. Dream analysis was based on the idea that unconscious desires would manifest themselves in dreams. Therapy involved patients recalling their dreams and Freud offering detailed analyses of these in terms of psychodynamic ideas. These interpretations centred on symbolism, that is, characters and situations in the dreams were seen as representing other things. For example, a woman dreamt that her child was sent away by the child's grandmother before the mother and grandmother boarded a train that subsequently ran the child over. The woman reproached her mother for having sent her child off alone. This was interpreted as the child representing the woman's genitals and the rapprochement of her mother represented her resentment at being 'expected to live as though she had no genitals' (Freud, 1954: 363). In other words, she was annoyed at her mother for wanting her to live a sexless life. A literal translation might alternatively be that the woman was just anxious about her daughter being harmed!

Therapies involving these kinds of techniques can last for years, and quite obviously involve huge amounts of subjective interpretation and guidance on the part of the therapist. The guiding principle though is that some deep-seated issues need to be unlocked by a therapist for a patient to be able to resolve these issues and move on.

Evidence for psychodynamic theories

The major problem with Freud's ideas is that they are unfalsifiable, that is, it is never possible to disprove them because the theory offers no predictions about behaviour. The theory was based on single case studies and so has little scientific basis, and stems often from Freud's own self-analysis. In terms of therapy, many have attempted to show the benefits of psychodynamic approaches. Smith and colleagues (1980) famously summarised the studies that had been conducted and concluded that psychotherapy was consistently beneficial in numerous ways. However, Eysenck (1985) went through these studies with a fine-toothed comb, and found that they often had major flaws such as not employing control groups who did not undergo therapy, or failing to include those who dropped out of therapy on the rather dubious assumption that they would have got better had they continued in therapy!

What does Freud have to offer?

We've only scratched the surface of Freud's ideas, but we hope to have shown that these are difficult to test and arguably have led to therapies with little demonstrated clinical efficacy.

Does this mean Freud has nothing to offer? Well, no, in a sense he did an amazing amount for psychology in identifying the unconscious, the important role played by early-life experiences, and starting scientists thinking about alternative models. His lack of scientific rigour and experimentation also did much to expedite experimental psychology as critics rushed to produce scientifically testable alternative theories. However, Freud's often intuitively understood theories have also left psychology with scars to bear, in that most people's perceptions of therapy are probably based on psychoanalysis, which although still widely practised, is probably not an effective treatment.

Cognitive Behaviour Therapy

Cognitive Behaviour Therapy (CBT) was first developed in the mid-twentieth century, thanks to the efforts of a young psychiatrist named Aaron 'Tim' Beck.[1] He had been trained in the psychodynamic tradition, but felt that this approach was letting a lot of his clients down. Instead, when he talked to them about the thoughts that were running through their minds, he realised it was not surprising that they were distressed. For instance, he discovered that his depressed patients often thought things like 'I'm no good at anything, and I never will be'. It occurred to Beck that, if he had these sorts of thoughts, he would be depressed too. He also noticed that, in many cases, these thoughts were highly inaccurate. For example, the people who were thinking 'I'm no good at anything' were often high flyers who had experienced great success in their lives. Beck reasoned that if he could help these clients to correct some of these inaccurate thoughts and beliefs, then he could alleviate some of their suffering. Hence Cognitive Behaviour Therapy was born. Many chapters of this book contain extensive discussions of CBT, so we will not go into great detail about how it works in this chapter. However, in summary, CBT works by changing people's inaccurate, negative beliefs (their 'cognitions') and by also changing the behaviours that maintain these. It is fair to say that CBT is the predominant paradigm in British clinical psychology today. It is based on a sound scientific understanding of the psychological processes that underpin human mental health difficulties, and most psychological research nowadays is based on its principles. CBT is usually considered to be a short-term therapy, with the intention of developing a client's skills for managing their difficulties, so that they can manage on their own as soon as possible.

Treatment of different client groups

The principles that we discuss in this book are largely those that have been developed for working with adults with no intellectual difficulties. The research literature has focused heavily on the needs of this group, and our understanding of psychological problems – and our knowledge of how to treat them – are far greater for this group than for any other.

---

[1] Tim Beck is the nearest thing that clinical psychology has to a superstar. At conferences, he can often be spotted signing autographs and surrounded by adoring fans ...

49

However, researchers are beginning to study cognitive processes in psychological disorders in other groups, and by and large we are finding that there are no great differences. Likewise, the treatment approaches that are found to be useful with adults are, with some modifications, probably useful for different groups too.

Children   We know relatively little about psychological distress in children compared to what we know about it in adults. However, this situation is changing, and part of the purpose of this book is to bring a developmental perspective to the study of psychological disorders in adults. As you might expect, because we know less about psychological disorders in childhood, we are also less adept at treating such disorders. Whilst there are thousands of randomised controlled trials of psychological treatments for adult disorders, there are probably no more than a few hundred good trials of treatments for childhood conditions.

That said, this does not stop psychologists from attempting to treat the children who sit in front of them with distressing psychological symptoms. Our descriptions of the processes of therapy that appear in this chapter and in those that follow are generally just as applicable to children as they are to adults. Yet there are a few additional things that a psychologist working with children needs to take into account:

- Psychologists working with children must take account of the *system* within which the child operates. Children have much less control over their lives than most adults. Instead, the actions of their parents, other carers, relatives, teachers, friends, neighbours, health professionals, and a multitude of others, have a big impact on the emotional life of the child. Most psychologists would not attempt to treat a child in isolation without trying to work out the role of these other agents, that is, the role of the system. See Box 2.6 for a case example to illustrate this role.

Box 2.6   Essential experience

Kayleigh's system

Kayleigh was eight years old and referred to a psychologist because of her refusal to attend school. Whenever she was taken to school she just screamed and clung to her mother and was absolutely terrified of being there. The school nurse had attempted to get her to come back to school using some sensible strategies. She had offered for Kayleigh to just come in for some half days at first, and said that she didn't have to do any lessons that she did not like. She also said that she could sit next to whomever she wanted, and did not have to do her homework. All very sensible stuff, but it just didn't work. When the psychologist (Stewart) met Kayleigh, they sat down and talked about school. Stewart also went into Kayleigh's school and talked to some of her classmates and her teacher, and

---

carried out an assessment with her mother in which he talked to her about her feelings about Kayleigh going to school, and how she managed her school refusal. As a result of this assessment, the psychologist worked out that two major parts of Kayleigh's system were probably at the core of her school refusal. The major causal factor turned out to be some severe bullying that she had experienced at the hands of a boy in her class. In addition, Stewart found a 'maintaining factor'. He discovered that Kayleigh's mother was very anxious herself. Although she very much wanted her daughter to return to school, she was extremely anxious about this. Her interactions with Kayleigh betrayed these fears loud and clear. Even when Mum was trying to encourage her to go to school, she did it in a tone of voice that made it sound as if she was sending Kayleigh to the dark side of the moon, rather than a nice little village school. Although this hadn't caused Kayleigh's problems, it was stopping her from getting over them. She had picked up on her mother's anxiety, and was clearly thinking 'Well if Mum thinks that school is a worrying place to go, then it really must be … '

Stewart used his formulation to develop an intervention for Kayleigh, and actually, because he had decided that most of the causal and maintaining factors lay in the *system*, the actual treatment hardly involved Kayleigh at all. Instead, he arranged for the teachers to keep a very close eye on the boy who had been bullying Kayleigh, and to make sure that he was not allowed near her at any time (he was eventually transferred to a different class). Stewart then helped her mother to come up with some strategies for managing Kayleigh's anxiety in a much more confident and assertive way. Together with the school nurse's techniques for gradually introducing Kayleigh back into school, Stew's intervention worked a treat, and within weeks she had returned to school and was having a great time.

- Children, even older children and teenagers, just don't have the same intellectual abilities as adults, so any therapy needs to take this into account. As psychologists, we need to be aware that we can't just do exactly what works with adults. We often have to turn our clinical techniques into a little game. It also helps to have fun materials, such as worksheets to fill in, and to remember that we can't expect children to keep concentrating for long periods of time. Because of this, sessions with children are usually shorter than those with adults.

Clients with learning disabilities Many psychologists work with people who have learning disabilities, and once again the issues of the system and intellectual capacity are very important. People with learning disabilities (depending on their impairments and their strengths) do not generally lead independent lives, and are very vulnerable to events going on in their system. Many different people may be involved in their lives, and a psychologist needs to check whether any of these people's actions could be causing or maintaining a client's difficulties.

Again, it is often inappropriate to expect a person who has a learning disability to sit with a psychologist for 50 minutes of talking therapy. Concentration spans will need to be assessed and taken into account, as will the person's ability to cope with the therapy. Therapies such as CBT often require an individual to manipulate complex ideas intellectually, and while there is some evidence that many people who have mild to moderate learning disabilities can do much that is required for CBT, this needs to be carefully assessed by the psychologist. Dagnan and colleagues (2000) devised a number of simple tasks to test the key skills that are required to undertake cognitive therapy, that is, an ability to see the links between emotions, events and beliefs. They found that many people with learning difficulties managed these tasks easily, and were therefore likely to benefit from CBT.

Older adults   Psychologists working with older adults often have very varied roles. Many will carry out therapy for psychological disorders, such as those described in this book. However, many will also have to deal with psychological problems that are specifically or primarily a problem for older people. In particular, psychologists working with this age group may specialise in diagnosing dementias and helping clients and their relatives to cope with these conditions. Many psychologists working with this group find that they become very experienced in working with issues around loss: not just the loss of friends and loved ones, but also of abilities (physical and mental) and independence. Issues that are specific to this age group will not be covered in detail in this book.

Other groups   Increasingly, you will find psychologists plying their trade all over the place:

- *Psychologists in physical health settings* As well as working in standard mental health settings, you will often find psychologists working in physical health settings. Physical health professionals (e.g. doctors, nurses) are starting to realise that health and illness are mental as well as physical phenomena. There is now much evidence that psychological interventions can be useful for helping people to cope with some apparently physical conditions (e.g. back pain) and medical interventions (e.g. drugs or surgery).
- *Neuropsychology* Many psychologists now use their skills to help diagnose and manage conditions that arise from brain damage or dysfunction, such as might be the case after a head injury or a stroke.
- *Psychologists in forensic settings* More and more psychologists are being employed in the criminal justice system. This may be in order to help clients with the standard range of mental health problems (which are extremely common in such settings) or to run programmes that will help rehabilitate offenders.

Although we will not be discussing the specific skills that are required by these sorts of psychologists, most psychologists working in these sorts of settings will base their work around the fundamental principles that are outlined in this chapter and those that follow.

Section summary

In this section, we have seen that psychologists work in a very wide range of settings and in a number of different ways. In the next section we will focus on what is probably the most common way of working – with individual, adult clients, using a CBT framework.

Section 4: How CBT works

Here we will see how a typical psychologist uses cognitive behaviour therapy to help an adult with a simple psychological disorder. We will also see that the intervention includes a set of standard components, tailored to the needs of each client: assessment, measuring progress, goal setting, formulation, intervention (using both cognitive and behavioural techniques) and homework. We will then go on to discuss some of the realities of carrying out cognitive behavioural therapy, focusing on some of the key difficulties that psychologists and their clients face.

Assessment

The beginning of any good psychological treatment is always a thorough *assessment*. During this assessment, the psychologist has two main aims: first, to get a good baseline measure of how the client is doing at the start of therapy. This measurement will then be repeated throughout the course of treatment, to make sure that things are progressing (and if not, so that the psychologist can take some action). The second aim is to try to find out all of the factors that might be involved in the difficulty with which their client is presenting, and to draw up a *formulation* (see below).

Measuring progress

Returning to the measurement of how a client is doing, a psychologist has a number of options. Most psychologists like to use a combination of standardised, well-validated questionnaires that measure the symptoms of psychological disorder, and idiosyncratic measures that are designed specifically for their client.

Well-validated measures

These are 'off the shelf' measures that have been designed specifically for measuring the symptoms of psychological disorders. These measures will have been through a rigorous process of research to make sure that they are:

- Reliable (i.e. that they consistently measure what they set out to measure). So for instance, if I use the Beck Depression Inventory (the BDI – perhaps the most widely used measure of depression symptoms for adults), I want to know that if you score as 'moderately depressed' today, you will also show up as 'moderately depressed' when I administer it tomorrow (unless I have effected some kind of miracle cure in the interim).

- Valid (i.e. that the measure measures what it is supposed to measure). So, if I am giving you the BDI to see how depressed you are, I really want to know that this is exactly what it is measuring. A good measure will have been exhaustively researched, to check that it correlates with clinicians' judgements of how a patient is doing, and that it also correlates with other questionnaire measures for similar symptoms.

Idiosyncratic measures

The advantage of well-validated measures is that you can be sure that they are both reliable and valid. In addition, the publishers will usually have lists of 'norms' that will tell you exactly how you would expect different populations to score on the measure, and so you can see how your client compares. However, the disadvantage here is that they might not measure quite the same thing that you want to measure. So, for instance, you may wish to measure exactly how scared of candy floss your client is, but you are unlikely to find a ready-made questionnaire that can do this for you. In these situations, you may wish to devise you own 'idiosyncratic' measure. An idiosyncratic measure can be anything that you want it to be. It might just be a simple question, such as 'Today, on a scale of 0–10, where 0 is not scary at all, and 10 is completely terrifying, how scary do you think candy floss is?'. However, you may find that your client is not very good at reporting their symptoms just by using pen and paper. Instead, you might think that you want to see their symptoms in action. Therefore you might decide that a better way to look at the candy floss phobia may be to show your client some candy floss and see how they react. However, in this situation you will need some way of coding how they do so. So, for instance, you might put them in a room with some candy floss and ask them to walk as close to it as they can, and then measure this. This is known as a 'behavioural approach test', and is widely used as a measure of fears.

Box 2.7   Essential research

Measuring the impact of a brief intervention for agoraphobia

In this study (by Salkovskis and colleagues, 1999) the authors were testing part of a new psychological treatment for agoraphobia. In order to do this they decided to assess their participants' agoraphobia before and after treatment. They gave out the usual array of scales and questionnaires, but they also wanted to gain a real behavioural measure of their participants' fear, so they devised a 'behavioural walk'. The intention was to make the participants do something that they found anxiety-provoking, and see how much they could manage. The participants were told that they were about to be asked to do something very difficult, and they should just try to complete as many steps as they could, but that they could turn back at any point.

The behavioural walk began with a psychologist walking a client to that psychologist's car. They then drove into the local town. The participant was then asked to get out of the car and walk down a quiet street, then through a marketplace, into a crowded shopping centre, and up to a bus stop, before getting on a bus and riding back to the start point. These steps were in an order of increasing difficulty for most agoraphobic participants, and by using this 'behavioural walk' the psychologists could get a really good measure of how troublesome the agoraphobia was. By asking the participants to rate their level of anxiety at various points along the way, the researchers were also able to establish how much distress they were experiencing before and after treatment.

Formulation

The second main aim of the assessment period is to develop a formulation of a client's difficulties. In order to draw up this formulation, the psychologist will want to find out: How did the problem start? What triggers the symptoms now? What does the client think and feel when they get these symptoms? What do they do when they get these symptoms? Does anyone else do anything that helps or hinders?

A very simple formulation of a client presenting with depression is reproduced in Box 2.8.

Box 2.8   Essential experience

Mike's formulation

Background factors	Resulting beliefs
Born with a sensitive disposition	I am not a worthwhile person
Bullied at school	I am unlovable
Mike's mother was often depressed when he was young, and he sometimes experienced mild emotional abuse and neglect as a result	

(Continued)

(Continued)

Trigger
Mike was made redundant from his job, and six months later was still struggling to find a new one
Mike's relationship with his wife was deteriorating

Thoughts
I am no good at anything
The whole world is against me
I will never find a job

Behaviour	Feelings
Sitting on sofa all day, not going out	Hopelessness
Critical towards wife	Misery
Given up applying for jobs	Helplessness

Mike was a 52-year old man who had been referred to his GP by the Job Centre. He had been unemployed for six months, but was at risk of losing his benefits because he was failing to turn up to Job Centre appointments, and was not actively trying to get a new job. His GP suspected that Mike was seriously depressed and referred him to the local mental health services, where he was seen by a clinical psychologist called Poppy. Poppy carried out an assessment, and together with Mike, drew up the simple formulation shown in Box 2.8.

Background factors

Although Poppy and Mike did not talk in great detail about his early life (Poppy was a cognitive behaviour therapist, so liked to focus on the here and now) they ascertained that Mike's mother had often been depressed when he was a child. Depression often runs in families, partly because of the effect that depression has on people's parenting skills (see Chapter 5). In Mike's case his mother had often been very withdrawn, and he experienced periods when his basic needs (food, warm clothing, cuddles) were not adequately met. His mother's depression often meant that she was angry and irritable, and at these times Mike experienced some emotional abuse from his mother (e.g. telling him he was a waste of space, and that she wished she had never had children). Mike described himself as 'hot-headed' as a child. He was often in trouble at school and described having been frequently bullied; he left at 15 without any qualifications. As a result of his temperament, and in all likelihood his genetic propensity towards depression, and as a consequence of these early life experiences, Mike had developed a set of negative beliefs about himself. He felt that he was not a worthwhile person, and that he was essentially unlovable. Despite this difficult start, Mike had gone on to do well. He began work as an unskilled labourer in a car factory, but due to hard work and natural ability, he rose up the ranks and eventually became a factory foreman. He met a lovely woman, Carol, who went on to become his wife, and they had two children.

The trigger for Mike's depression came when, owing to a transfer of much car production overseas, he was made redundant. He tried applying for a few similar jobs, but of course they were swamped with applicants at that time and he was unsuccessful. Although his beliefs about being unloveable and unworthy had lain dormant for many years, they began to resurface. He started to have thoughts that he would never work again. Although he had been skilled at his car factory job, he could think of no other job that he would be good enough to apply for. The rejection letters that he received triggered thoughts that the world was against him. These thoughts led to feelings of misery, hopelessness and helplessness. And these thoughts and feelings together resulted in a set of behaviours that made things even worse: Mike stopped applying for jobs, and started to miss Job Centre appointments (thus meaning that there was absolutely no chance that he would find a new job, and thereby confirming his thoughts and beliefs). In fact he stopped doing almost everything. He had once had an active social life, seeing friends with Carol every Saturday evening and friends in the pub two or three times a week, going to the cinema a couple of times a month, and to a cycling club once a week. This had now all stopped. Mike spent all day in his pyjamas on the sofa, watching daytime TV and ruminating on his dreadful life. His low mood also made him irritable and he had become increasingly critical and snappy with Carol. Poppy met Carol at a later session and discovered that although she had been understanding to begin with, she was now getting very frustrated with Mike, as she could see that he was 'his own worst enemy'. She also felt that she had to 'walk on eggshells' around him. The relationship between Carol and Mike was very fragile, and Mike was taking this as yet further indication that the whole world was set against him.

Can you see how Mike had got into a vicious cycle of depression? His behaviour was acting in a way that reinforced his negative thoughts, which in turn made him even more miserable, and also made these problematic behaviours yet more likely. Poppy had to find a way to break into this vicious cycle.

Establishing goals

A final main aim of assessment is to establish the goals of therapy, and the psychologist and the client must work these out together. In this case, by the end of the intervention, Mike and Poppy hoped that he would be feeling more cheerful, and would either have a new job or be applying for jobs again.

However, therapy goals can be much more complex than this, as we will see in the coming chapters. What is important, no matter how complex the goals are, is for the psychologist to try to ensure that they are measurable, so that client and therapist can tell whether they are achieving them or not.

Having completed some baseline measures, developed a formulation and established some goals, the formal assessment period is almost complete. However, for a good psychologist an assessment will never truly be over until the client is discharged. The psychologist should revisit the formulation at every session to incorporate any new information that has been gleaned. Sometimes, very important bits of information will not come out until many weeks into therapy. Perhaps a client did not think the information was important, or often they needed to feel that they could trust the psychologist before they were able to divulge some difficult or sensitive information. Sometimes, as in this case, another person (Carol) will shed extra light on what has been going on.

The intervention

By the end of the assessment, the intervention has already begun. In Mike's case, during the assessment sessions whilst drawing up the initial formulation, Poppy had been working hard to explain to Mike what was causing his depression. So by the start of the intervention, Mike was already aware of where the problems lay, and had a good idea of what he needed to do to sort out the problem.

At the start of the intervention, the psychologist will have a plan of action. This is never set in stone, and will evolve along with the formulation. For Mike, the initial plan was as follows:

Use cognitive techniques to unpick some of his beliefs about himself, the world and the future.

Use behavioural techniques to get him active again (and also to test out some of his beliefs about himself, the world and the future).

Cognitive techniques

As we have seen, during the assessment, the psychologist, Poppy, found that some of Mike's beliefs were very important. As is often the case in depression (see Chapter 5), Mike had negative beliefs about himself, the world and the future. These beliefs were internal (i.e. that he was flawed and incapable of finding a job/being loved), global (i.e. that he was completely unworthy as a person, rather than just a bit shaky in a few areas) and stable (i.e. that he would *never* get a job and *never* be worthwhile or lovable).

Being a good psychologist Poppy was constantly measuring Mike's progress, so she asked him to rate how much he believed these thoughts on a scale of 0% to 100%. His ratings for each of the key beliefs are reported in Box 2.9.

Box 2.9   Essential treatment

Mike's beliefs at the start and end of the first
treatment session

Belief	Rating (0–100%) at start of session	Rating (0–100%) at end of session
I am no good at anything	100	80
I am unlovable	90	60
The world is against me	90	50
I will never work again	100	99

Poppy decided that the first task was to try to loosen some of Mike's beliefs just by talking about them. They began by talking about the beliefs, and discussing whether Mike had any evidence that these were true. Poppy asked gentle questions of Mike, such as:

Tell me about the people love you – Carol, your children.

Tell me about the people who are on your side, and who have tried to help you.

Tell me about times in your life when you have done well.

Have any of the people who were made redundant at the same time as you found jobs?

Poppy asked these questions in a kind and unthreatening manner. Her aim was to prompt Mike to begin questioning whether his beliefs were totally accurate. So in answer to the questions listed above Mike realised that not quite the whole world was against him (his wife and some of his old friends had really tried to help, as had his GP, the lady at the Job Centre, and some others). He also realised that he couldn't be totally unlovable. His wife clearly loved him, even if she didn't show it as much as usual at the moment. His children loved him very much and were clearly worried about him. Although he still felt that he would never work again, he admitted that some of his ex-colleagues, who were no more skilled than him, had managed to secure okay jobs. He also realised that although he didn't use his skills at the moment, over the course of his career he had done very well, and had become respected for his ability to quickly sort out problems on the factory floor.

At the end of the first treatment session, Poppy asked Mike to re-rate how much he believed each of these key beliefs. As you will see from Box 2.9, his conviction in each of the beliefs had dropped away a little bit, but there was still quite a way to go.

Behavioural techniques

Although the first session had gone well and she intended to keep going with the cognitive techniques, Poppy knew that the only way to really crack Mike's depression was to get him back to engaging in his normal activities. People who are seriously depressed are usually very inactive, and getting them going again (otherwise known as 'behavioural activation') is critical to their recovery. However, this usually has to be done very gradually. Trying to go from doing virtually nothing to an active social life overnight would be overwhelming for a depressed person and would almost certainly result in failure. Therefore, Poppy asked Mike to choose one activity that he would agree to take up again. Mike, reluctantly, chose returning to his cycling club. He agreed that he would go along again this Thursday evening, and promised Poppy that he would do this, even if he didn't feel like it. Poppy asked him to tell her how he felt about this. Mike said that he felt very anxious about going back. He was worried that everyone would quiz him about why he had not been for so long and he wouldn't know what to say. Poppy felt that this concern was reasonable – as people would be wondering where Mike had been – so she and Mike practised some answers to this question. Poppy then got Mike to rate how much he thought he would enjoy going to the cycling club and how much 'mastery' he expected to feel after it, that is, how much he would feel that he had achieved something in going. Mike said that he thought he would enjoy it 0% and would feel 5% 'mastery' as a result of going.

The next week Mike returned to see Poppy and seemed a little better. He reported that he had been to the cycling club and had really enjoyed it. People had asked him why he hadn't been for a while, but he just gave the simple answers that he and Poppy had rehearsed and it was fine. Afterwards, he felt as if he had really taken some steps forward and had done something good (both for his fitness and his mental health). He also rated his pleasure in going at 70% and his 'mastery' in going at 80%. Poppy used the discrepancy in Mike's pleasure and mastery ratings before and after the visit to the cycling club as a basis for a discussion about how depression negatively influences your predictions about things, and about how activity lifts your mood.

Poppy then asked Mike to add another activity into the following week, and he chose going to the pub with mates one evening. Poppy asked him to rate his predicted pleasure and mastery in doing this, as he had done before.

Each week Poppy asked Mike to add in another activity, until by the end of therapy, his social life was almost as busy as before he became depressed. Each time he went out he rated how much 'pleasure' and 'mastery' the trip gave him, and soon came to see the powerful positive effect that activity had on his mood.

Over the course of their sessions Poppy and Mike worked further on his negative beliefs, gathering evidence to test whether these were true or false. For example, one week Poppy got Mike to carry out a 'mini-survey' of his mates to test out his belief that 'there are no jobs for someone of my age'. He had to ask 10 friends, in the pub for instance, whether their employers ever took on people of his age. He predicted that they would all say 'never'. In fact eight said that their employer had recently taken on someone of Mike's age or older, and one even said that his boss preferred employing people with a bit of life experience and common sense.

Together with Mike's contact at the Job Centre, Poppy and Mike put together a plan for him to start applying for jobs again. He had come to accept that he did have useful skills, and that if he was willing to be flexible he might find something roughly suitable if not exactly like his old job. And sure enough, within a month of starting applying he was offered a job. It wasn't quite the same as his old job, and didn't use all of his skills. It was also slightly less well paid. But Mike grabbed it, and threw himself into it wholeheartedly. Within six months his ability and hard work had been spotted, and he was promoted to a job that he loved and which paid as much as his previous one. His improved mood meant that he was much nicer to his wife, and because he was now at work all day he wasn't getting under her feet quite so much. Their relationship improved markedly, and at a follow-up appointment with Poppy six months later they were planning a party to celebrate 25 years of marriage.

Homework

Homework is a critical part of almost every psychological intervention. It may not be homework in the way that you remember it from school. In fact, the further away we can get from giving clients written homework, the better.

Homework is used to reinforce the most important messages from the therapy session. It is also used to help move things on between sessions, as well as help a client generalise what they have learnt in the psychologist's office to be of use in the outside world. There is no point a client being happy and confident when they are with the psychologist, if this evaporates the moment they walk out of the building.

For homework Poppy asked Mike to engage in a new activity every week, and to rate how much 'pleasure' and how much 'mastery' this gave him. Sometimes she also asked him to complete a 'thought diary'. A thought diary is used to write down negative thoughts that can then be discussed in therapy. It also helps to identify the triggers to such thoughts, and over time, for the client to practise coming up with more positive ways of thinking.

Maintenance and generalisation

Although many clients do well in their therapy, relapse is a big problem. After the initial buzz of improvement, and the resulting motivation to try really hard, things can start to slow down. Eventually, despite marked initial improvements, many clients' symptoms will begin to creep back. There are two main reasons for this:

1. Therapy is too restricted, and although the patient is fine in the psychologist's office or in their own home, when they have to cope in a new situation they lack either the skills or the confidence to do this.
2. The client forgets to keep practising their new behaviours and ways of thinking, and the old difficulties gradually creep back.

To minimise the chances of this happening, Poppy and Mike drew up a 'first aid kit' of 'tools' that he could use if he ever felt his mood slipping again. This included all of Mike's thought diaries and handouts from therapy, and a list of activities that could reliably be used to lift his mood.

Finally, Poppy carried out a last assessment to do a formal check on how he was doing. The questionnaires all showed that Mike's symptoms of depression had reduced dramatically and were now well within the normal range.

The realities of treatment

What we have presented here is a very simple and idealised case. Most practising psychologists will never see a case as simple and as straightforward as Mike's. We have presented this here so that we can explain the fundamentals of psychological therapy, unclouded by the complexities that often arise. So what are the main difficulties that psychologists face in their work? We will give a brief overview of these next, and return to them in more detail throughout subsequent chapters.

Comorbidity

We presented Mike as someone who had a fairly simple mood disorder. However, such an individual is quite rare. Many people who present with depression also have anxiety disorders, or personality disorders, or intractable 'life' problems such as serious health concerns or debts.

Moreover, when some people have problems they can attempt to solve these in maladaptive ways. We know that many (but certainly not all) people with mood disorders use alcohol or drugs to help ease their symptoms. If this gets out of hand then they can end up with a substance use disorder (see Chapter 9) on top of their mood disorder.

As a result, having a minor disorder can snowball until a client has multiple layers of difficulty. We're sure that we don't have to explain how much this complicates therapy. Unfortunately, since there are (and probably always will be) too few psychologists to go around, it is usually only those with the most severe or complex disorders that can access therapy.

Motivation

The clients described in this book are largely individuals who have come willingly to therapy and are motivated to try hard and get better; however, this is not always the case. Many of the clients that psychologists see do not finish therapy, or if they do they are unable to really give it their best shot. There are a number of common reasons for this. Although many adult clients will have asked for therapy and will be coming along willingly, other clients will not. Many child clients, for instance, have been taken to see a psychologist against their will. Likewise, some of the adults that psychologists work with will have been forcibly detained in hospital under the Mental Health Act. In such cases the psychologist's job is that much harder as a result. The first thing they have to try to do is build a relationship with that client (not always easy, as you can imagine) and then to work on that person's motivation to change.

In the past, motivation was seen as the client's problem. If they didn't want to come to therapy, or make an effort when there, tough! However, in recent years, in the UK at least, there has been a move towards 'assertive outreach'. Those most in need of psychological assistance are now often identified and then sought out by services, who will do all they can to meet those clients' needs, which might mean going and seeing them in the community rather than expecting them to attend a clinic, allowing them to miss sessions without discharging them, and so on.

When motivational techniques and assertive outreach fail, however, there is little that a psychologist can do other than put some work into improving that client's 'system'.

External factors

Sometimes it can be just people's lives that get in the way of them benefiting from therapy. It is difficult to concentrate on making subtle changes to our thinking style, or making scary changes in our behaviour, when we haven't got enough to eat, are about to be evicted, or we live in constant fear of violence. Unfortunately, many, many British people still have to cope with this sort of situation, and not surprisingly, it is those same people who have the most mental health difficulties. However, working psychologically with someone who is living in such difficult circumstances is very hard. The sad fact is that therapy in these situations is much less likely to be successful, and psychologists working for long periods of time with such client groups need to take special care of themselves if burnout is to be avoided.

Relationship and personality factors

Many of the clients that you meet as a psychologist will be lovely, easy people to get on with. However, it would also be a rare psychologist who has never come across a client that they just could not warm to. Sometimes this will just be a 'personality clash' and the psychologist should then use 'supervision' (this is the mandatory, regular, scheduled sessions with a colleague where the psychologist critically discusses their practice) to help manage this, or could, in serious cases, consider transferring that client to someone else. However, in some instances it can be very difficult to build a trusting therapeutic relationship with a client because they have what is known as a 'personality disorder'. Now there is a great deal of controversy around personality disorder, and this will be covered in greater detail in Chapter 11, but just to summarise briefly, some psychologists believe that certain people have a damaged personality structure which means that it is difficult for them to develop meaningful, trusting relationships. There are a number of different personality disorders, and each brings with it specific problems. However, the evidence suggests that psychological therapies are less successful when they are attempted with clients who have comorbid personality disorders. In part this is likely to be because the client and their psychologist find it difficult to trust each other and get along. However, it is also likely to be because people with personality disorders usually have difficulty building and maintaining fulfilling relationships in the outside world too. It is not difficult to see how therapy is less successful for someone who only has precarious relationships to lean on in times of need.

Section summary

In this chapter we have looked at the main components of CBT. We know that when CBT contains all of these components, it is more likely to succeed than when some of them are missing. We have also seen that therapy does not always run smoothly, and have outlined some of the main reasons for this.

Section 5: The ethics of psychological therapy

Psychologists working with members of the public (whether as researchers, lecturers or therapists) can be in a very powerful position. In response to the risks associated with this power, all UK psychologists are bound by a code of conduct published by the British Psychological Society (*Code of Ethics and Conduct*, 2009 (August)). All psychologists are bound by these guidelines, but the key aspects for those who are delivering therapy are outlined in Box 2.10.

Box 2.10   Key guidelines for psychologists delivering psychotherapy

The following guidelines have been adapted from the British Psychological Society's *Code of Ethics and Conduct* (August 2009):

Respect

- Psychologists should respect the differences between individuals, and be non-discriminatory in their work.
- Psychologists should endeavour to protect clients' privacy and confidentiality, except where doing so puts a client or someone else at risk.
- Psychologists should always seek to obtain informed consent for their interventions.

Competence

- Psychologists should be familiar with the *Code of Ethics and Conduct*.
- Psychologists should recognise the limits of their own competence.

  - They should not offer interventions for disorders or client groups for whom they are not adequately trained or experienced.
  - They should endeavour to keep up to date with new developments, using a formal system of 'Continuing Professional Development'.

- They should get regular supervision on their practice from another qualified practitioner.
- They should be aware that sometimes their own problems and functioning can impair their ability to deliver therapy to the highest standard. In these situations they should seek appropriate supervision from colleagues, and consider suspending their own practice temporarily.

Responsibility

- Psychologists should avoid engaging in any behaviour that might harm their clients.
- Psychologists should avoid personal and professional misconduct that might bring the profession into disrepute.
- Psychologists should be mindful of the risks to themselves.

Integrity

- Psychologists should keep very tight boundaries on their relationships with their clients. It is viewed as highly inappropriate to develop a romantic relationship with any client, past or present.
- Psychologists should think very carefully before attempting to provide therapy for friends or family.
- Psychologists should be aware of the powerful position that they are often in with clients, and should be careful never to abuse this position for their own gain.

These guidelines are particularly relevant to psychologists engaged in therapy. The full code, which applies to psychologists generally, is available at www.bps.org.uk/ethics

All psychologists should strive to meet these standards at all times, but in practice there is room for considerable interpretation in some of these guidelines, and others can be tricky to follow. For instance, one of the key ethical standards, which is drummed into all trainee psychologists from Day 1, is the need to respect client confidentiality. Clients need to know that they can trust their psychologist in order that they can share difficult information with them. To encourage this, a psychologist – usually at the first session, and then repeatedly throughout therapy as necessary – reminds the client that whatever they say will be treated in confidence. However, there are times when this trust must be broken. Some of these times are clear cut: for example, if a client tells you that they plan to leave the session and kill themselves, and that they have a clear plan of where, when and how they will do this, then as their therapist *you must act on this information* (usually by ensuring that the client gets to the nearest hospital as soon as possible). Likewise, for example, if a client tells you that they have sexually abused a child, *you must alert social services/the police as a matter of urgency*, regardless of your responsibility to keep that client's information confidential.

There are situations, however, that are less clear cut. What if a client says they have had thoughts of killing themselves, have given some consideration as to how they might do it, but haven't got a clear plan yet? You try to persuade them to take themselves to hospital but they are not keen. You know that if you call their GP to pass on this information this may ensure their safety for now, but it will ruin their relationship with you and they will probably never return to therapy. Similarly, it is technically illegal to hit a child in the UK, but the law is vague, and in many areas of the country social services will not take an interest in parents who hit their children unless they are doing physical harm, or there are other significant parenting issues as well. So if a parent tells you that they regularly smack their child … what do you do? In other respects, they are not terrible parents … and you are optimistic that if you can keep them in your parenting group for just a few more weeks, they will learn some better strategies for managing their children, and family life will become happier for all concerned. On the other hand, if you alert social services they will probably do nothing beyond a brief assessment, and you will almost certainly lose the family from your group.

In order to manage this situation, most psychologists would say something like the following when they first meet a new client: 'Everything you tell me here is private. I won't tell anyone else. The only exception is if you tell me something that makes me very worried about you or about someone else. In that case it's my duty to act to make sure that everyone stays safe. Is that okay? If I have to do this, I will do my very best to get hold of you and tell what I'm going to do first.'

Section summary

We have learnt that psychologists are bound by codes of conduct that dictate minimum levels of competence and integrity, and set out the framework of respect that all psychologists should show for their clients.

Essential questions

- What are the main stages in the psychological treatment of a psychological disorder?
- Should medications ever be prescribed for the treatment of psychological disorders?
- How are new psychological treatments evaluated? What are the difficulties in evaluating new treatments?

Further reading

Bennett-Levy, J., Richards, D., Farrand, P., Christensen, H., Griffiths, K., Kavanagh, D. et al. (2010) *Oxford Guide to Low Intensity CBT Interventions*. Oxford: Oxford University Press. (This book will give you an idea of how basic CBT works, in the reality of the NHS.)

British Psychological Society (2009). *Code of Ethics and Conduct*. London: BPS. (This is the full version of the *Code of Conduct* that is outlined earlier and is important reading for anyone considering a career as a psychologist.)

Wilson, P., Rush, R., Hussey, S., Puckering, C., Sim, F., Allely, C. et al. (2012). How evidence-based is an 'evidence-based parenting program'? A PRISMA systematic review and meta-analysis of Triple P. *BMC Medicine*, 10(1): 130. (This is a systematic review of the research published about the Triple P Parenting Programme. This is a very critical paper, and highlights the many difficulties of doing research on psychological interventions.)

www.thementalelf.net/ (This website provides very useful summaries of individual studies and meta-analyses of treatments for psychological disorders. The summaries are brief and appropriately critical, and also a good way to 'dip into' a topic before you turn to look at articles published in scientific journals.)

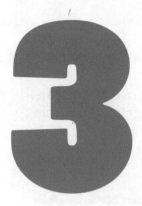

CHILDHOOD DISORDERS

General introduction

In this chapter, we look at how children's clinical psychologists go about their work. Children can experience most of the disorders that adults experience, so child psychologists have to know all about those. However, there are a set of additional disorders that usually appear first in childhood, such as behaviour problems and autistic spectrum disorders, which make up a lot of the general child psychologist's caseload. Clearly, we cannot cover all of these in one chapter. Instead, we will look at how two very common disorders in adults – anxiety and depression – manifest in children. We will then look at behaviour disorders, which are extremely common in children's mental health services. In each case, we will focus on the symptoms that children present with, the causes of disorder and how children are treated.

Assessment targets

At the end of the chapter, you should ask yourself the following questions:

- Can I explain the key diagnostic criteria for childhood and adolescent anxiety disorders, depression and behaviour problems?
- How are childhood and adolescent anxiety disorders, depression and behaviour problems treated? Is there any evidence that these treatments are effective?
- What are the roles of genetic and environmental factors in the aetiology of childhood and adolescent anxiety disorders, depression and behaviour problems?
- Do parents cause childhood and adolescent psychological disorders?

Section 1: Anxiety disorders of childhood

Diagnosis of anxiety disorders in childhood

Children can be diagnosed with any of the anxiety disorders that adults are diagnosed with, including those discussed in this book such as Generalised Anxiety Disorder (sometimes called Overanxious Disorder in children; see Chapter 6), specific phobias (Chapter 7) and Panic Disorder and Social Anxiety Disorder (Chapter 8). However, it is important to take the child's age and developmental stage into account when making such diagnoses, because it is normal for children to have heightened fears (e.g. animals, separation, the dark) at certain stages in their development.

Although children can get all of the same anxiety disorder diagnoses as adults, there is one additional diagnosis that is only available to children in the *ICD*-10 classification system (although, interestingly, in the latest version of the *DSM* adults can get this diagnosis too). This is Separation Anxiety Disorder, and the *ICD*-10 diagnostic criteria are shown in Box 3.1, followed by a case study which is described in Box 3.2.

Box 3.1   Essential diagnosis

ICD-10 separation anxiety disorder (World Health Organisation, 1992)

A. At least three of the following:

    (1) Unrealistic and persistent worry about possible harm befalling major attachment figures or the loss of such figures (e.g. fear that they will leave and not return or that the child will not see them again) or persistent concerns about death of attachment figures.

    (2) Unrealistic and persistent worry that some untoward event will separate the child from a major attachment figure (e.g. as by the child getting lost, kidnapped, admitted to the hospital, or killed).

    (3) Persistent reluctance or refusal to go to school because of fear over separation from a major attachment figure or in order to stay at home (rather than for other reasons such as fear over happenings at school).

(Continued)

(Continued)

(4) Difficulty separating at night as manifested by any of the following:

  (a) persistent reluctance or refusal to go to sleep without being near an attachment figure;

  (b) often getting up during the night to check on, or to sleep near an attachment figure;

  (c) persistent reluctance or refusal to sleep away from home.

(5) Persistent inappropriate fear of being alone, or otherwise without the major attachment figure at home during the day.

(6) Repeated nightmares about separation.

(7) Repeated occurrence of physical symptoms (such as nausea, stomach ache, headache, or vomiting) on occasions that involve separation from a major attachment figure, such as leaving home to go to school or on other occasions where anticipating a separation (holiday, camps, etc.).

(8) Excessive, recurrent distress in anticipation of, or during, or immediately following, separation from a major attachment figure (as shown by: anxiety, crying, tantrums; persistent reluctance to go away from home; excessive need to talk with parents or desire to return home; misery, apathy or social withdrawal).

B. Absence of generalized anxiety disorder of childhood.

C. Onset before the age of six.

D. The disorder does not occur as part of a broader disturbance of emotions, conduct, personality, or of a pervasive developmental disorder, psychotic disorder, psychoactive or substance use disorder.

E. Duration of at least four weeks.

Box 3.2   Essential experience

Anxiety disorders in children

Jack is nine years old and has been diagnosed with generalised anxiety disorder, separation anxiety disorder and social anxiety disorder. He has a number of symptoms that make life difficult for him and his family. Although he now manages to go to school reasonably well (he used to cry and cling to his dad at the school gate every morning) he refuses to go to after school club, which means that his mother has had to give up her full-time job and find a part-time one so that she can collect him after school every day. He worries a great deal, even about things that you wouldn't expect a young child to worry about, such as war breaking out and his family's financial situation. He refuses to stay over at anyone else's house, and doesn't even like going to friends' birthday parties, which means that he misses out on a lot of social life. He hates it when his parents go out for the evening, and will only just about tolerate this if his grandparents come to babysit, but they live miles away, so Jack's parents don't get out much any more. His sleep has improved a bit of late, but he still finds it difficult to sleep at night, and also still sleeps with his parents most nights. All of this is starting to make Jack stand out at school. His friends are beginning to get quite independent. They go to football club and cubs, but Jack won't go. He also won't go to sleepovers, which are very common now. One of his friends found out that he sleeps in his parents' bed, and now he is being teased about it. It is also taking its toll on his parents' marital relationship. The lack of privacy in the bedroom and the lack of time out together have caused some friction, and arguments are becoming common.

How common are anxiety disorders in childhood?

As is usually the case, it depends on who you ask. A systematic review of the area by one of the authors of this book found prevalence rates ranging between 2% and 40% (Cartwright-Hatton et al., 2006). If you read this paper it outlines some of the reasons why these rates are so very varied. However, a group of British psychiatrists set out to find out how common psychological disorders are in British children (Ford et al., 2003). They did this really properly

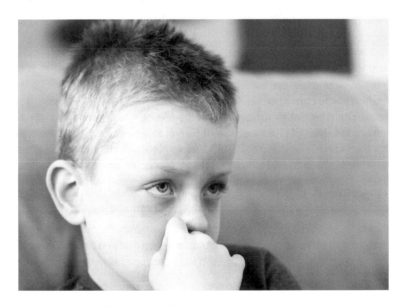

Figure 3.1   Jack (portrayed by an actor)

and carefully (see Box 3.3), surveying a huge sample of children, and found that around 3% of 5 to 10 year olds had an anxiety disorder (about the same numbers of boys and girls), as did 4.6% of 11 to 15 year olds, but in this age group, anxiety was more common in girls (5.3%) than boys (3.9%).

Box 3.3   Essential research

Measuring the prevalence of psychological disorders in children

Epidemiological research is the type of research that is used to estimate how common something is in a population. Good epidemiological research has a number of features:

1. It has a very large sample, to make sure that a wide range of the population are represented.
2. It tries to get a representative sample, so that all sectors of society are represented.
3. It tries to obtain a very high response rate. People who take part (and don't take part) in surveys are not random. We know that certain groups in society (e.g. the less highly educated and males) are less likely to take part in research, and therefore they are also less likely to be represented by the results of research. In order to make sure that everyone is represented, good epidemiological research tries to get a very high response rate from all sectors.
4. It tries to get accurate information if possible, and also appropriate information, from a number of sources.

The Mental Health of Children and Adolescents in Great Britain (Ford et al., 2003) was the first proper, large-scale epidemiological survey of children's mental health in the UK, and this is how it was carried out.

   The researchers set out to survey not just the prevalence of mental health difficulties in children and adolescents, but also the impact of these on them, and the burden this caused for their families and society. They also wanted to understand how children with mental health difficulties used services so that these could be planned more effectively for the future. They aimed to obtain a very large sample, so they sent invitation letters to over 14,000 families. In order to ensure that these families were representative of the entire population, they selected families from the child benefit register. Almost every child in the country (at that time) received child benefit payments, no matter what their background was, so this was a very good way of making sure that just about every child in the country had a chance to participate. Children from this register were selected at random, although the researchers made sure that there was a very wide and even geographical spread across the country. They then worked hard to make sure that they got a very high response rate. They gave people the chance to 'opt out' of the research when they were first invited to participate, but if they did not hear from the participants they got in touch to arrange a visit. In the end 83% of those approached took part in the research, which was an excellent response rate.

In some epidemiological studies, to save money, people will just fill in question-naires and return these to the researchers, who will then base their diagnoses on the responses to these questionnaires. However, this can result in mistakes, and can mean that disorders are missed or diagnoses are made when no real disorder is present. Sometimes, in order to check that the questionnaire is doing a good job, the research-ers will then go and interview a small subset of participants and assign a diagnosis that way, and then check that this matches with the questionnaire-based diagnoses that were given to this sample. This will usually show up some inaccuracies in the questionnaire, and the researchers will use these to adjust the results of their survey. However, this gives rise to quite a lot of guesstimation and less reliable results. So in their survey, Ford et al. (2003) chose to interview every single family in person. Clearly this was a very expensive and time-consuming task, but it did mean that the results were very reliable.

In some epidemiological studies only the child is asked about their symptoms, or only the parent. This produces biased results, with parents being more likely to report annoying behavioural symptoms, and children being more likely to report subtle emo-tional symptoms. Therefore Ford et al. interviewed both the parents and the children (only those aged 11 or over). They also sent questionnaires to teachers, in order to gain some additional, objective perspectives.

Finally, some epidemiological studies of mental health difficulties will just look at symp-toms, and if a participant has enough symptoms they will get a diagnosis. In their study, Ford et al. insisted that in order to get a diagnosis, children had to show *impairment* as a result of their symptoms. In other words, they had to be distressed by their symptoms, or their symptoms had to have a significant impact on their daily life. Taking this approach does reduce the prevalence rates of reported disorder, but it also makes sure that only people who actually have problems get diagnosed.

So what did this study find?

They found that around 10% of 5 to 15 year olds had a diagnosable mental health condition. This was higher in 11 to 15 year olds than 5 to 10 year olds, and was also higher in boys than girls, although the girls were starting to catch up by adolescence.

(Continued)

(Continued)

They also discovered that the likelihood of having a diagnosis was strongly associated with socioeconomic status, with those lower down the social hierarchy receiving more diagnoses. They also found that children with diagnoses were much more likely to be having educational problems at school, and were much more likely to report that they smoked tobacco or cannabis or drank alcohol. In relation to this point, this was a cross-sectional survey, so it was not able to tell us whether the mental health difficulties caused their alcohol and drug use, or vice versa, or whether some third factor caused all of these (see Chapter 9).

What causes childhood anxiety?

As is the case for every psychological disorder, childhood anxiety disorders are caused by a complicated concoction of heritable and environmental factors.

Heritability and genetics

Family studies, where relatives of people with anxiety disorders are studied, show that anxiety definitely runs in families. For instance, Hettema (2001) showed that first-degree relatives (the parents, children and siblings) of people with panic disorder were around five times more likely to have panic disorder themselves than people who did not have a first-degree relative with panic disorder. Similarly, Turner et al. (1987) found that children of anxious parents were seven times more likely to have an anxiety disorder than children who did not have a parent with an anxiety disorder. However, this in itself does not tell us whether anxiety is heritable. It could be that anxious people behave in a way that means that their relatives are more likely to become anxious. Or it could mean that an environment that is shared between the relatives makes them all more prone to anxiety (see Box 1.8 in Chapter 1). So in order to untangle this, researchers have used twin and adoption studies to estimate the heritability of anxiety disorders in children. In one study of anxiety in six year old twins, the heritability of separation anxiety disorder was estimated at 73% (Bolton et al., 2006). Using an adoption study, Daniels and Plomin (1984) showed that shyness in young children was related both to shyness levels in their biological mothers, indicating a genetic contribution to the trait, *and* to low sociability in their adoptive mothers, indicating an environmental contribution too. A broader review of twin studies that investigated the heritability of anxiety disorders in children (Hettema, 2001) reported that 30% to 40% of the variance in panic disorder could be attributed to heritable influences. The heritability estimate for generalised anxiety disorder was 31.6%, and for phobias (including social anxiety disorder) it was 20% to 40%.

These figures should be interpreted with caution, however. Gregory and Eley (2007) point out that these heritability estimates could be influenced by a wide range of variables, including the severity of the anxiety that is being studied (is it 'normal' anxiety, or anxiety disorders?), the type of anxiety that is being studied (e.g. social anxiety, or GAD), who reports on the level of anxiety (e.g. the parent or the child), and the age of the participant (genetic heritability estimates seem to get higher as people get older). However, in concluding their review of genetic studies they state that '… environmental factors are at least of equal importance … [to genetic factors]'. In Chapter 1 we discussed the importance of studying gene × environment interactions, and an important example of this in relation to psychological disorders is discussed in Box 3.4.

Box 3.4   Essential research

Orchid children: Are some children genetically wired to be extra sensitive to their environment? (Dobbs, 2012)

There is a gene, known as the DRD4 gene, which used to be thought of as a pretty bad lot. Having a particular version of this gene (the 7R version) had been shown to be associated with a whole load of Bad Things. From promiscuity to excessive drinking, from Attention Deficit Disorder (ADD) to conduct problems, poor old 7R has been blamed. Results were sometimes a bit inconsistent, and could not always be replicated, but all in all, everyone agreed that 7R was something you really didn't want. But then, something strange happened … it was discovered that children with this version of the gene were rather good at sharing, and were rather kind, and empathic. BUT this was *only* true for children who were being brought up by caring, sensitive parents.

The same has happened for a number of other genes that were once seen as 'risk' genes, and cropped up with monotonous regularity in mental health research. A gene controlling monoamine oxidase A (MAOA) activity and a couple of genes that control serotonin, which had previously been seen as synonymous with a vulnerability to psychological disorders, were showing up as actually being protective against these exact same disorders, but again, *only* in situations where the bearer had experienced warm and loving parenting in childhood.

Psychologists are now starting to think that instead of coding for mental illness, these 'orchid' genes might code for sensitivity to one's environment. And indeed, early investigations of this hypothesis do appear to confirm that having a lot of these genes, and also having a happy childhood, far from producing children who experience high levels of mental illness, instead produces children with very good mental health (Belsky & Beaver, 2011). On the other hand, children who have lots of these variants but have a stressful childhood are at high risk of psychological difficulties. Children who do not have many of

(Continued)

(Continued)

these orchid variants, the so-called 'dandelion' children, seem to do pretty much equally well regardless of their environment. In other words, it may be that having a lot of these 'orchid' variants means that a child is particularly sensitive to the parenting that they receive. Indeed, some early research looking at parenting interventions shows that children with the dreaded 7R variant of the DRD4 gene benefit more from clinical parenting interventions than their peers with different variants of the gene.

Environment

Environmental influences on mental health in childhood are many and varied. They can include parents, grandparents, other family members, the neighbourhood, friends, school, diet, and numerous other things. We have recently realised that the pre-natal environment is particularly important. However, the area of environment that has received the bulk of the research is parenting after a child is born, and that, therefore, is what we will focus on here.

Do parents cause anxiety in children?

In the vast majority of cases the answer to this question is no. Although, as you will see, there is some evidence that parents of anxious children behave in a different manner from that of parents of less anxious children, there is precious little evidence that this relationship is causal. That is, it may well be that anxious children cause their parents to act in this way, rather than the parenting causing the original anxiety (see Box 3.11 later). However, as we will see, once this parenting style starts, it may well be instrumental in *maintaining* an anxiety disorder in a child.

Summarising the research in this area is complicated by the fact that the literature tends to use different terms to describe overlapping concepts. However, two main parenting styles have been associated with anxiety in childhood: harshness/a lack of warmth, and overcontrol/overprotection.

Overcontrol/overprotection   There is some evidence that the parents of anxious children may be rather overprotective (Hudson & Rapee, 2006). For example, Edwards et al. (2010) measured overprotection in the parents of preschoolers, and then measured the children's anxiety a year later. The parents' overprotection at the first measurement point predicted the children's anxiety a whole year later, suggesting that it may have had some role in the appearance of the anxiety. A review of the area confirms this relationship (Van der Bruggen et al., 2008). It is easy to see how overprotection could be a problem for children, particularly those who are genetically a bit sensitive and cautious: the overprotected child gets fewer chances to develop skills than a child who is gently encouraged to participate in a range of activities. The overprotected child does not find out that they can take risks and succeed.

Likewise, they do not find out that they can take risks and fail, and that this is okay too. If a parent is overprotective the child can pick up subtle messages that they cannot cope on their own, and that the world is a dangerous place, and that the best thing to do when they are scared is to avoid (and this avoidance, as we will see in subsequent chapters, is Not A Good Thing).

Harshness/lack of warmth   There is also some evidence that the parents of anxious children might use harsher punishment techniques and fewer gentle ones. For example, research from one of your authors has shown that parents of anxious toddlers (Robinson & Cartwright-Hatton, 2008) and parents of anxious pre-adolescents (Laskey & Cartwright-Hatton, 2009) report higher levels of smacking and shouting than other parents. High trait anxious adolescents are also more likely to report that their parents used a harsh, over-reactive parenting style in the past (Gallagher & Cartwright-Hatton, 2008). Again, it is not difficult to see how, for a vulnerable child, these harsh parenting styles can create a fertile environment in which anxiety may grow.

A systematic review of this research (Wood et al., 2003) confirmed these findings, namely, that parents of anxious children are more overprotective and more likely to be harsh with them. However, it also showed that these parenting behaviours only accounted for a tiny 4% in the variance of child anxiety. Yet given recent research into 'Orchid children' (see Box 3.4) it is possible that this figure is much higher for those who are particularly sensitive to parenting.

Finally, we should point out that although these relationships between parenting and child anxiety have been demonstrated, no one has been able to show, beyond reasonable doubt, that the parenting causes the anxiety. It is equally likely that anxious children cause their parents to act differently. After all, if your child is very sensitive, becomes upset easily and is difficult to console … isn't that going to make you want to protect them from life's ups and downs? And if you have a child who, like Jack described in Box 3.2, has symptoms that make life very difficult for you, is it not surprising if you sometimes crack and indulge in a bit of shouting?

Treatment of childhood anxiety disorders

The two main treatments that have been used for childhood and adolescent anxiety disorders are Cognitive Behaviour Therapy (CBT) and Selective Serotonin Reuptake Inhibitors (SSRIs). A recent review of the psychological treatment literature (Reynolds et al., 2012) found a total of 55 trials where anxious children had been treated – most of them with some sort of CBT. Overall, they found that, when you looked at all of the studies together (i.e. a meta-analysis), the effect of CBT was moderately good, compared to doing nothing. In the studies that compared CBT to a placebo treatment, the effect was smaller but still good. This paper found that treatments targeted at a specific disorder (e.g. social anxiety disorder) were better than those targeted at a range of anxiety disorders. Finally, one-to-one treatment came out as better than group treatment, and adolescents seemed to fare better than younger children. However, the authors had a number of complaints about the material that they had to work with. Although they found that the quality of the trials that they were assessing had improved over the years, they also found that many of the studies were far too small to really make proper comparisons between groups, and very few followed their participants up for long enough to judge whether the treatment effects persisted in the long term.

But should anxious children and adolescents be given better access to medication? The largest trial (by a long way) of treatments for child and adolescent anxiety had a good go at answering this question. Walkup et al. (2008) divided 488 anxious 7 to 17 year olds into four groups. One group received just CBT. Another group was given just Sertraline, which is an SSRI medication. Another group got both CBT and Sertraline, and a final smaller group was given a placebo pill. At the end of 12 weeks of treatment (or placebo) all of the active treatment groups had done well, but the clear winner was the group of kids who had received both CBT and Sertraline. Critics of the study will point out that there was no follow-up, and if it follows the pattern of many adult studies, children who had medication (either with or without CBT) will do worse in the long run, particularly if they stop taking the drugs. However, in the short term it did seem that having both CBT and medication was the most effective treatment.

In line with the findings from the meta-analysis described above, the National Institute for Health and Care Excellence (NICE) guidelines for social anxiety disorder, which included a section on children (it has not included children in other anxiety guidelines), recommend that children should be offered CBT for their condition, and that this should preferably be CBT focusing on social anxiety symptoms (rather than 'transdiagnostic' CBT focusing on the general symptoms of anxiety) (NICE, 2013a). These guidelines recommend that medication should only be offered as a last resort. The UK has traditionally been much more cautious about prescribing medications for all psychological disorders of childhood than the USA, where the Walkup et al. study took place. And in recent years, everyone has been much more cautious about prescribing SSRIs because of some evidence that children taking these were more prone to having suicidal thoughts than those on placebos. There has been no evidence of children actually taking their own life because of SSRIs, but everyone, including NICE, is now very edgy about the issue. Interestingly, in the Walkup et al. (2008) study, there was no evidence of increased suicidality in those taking the Sertraline, compared to those taking the placebo.

Section summary

In this section, we have seen that children can suffer from a range of overlapping anxiety disorders. We have also seen that both genetic and environmental factors contribute to childhood anxiety, and that often these interact with each other. We do have some effective treatments for anxiety disorders of childhood, but much more research into these is needed.

Section 2: Childhood depression

In this section, you will learn about the symptoms of depression in childhood and adolescence and see how these might differ from those in adults. You will also study the epidemiology of depression in youth. We will briefly cover the basic genetic and environmental causes of depression, before discussing the effectiveness of psychological and drug treatments.

Box 3.5   Essential diagnosis

Diagnosis of depression in children and adolescents

The diagnosis of depression in children and adolescents is similar to that for adults (see Chapter 5), although some of the symptoms will look a bit different in children. For example, instead of looking sad children can be irritable, or complain of aches and pains, and sometimes they will act out their distress and appear to have behaviour problems. Instead of losing weight, a child may fail to gain weight as expected.

Box 3.6   Essential experience

Ruby

Ruby is 13 and has been diagnosed with major depressive disorder. The problems probably began shortly after she moved to secondary school when she was 11. At first she did well academically, but then she experienced bullying from some other girls in her class. Her school grades started to decline and she began missing school, either complaining of vague stomach aches or headaches, or just not turning up. Now she does not go to school at all. She lives at home with her mum, who is unemployed and has experienced significant depression in her own life. The psychologist's first assessment with Ruby is a rather one-sided affair, as Ruby barely speaks. She occasionally nods or shrugs in response to questions, but says very little. However, from her mother the psychologist determines that Ruby is very miserable. She is often tearful, and tells her mum that she feels ugly and stupid and that no one loves her. Ruby used to hang out with her friends at the weekends, and go to Girl Guides and cheerleading club every week, but now she has stopped all of this. In fact she only leaves the house if she is dragged along by her mother. When she is at home she often spends the days in her pyjamas, watching TV or just lying in bed doing nothing. She complains of feeling exhausted, but often has serious trouble sleeping at night. The relationship between Ruby and her mother is fragile. Mum is exasperated by her daughter's refusal to do anything, and Ruby is very irritable, meaning that arguments are frequent. Mum is also being hassled by the authorities because of Ruby's refusal to go to school. They are threatening to fine her, and she cannot afford to pay this, but Ruby says that she can't go back to school because of the bullies, and because she is so tired, and she's too stupid and can't do the work. Ruby's mother is also worried that she is looking very thin these days.

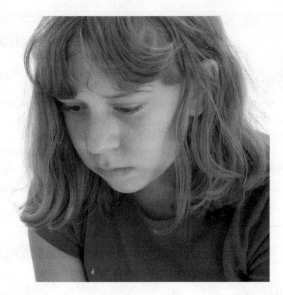

Figure 3.2   Ruby (portrayed by an actor)

How common is depression in childhood?

Depression is not very common before adolescence. Most studies that have looked at depression in this age group come up with figures of less than 1% of children having a diagnosable level of depression at any one time. However, at puberty, this figure increases markedly, particularly for girls, and by mid-adolescence around 2% to 3% of children will be experiencing a diagnosable depressive disorder (see Ford et al., 2003; McGee et al., 1992).

What causes childhood depression?

As for anxiety disorders, many, many causes of childhood depression have been identified. We will consider heritable and environmental influences in this section. Within environment, we will focus on parenting and family factors, because these are things that psychologists have some ability to change.

Heritability and genetics

Depression in adults and adolescents is thought to have a moderately large genetic component (see Chapter 5). However, it is starting to look like that might not be the case for depression earlier in childhood. Whilst depression definitely runs in families for adolescents and adults (e.g. adolescents with depressed parents are two to three times more likely than other adolescents to be depressed themselves; see Lieb, 2002), it seems that the role of genetics is different for children. For adolescents, twin and adoption studies show that around 40% of the variance in the disorder can be accounted for by genetics. However, for preadolescent children the role of genes appears to be negligible (see Rice, 2010, for a review).

And once again, gene–environment interaction raises its befuddling head. Kaufman et al. (2006) showed that adolescents with a combination of two particular gene variants were at increased risk of depression, but only if they had experienced maltreatment. Children who had this genotype but had not been maltreated were not at increased risk of depression (but for a critique of similar studies in adults, see Box 5.4 in Chapter 5).

Environment

As for the other disorders discussed in this chapter, it seems likely that the environment is at least as important as genes in dictating which children and adolescents become depressed. And as for the other conditions, there are very many aspects of the environment that have been shown to have an impact – for example, bullying from peers and siblings, poverty, parental mental health, diet, even your mother's state of mind when she was pregnant, and possibly even your maternal grandmother's! And you won't be surprised to hear that all of these factors overlap and influence each other. However, we will, as previously, focus on the role that parents have to play because this is likely to be key, and it is one that psychologists can (sometimes) do something about.

Do parents cause childhood depression?

Particularly for younger children, as outlined above, there is evidence that genetic factors may not be that significant. So attention has turned to environmental factors, particularly parents, and there are now quite a number of studies looking at the role of parenting in depression. So what do these show? Well they are, as always, a bit of a hotch-potch, using different measures of depression, and different age groups, and different informants (kids, parents, observers), and measuring different aspects of parenting, and doing all this measuring in different ways, so it's difficult to get a clear idea of what is going on. However, three brave American souls decided to have a go. McLeod et al. (2007) scoured the literature to find all the research that had looked at the association between depression in childhood or adolescence and parenting. After throwing out studies that used retrospective reports of parenting[1] they had 45 left. These measured a real mix of what the individual studies considered to be 'parenting', but McLeod et al. managed to categorise these studies into two large clusters, one measuring 'rejection' and one measuring 'control', plus a number of subcategories. They classed a study as measuring parental 'rejection' if it measured (a) parental withdrawal (a lack of involvement between parent and child, a lack of interest in the child's activities, or a lack of emotional support); (b) aversiveness (parental hostility towards the child); or (c) warmth (a sense of positive regard expressed by the parent towards the child). They classed a study as measuring parental

---

[1]A bit dodgy, but they reasoned that memory biases come into play when you ask people how they (or their parents) parented years ago – and this did cut their studies down to a manageable number.

'control' if it assessed parental interference with the child's autonomy or emotional independence. When they looked at all of the studies together, they found that parenting accounted for 8% of the variance in depression in children, which is classed as a medium effect size. When looking at parental rejection, this also accounted for 8% of the variance in depression, giving a medium effect size. However, parental control only had a small effect size, accounting for 5% of the variance in depression scores. One of their subcategories of parenting ('aversiveness'), however, seemed to be particularly powerful on its own. This style of parenting accounted for 11% of the variance in depression. In all cases, the relationship of parenting to depression was as expected, that is, the more negative the parenting, the worse the depression. However, the authors noted that there were no studies at all that would allow us to conclude that parenting *caused* depression. In all cases the association was purely correlational, and could have arisen because depressed children cause their parents to act differently, or because of some third variable (e.g. poverty) that caused changes in parenting and also childhood depression. As in the previous section (on childhood anxiety disorders), interpreting these parenting studies is far from straightforward.

Treatment of childhood depression

NICE published a guideline on the treatment of depression in children and adolescents in 2005.[2] This pulled together all of the available evidence and recommended the following.

Mild depression   This recommended 'watchful waiting' for four weeks. Here, someone (e.g. the GP) keeps an eye on the child for four weeks. This is based on evidence that lots of children and adolescents will have spells of low mood that will recover fairly quickly without needing any intervention.

If the mild depression is still present after four weeks, the young person should be offered either 'Supportive Therapy', which is basically an opportunity to talk through problems with a sympathetic adult, or Group CBT or Guided Self Help, which is where the client follows a book or a computer program, with a small amount of help from a clinician.

NICE states quite clearly that medication should not be prescribed for mild cases of depression in children or adolescents.

Moderate to severe depression   Clients diagnosed with moderate to severe depression should be offered either individual CBT, or interpersonal therapy (which is a bit like CBT but focuses on improving relationships with the people around you) or short-term family therapy (which aims to improve relationships in the family).

If the young person is still depressed after four to six sessions they should be offered another therapy from the list above, or if they are aged 12 to 18 they could be prescribed the SSRI fluoxetine (otherwise known as Prozac). Children aged 5 to 11 can also be prescribed fluoxetine if they are not responding well to therapy, but this should be done very cautiously.

---

[2]NICE is reviewing this guidance in 2015, and may issue more up-to-date guidance soon.

If the depression does not resolve with these steps, then the young person should, as a last resort, be offered more intensive and longer-term family therapy, or individual child psycho-therapy (which is based on the psychodynamic model).[3] Alternatively, the young person could be offered a trial of a different SSRI medication.

In very severe depression, particularly if the young person is judged to be at risk of suicide, inpatient treatment should be considered.

A recent meta-analysis of the area by Cox et al. (2012) concluded that whilst CBT and SSRIs both look moderately effective, they could not conclude which of the two, or a combination of them, was better, as there was not enough research and the results were confusing and conflicting.

Section 3: Childhood behaviour problems

If you ever go to work in a general Child and Adolescent Mental Health Service (CAMHS), you will probably find that the bulk of your cases relate to behaviour problems. This isn't to say that behaviour problems are the most common disorder of childhood (that accolade probably goes to anxiety disorders), but they are the disorder that is most likely to be referred, by exasperated teachers, parents and social workers. In this section you will learn about the symptoms of two major childhood behaviour problem diagnoses, namely Oppositional Defiant Disorder (ODD) and Conduct Disorder (CD). You will also study the epidemiology of behaviour problems in youth, and learn about the genetic and environmental causes of these. Finally, we will discuss the outcomes of behaviour problems in the young if these are not treated, and learn how effective drug and psychological treatments are.

Box 3.7 Essential diagnosis of behaviour problems in childhood

Conduct Disorder (CD) and Oppositional Defiant Disorder (ODD)

The *ICD*-10 (World Health Organisation, 1992) criteria for these disorders are detailed below.

(Continued)

---

[3]This was a bit controversial, as many people did not think that psychotherapy had enough evidence to be recommended at all.

(Continued)

Conduct disorder

A. Does not meet the criteria for dissocial (antisocial) personality disorder, schizophrenia, mania, depression, pervasive developmental disorder, or hyperkinetic disorder. (If criteria for emotional disorder are met, diagnose "mixed" disorder of conduct and emotions).

B. Presence of three or more symptoms from the criterion list below, of which at least three must be from items 9–24.

C. At least one of the symptoms from items 9–24 must have been present for at least six months.

Oppositional defiant disorder

A. Does not meet the criteria for dissocial personality disorder, schizophrenia, mania, depression, pervasive developmental disorder, or hyperkinetic disorder. (If criteria for emotional disorder are met, diagnose "mixed" disorder of conduct and emotions).

B. Presence of four or more symptoms from the criterion list below, of which no more than two from items 9–24.

C. The symptoms in B must be maladaptive and inconsistent with the developmental level.

D. At least four of the symptoms must have been present for at least six months.

Criterion list

1. Unusually frequent or severe temper tantrums for the child's developmental level.
2. Often argues with adults.
3. Often actively defies or refuses adults' requests or rules.
4. Often, apparently deliberately, does things that annoy other people.
5. Often blames others for one's own mistakes or misbehaviour.
6. Often touchy or easily annoyed by others.
7. Often angry or resentful.
8. Often spiteful or vindictive.
9. Frequent and marked lying (except to avoid abusive treatment).
10. Excessive fighting with other children, with frequent initiation of fights (not including fights with siblings).
11. Uses a weapon that can cause serious physical harm to others (e.g. a bat, brick, broken bottle, knife, gun).
12. Often stays out after dark without permission (beginning before 13 years of age).
13. Physical cruelty to other people (e.g. ties up, cuts or burns a victim).
14. Physical cruelty to animals.

15. Deliberate destruction of others' property (other than by fire-setting).
16. Deliberate fire-setting with a risk or intention of causing serious damage.
17. At least two episodes of stealing of objects of value (e.g. money) from home (excluding taking of food).
18. At least two episodes of stealing outside the home without confrontation with the victim (e.g. shoplifting, burglary or forgery).
19. Frequent truancy from school beginning before 13 years of age.
20. Running away from home (unless this was to avoid physical or sexual abuse).
21. Any episode of crime involving confrontation with a victim (including purse snatching, extortion, mugging).
22. Forcing another person into sexual activity against their wishes.
23. Frequent bullying of others (i.e. deliberate infliction of pain or hurt including persistent intimidation, tormenting, or molestation).
24. Breaks into someone else's house, building or car.

Box 3.8   Essential experience

Josh

Josh is six years old and has been diagnosed with ODD. His parents report that he was always a 'handful' but now it is getting near impossible for them to manage him. He has a very hot temper – exploding at the slightest thing, especially when his parents ask him to do something that he does not want to do. He will normally refuse to carry out these tasks with a huge argument, even if they are relatively simple, such as 'put your bike away' or 'go and brush your teeth'. His parents say that he is 'attention seeking' and will go out of his way to deliberately annoy people, particularly his mother, his younger brother, and – especially when he is bored at school – other children in his class. Despite the bravado, Josh is actually quite a sensitive soul. He gets extremely upset when he is told off for something, and will usually try to lay the blame on someone else. He is often tearful and says that his parents love his brother more than him, and is resentful of any attention that they give his brother. His teacher is very concerned about his behaviour. He has no real friends and some children are quite scared of him, as he can sometimes be quite vindictive. His academic performance is well below what is expected of his age.

How common are behaviour problems in childhood?

Behaviour problems are very common. In a review of international epidemiological studies, Canino and colleagues (2010) showed that ODD was present in 0.47 to 8.7% of children, and

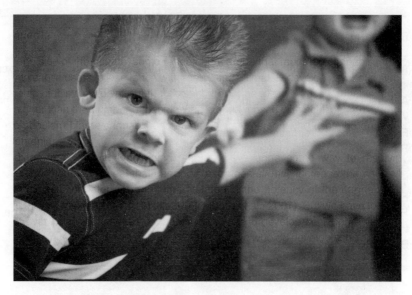

Figure 3.3 Josh (portrayed by an actor)

CD was present in between 0.33% and 11%, depending on the methods used by the study that was doing the measuring. In the large and carefully conducted British study that we describe earlier (Ford et al., 2003), ODD and CD (combined) were present in 6.5% of boys and 2.7% of girls aged 5 to 10. In adolescents aged 11 to 15 they were present in 8.6% of boys and 3.8% of girls. The pattern of behaviour disorders being much more common in boys than girls is a very consistent one, and is found across the world.

What becomes of children with behaviour problems?

There is a huge body of research showing that children with significant behaviour problems grow up to have an increased risk of difficulties in just about every area you can think of. For example, they are more likely to become a parent when they themselves are still very young; they are less likely to have a good job, or indeed any job at all; they tend to have poorer interpersonal relationships with both friends and family; they are at increased risk of substance use disorders (see Chapter 9), personality disorders during adulthood (Chapter 11) and suicide; and they are far more likely to engage in criminal activity. One large British study has been following a group of 3,652 teenagers who were first studied when they were 13 to 15 years of age. They recently reported on how these children were getting on at the age of 53 (Colman et al., 2009). Within this sample, the researchers identified a group (about 9.5% of the total) whose teachers had identified them as having a severe externalising disorder (another term for behaviour disorders) when they were teenagers. Forty years on, at the age of 53, this group of severely behaviour-disordered teenagers was around 20% more likely than those with no behaviour problems to abuse alcohol. They were about twice as likely to have experienced an episode of depression. They were three times more likely than their well-behaved peers to have no qualifications, and twice as likely to have had a child of their own before the age of 20. Finally, they were 50% more likely to have had problems in relationships with other people.

Of course, these are just group averages, and many children with behaviour problems turn out just fine. Maybe you were a bit of a tearaway, and yet here you are now, studying hard for your degree. The data show that children who first develop behaviour problems in their teens are more likely to be fine in the longer term. Children who had significant problems before their teens are more likely to continue having difficulties, such as those outlined above, for the rest of their lives.

What causes childhood behaviour problems?

This has been heavily studied, and a whole host of variables have been implicated. In particular, being born into socioeconomic disadvantage is a very big risk factor, and there is some evidence that alleviating poverty goes a long way to reducing behaviour problems. There is a role for genetics too, and we will touch on this. However, unfortunately, as psychologists there is very little that we can do to alleviate poverty and disadvantage, and absolutely nothing we can do to alter our clients' genes. So we tend to focus on the things that we can change, for example parenting practices. For this reason, we will focus on the role of parenting here.

Heritability and genetics

All of the behaviour disorders run in families. However, this does not prove that there is a genetic component, as it could be the environment that causes different members of the same family to experience similar symptoms (see Box 1.8 in Chapter 1). But a number of twin and adoption studies suggest that these disorders are in fact highly heritable, that is, that they have a strong genetic component (e.g. Slutske et al., 1997), particularly in children who have high levels of 'callous unemotional' traits (Viding et al., 2005; see Chapter 11). And the studies looking at the different candidate genes keep coming up with inconsistent data – some saying that a particular gene is involved, others saying that it is not … Perhaps part of the problem here is the issue that we discussed earlier, namely that of gene–environment interaction. Indeed, it seems likely that children with a gene coding for low levels of MAOA activity are at risk of behaviour problems, but only if they also experience early maltreatment (Kim-Cohen et al., 2006). Children with this genetic profile who have happy, well-supported childhoods do not seem to be at excess risk of developing problems.

Environment

Although there is a large role for heritable factors in these disorders, there is also a substantial role for the environment. In particular, the parenting received by children with behaviour problems has come under scrutiny, and a number of common problems have been identified.

Do parents cause childhood behaviour problems?

A large body of research now exists showing that there is a role for parenting in the development and/or maintenance of behaviour problems. In particular, it is widely recognised that parents of children with behaviour problems are less likely to use strategies of positive reinforcement (i.e. praise and reward) to encourage good behaviour than parents of average children (Webster-Stratton, 1985). There is also substantial evidence that parents of children with behaviour problems set household rules less effectively than parents of other children and are then less likely to enforce those rules (e.g. Forehand et al., 1978). However, although parents of children with behaviour problems have been shown to give less attention to good behaviours than other parents, it seems that they give significantly more attention to unwanted behaviours (such as arguing with siblings, moaning, whining), often in the form of shouting, hitting or nagging (Dumas et al., 1995; Patterson & Stouthamer-Loeber, 1984). Some children, particularly those who do not get all the attention that they need through other avenues (e.g. by getting praised for good behaviours), will actually engage in negative behaviours as a means of getting the adult attention that all children need. There is now much evidence that parents of children with behavioural difficulties tend to use more punishment than other parents, and when they do, it is harsher and used less effectively (e.g. Patterson & Stouthamer-Loeber, 1984: see Box 3.9). This is problematic for a number of reasons. First, it means that children get lots of attention for unpleasant behaviour, and in conjunction with the limited attention that they get for desirable behaviour this can encourage the child to invest their efforts in undesirable behaviour. Second, when parents use harsh, frightening disciplinary strategies, this has been shown to impair children's learning of the very behaviour that the parent is attempting to teach (Abramowitz et al., 1988; Acker & O'Leary, 1988) and this is particularly the case for physical punishment (Power & Chapieski, 1986). Finally, it damages the parent–child relationship, making all of the above much more likely.

Box 3.9   Patterson's Coercive Cycle (Patterson, 1982)

When looking at children with behaviour problems, and the way that their parents manage them, it is easy for the outsider to say 'Why don't the parents just put their foot down?'. Patterson's Coercive Cycle goes some way to explaining why this does not happen.

In this cycle, the parent issues a command, such as 'Tidy your toys away'. The child refuses, perhaps using an aversive behaviour (e.g. whingeing, shouting, hurling abuse at the parent), and the parent gives the command again, throwing in some aversive behaviour of their own, for example shouting, or threatening to smack the child. Sometimes the child will comply at this point, which reinforces for the parent their use of shouting and threats of aggression. However, much of the time the child ups the ante, perhaps deploying a full-blown tantrum. The parent, often exhausted by repeated experiences of this nature, and by other life stresses, gives up, and does not insist that the toys are put away. The child has learnt that by displaying *coercive* behaviours, they can avoid complying with their parent's commands. If these coercive patterns of behaviour persist over time, they can often become internalised and have long-term effects on the child's behavioural and emotional development. Worryingly, the child can transfer these coercive techniques outside of the home, and use them, with negative consequences, with teachers, other authority figures, and peers (Dishion et al., 1992). For this reason, helping parents to set and enforce commands is a central part of most standard Parenting Skills Training Programmes, and once parents give commands in this way, compliance rises substantially (Roberts et al., 1978).

Treatment of childhood behaviour problems

The National Institute for Clinical Excellence (2013b) has issued a guideline on the management of antisocial behaviour and conduct disorders in children and young people. They state that for 3 to 11 year olds who have CD or ODD, or are at risk of developing either disorder, their parents or guardians should be offered a parent-training intervention. These interventions attempt to address the parenting difficulties outlined above, that is, they give parents a warm, calm, clear and consistent way of managing difficult behaviour in their child. They recommend that for children aged 9 to 14 years the child should also be offered a group-based course for themselves, based on a cognitive-behavioural problem-solving model, which helps that child to manage their emotions, and the behaviours that flow from them, a bit better.

Box 3.10   Essential treatment

Parenting skills training programmes

These programmes for managing behaviour problems typically run for a couple of hours a week for six to ten weeks. They are usually run by two psychologists, with a group of six to eight sets of parents, although they can be run with individual clients. A large number of different Parenting Skills Training Programmes are in existence, but they tend to use a similar core of techniques that aim to address the parenting difficulties that are identified above.

(Continued)

(Continued)

Relationship-building play Often, by the time they reach the clinic, the relationship between the parent and the child has become fraught. To help repair this, and to ensure that children are getting some much-needed positive attention from their parents, most programmes begin by encouraging parents to spend some quality time with their child every day.

Positive reinforcement of good behaviours Parents are taught to praise their child whenever possible, in response to good, prosocial behaviours seen in the child. Parents are also taught to praise in ways that will maximise their impact, as believe it or not, it is possible to do praise wrong![4] Parents are taught, as well, to use small rewards to help their children develop new, positive behaviours.

Setting limits Parents are taught how to think up sensible rules for their children, and how to communicate these to their children.

Withdrawal of attention Parents are taught how to reduce the amount of attention that they pay to minor annoying behaviours such as moaning, whingeing and whining. This, basically, amounts to 'ignore the bad behaviour', but is actually quite complicated to do, and the course leaders will spend some time practising and doing role plays with parents.

Punishment/consequences and time out This is usually taught at the end of the course, as the idea is that parents will get used to using all of the more positive techniques first. Parents are helped to devise simple, clear, gentle, non-physical punishments, which are delivered rapidly.

Behavioural parent training programmes have been used in many countries, for decades, and there is a huge quantity of evidence to suggest that they work in treating behaviour problems (Dretzke et al., 2009). There is also evidence that the effects of these programmes last in the long term: Webster-Stratton and colleagues (1989) showed that improvements were sustained when they assessed families five years after they had received a behavioural parent-training intervention. A recent economic analysis estimated that a parenting intervention, given to families of five year olds at risk of developing conduct disorder, would save over £16,000 per family in costs to society (such as extra mental health care costs, criminal justice system costs) compared to the cost of an intervention of around £1,000 to £2,000 per family (see Bonin et al., 2011).

---

[4]"Matt, I really like the Chapter on Mood Disorders that you just sent me. It's a pity you can't always put that much effort in'. (Which bit of this praise is Matt going to remember, and do you think it will motivate him to try harder next time … ?)

Box 3.11 Essential debate

Do parents cause childhood psychological disorders?

Let's be honest, this is what most lay people think … but is it true?

No, leave the poor parents alone!

- As you will see in this chapter, the meta-analyses of parenting studies are not that convincing: Wood et al.'s (2003) anxiety study showed that only 4% of the variance in child anxiety could be attributed to parenting; McLeod et al.'s (2007) meta-analysis showed that parenting accounted for 8% of depression symptoms; and Rothbaum and Weisz (1994) showed that parenting accounted for just 6% of behaviour problems.
- What is more, most of the studies have been quick and dirty ones, done on the cheap. These studies often have flaws, such as 'shared method variance' where the same person reports on the symptoms and the parenting, which can lead to inflated estimates of any association between the two.
- We have very little data showing that parenting *causes* these mental health difficulties. It could be that having a child with a psychological disorder makes your parenting go a bit wrong. It's also quite likely that another factor (e.g. genes, or living in poverty or in a bad area) causes both the poor parenting *and* the child's difficulties.

Yes, blame the parents!

- Remember that gene–environment interaction thing? It has shown, repeatedly, that some children, with particular genotypes, are more sensitive to parenting than others. Although the meta-analyses come up showing that parenting only accounts for small amounts of symptom variance, these are looking at *all* children. Some of these children may have been relatively insensitive to parenting, whereas others may have been much more sensitive. For these sensitive children, the amount of variance explained by parenting may have been much higher.
- Other factors will almost certainly moderate the results, so that some children will be much more affected by parenting than others, meaning that these low figures are not representative of all groups. We have barely begun to scratch the surface of what these other factors might be, but McLeod et al. (2007), for example, found that parenting explained much more of the variance in depression in children of highly educated parents, as compared to less well-educated parents (you'll have to read their paper to see why they thought this was!).

(Continued)

(Continued)

- Back to the quick and dirty thing. This could work both ways. The best way of measuring parenting is generally agreed to be by observation, that is, a neutral observer goes and watches what the parents do. However, most of these studies measured parenting using questionnaires that were given out to the parent or the child. We know that questionnaire studies generally find lower associations between parenting and mental health than observation studies, and this could account, in part, for the low levels of variance explained.
- Are we measuring the right bits of parenting? If you yourself are a parent, you will know what we mean when we say that parenting is … complicated. There are a simply enormous number of behaviours, thoughts and attitudes that every parent could display. When we measure parenting, we have almost certainly only scratched the surface of what there is to measure. So is it possible that we have not yet measured all of the right things? We'd put money on it.
- Parenting interventions work. We have some evidence (okay, virtually all for behaviour problems rather than the other disorders) that changing parenting (in a positive direction) results in reduced problems for the child. This isn't totally clear-cut evidence that the parenting causes the child's difficulties in the first place, but it is a strong clue that parenting is at least involved in maintaining the disorder.

Essential questions

- Are childhood psychological disorders heritable?
- How common are psychological disorders of childhood, and what are the difficulties in measuring this?
- Can we effectively treat childhood psychological disorders? What are the difficulties in evaluating the treatments?
- What do we need to consider before we 'blame the parents' for psychological disorders in children?

Further reading

Dobbs, D. (2012). Orchid children: How bad-news genes came good. *New Scientist*, 2849: 42–45. (*New Scientist* is a great source of entertainingly written and up-to-date overviews of many areas of psychology. This article unfolds the story of how genes and environments interact to determine our mental health.)

Epigenetics and Stress in Pregnancy: Baby Blues. www.economist.com/node/18985981 (This is a nice, approachable article, written for a non-expert audience, about the effects of stress during pregnancy on the mental health of the child that is eventually born.)

Gregory, A. M., & Eley, T. C. (2007). Genetic influences on anxiety in children: What we've learned and where we're heading. *Clinical Child and Family Psychology Review*, 10(3): 199–212. (This paper gives a very readable overview of the research designs that are commonly used to determine how and why psychological disorders run in families. It outlines some of the strengths and weaknesses in each design, and issues that should be taken into account when interpreting their results.)

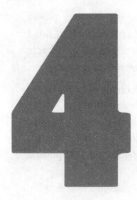

SCHIZOPHRENIA

General introduction

This chapter begins with an introduction to the diagnostic label of 'schizophrenia' and we discuss why some researchers and clinicians hotly debate the validity of this label. We then demonstrate that many different things can cause schizophrenia and focus on heritable influences, adverse events during childhood, and broader social factors. In the next section we discuss and evaluate theoretical models that are informed by studies of brain activity and cognitive function in schizophrenia. We show that the latest versions of these theories attempt to explain how the ultimate causes of schizophrenia lead to abnormalities of brain structure and function that underpin cognitive changes, which may in turn underlie the symptoms of the disorder. In the final section we discuss treatments for schizophrenia, which include taking a critical look at antipsychotic medications and a discussion of the very latest evidence on psychological therapies.

Assessment targets

At the end of the chapter, you should ask yourself the following questions:

- Can I explain the diagnostic criteria for schizophrenia, and is it appropriate to even call it a 'disorder'?
- To what extent are psychological theories of schizophrenia supported by evidence?
- Is there anything wrong with the brain in schizophrenia, and how does this relate to symptoms?
- How does family influence the likelihood of developing and recovering from schizophrenia?
- Can I evaluate the effectiveness of treatments for schizophrenia, and are psychological treatments more effective than drugs?

Section 1: What is schizophrenia?

The diagnostic label 'Schizophrenia' resides in the *ICD*-10 category of 'Schizophrenia, Schizotypal and Delusional Disorders', and the *DSM*-5 category of 'Schizophrenia Spectrum and Other Psychotic Disorders'. Both classification systems group it alongside related disorders such as Schizoaffective Disorder. This chapter is focused on schizophrenia so we won't be discussing the other psychotic disorders in detail, although we will mention them in passing because there is considerable overlap between all of the disorders within this category. Before we get started we need to correct some common misconceptions. First, schizophrenia is not the same as having a split personality. 'Multiple personality disorder' (termed 'Dissociative Identity Disorder' in *DSM*-5; see also Chapter 11) is viewed as totally distinct from all psychotic disorders, including schizophrenia. Second, despite portrayals in the media, people with schizophrenia are far more likely to be the victims of violence than to commit violent acts themselves. People with schizophrenia are (slightly) more likely to commit violent acts only if they are left untreated, particularly if they also have a substance use disorder (see Chapter 9) (Fazel et al., 2009).

Schizophrenia was first identified as a pathological condition by Kraepelin (1922) who described it in terms of a set of specific symptoms, originally subdivided into positive and negative symptoms. There is now agreement that 'disorganised' symptoms are an additional category, distinct from positive and negative symptoms (Liddle, 1987). You will frequently see these referred to as 'psychotic' symptoms, and a person who is experiencing them is said to be experiencing a 'psychotic episode'.

Positive symptoms

These symptoms are said to add something unusual to the patient's experience, and the most widely studied are delusions and hallucinations. 'Delusions of grandeur' mean that the person thinks that they are superior to other people and that they have power and influence over them, whereas 'delusions of persecution' (or paranoid delusions) mean that the person thinks they are being unfairly persecuted or threatened by other people or organisations (e.g. the CIA). Hallucinations are usually auditory rather than visual, and they commonly take the form of 'hearing voices' that command the person to do something, or offer a running commentary on their life. Although delusions and hallucinations are very common, there are enormous individual differences in the form that they take (see Box 4.1).

Negative symptoms

These symptoms are technically 'signs' of the disorder rather than symptoms, because a symptom is something that the patient reports, whereas a sign is something that can be observed by somebody else (usually a nurse or doctor). They are described as negative because they reflect something missing from the patient's behaviour and take the form of 'flat affect' (emotional reactions that are blunted or missing), 'avolition' (a lack of motivation, interest and energy), 'asocial' behaviour (withdrawing from the company of others), 'poverty of speech' (either they don't say much at all, or speech seems to be random and lacking in meaning) and 'anhedonia' (the inability to experience pleasure) (Crow, 1980).

Disorganised symptoms

These symptoms relate to disorganised or strange behaviours and actions, such as inappropriate emotional reactions (e.g. laughing when being told bad news), and disorganised thoughts that are reflected in speech that others cannot understand.

Box 4.1   Essential experience

The diversity of symptoms of schizrenia

Here are some examples of the types of positive symptoms that schizophrenic patients experience (taken from Mellor, 1970).

Delusions

Bodily sensations imposed from external agents 'X-rays entering the back of my neck, where the skin tingles and feels warm, they pass down the back in a hot tingling strip about six inches wide to the waist'.

Thoughts are being broadcast 'As I think, my thoughts leave my head on a type of mental ticker-tape. Everyone around has only to pass the tape through their mind and they know my thoughts'.

Hallucinations

Hearing voices A 35 year old painter heard a quiet voice with an 'Oxford accent' which he attributed to the BBC (i.e. the radio or television). The voice would say 'I can't stand that man, the way he holds his brush he looks like a poof'. He immediately experienced whatever the voice was saying as his own thoughts, to the exclusion of all other thoughts. When he read the newspaper the voice would speak aloud whatever his eyes fell on.

Box 4.2 describes a case study of a young man with schizophrenia, which illustrates how the different types of symptoms can co-occur.

Box 4.2   Essential experience

The case of Nigel (National Prescribing Centre, 2010)

Nigel is 19 years old. He started at a local university six months ago to do a course on Computer Science, but failed to attend lectures after the first few weeks. He began to suffer from periods where he would not get up in the morning, didn't seem to care whether he went to university or not, and was unable to concentrate on any of his work. He became more and more withdrawn, and stopped going out with his friends. He neglected his personal hygiene, which was unusual for him as he had previously been careful about his appearance. He described strangers following him in the street, and one day after shouting that there were people installing hidden cameras in his bedroom to spy on him, he stormed out of the house. When he did not return that night, his mother and father went out to search for him and found him wandering the streets. With much persuasion they managed to get him to return home and next morning they contacted their doctor.

At first Nigel refused any help, and was convinced there was nothing wrong with him. However for the sake of his parents he agreed to be assessed by a psychiatrist, who subsequently assessed and diagnosed him as having a schizophrenic psychotic episode.

Diagnosis of schizophrenia

The *ICD*-10 criteria for schizophrenia are shown in Box 4.3. The *DSM*-5 criteria (American Psychiatric Association, 2013) are similar, and both require that the psychotic episode is associated with some degree of social or occupational impairment. Importantly, both the *ICD*-10 and *DSM*-5 specify additional exclusion criteria to eliminate psychotic symptoms that may arise as a result of drug or alcohol intoxication or dependence, other disorders with psychotic symptoms, and certain developmental disorders.

Box 4.3   Essential diagnosis

Schizophrenia

The *ICD*-10 (World Health Organisation, 1992) criteria for schizophrenia are as follows.
Either *at least one* of the following:

a) Thought echo, thought insertion or withdrawal, or thought broadcasting.
b) Delusions of control, influence or passivity, clearly referred to body or limb movements or specific thoughts, actions, or sensations; delusional perception.

(Continued)

(Continued)

c) Hallucinatory voices giving a running commentary on the patient's behaviour, or discussing him between themselves, or other types of hallucinatory voices coming from some part of the body.
d) Persistent delusions of other kinds that are culturally inappropriate and completely impossible (e.g. being able to control the weather, or being in communication with aliens from another world).

Or *at least two* of the following:

e) Persistent hallucinations in any modality, when occurring every day for at least one month, when accompanied by delusions (which may be fleeting or half-formed) without clear affective content, or when accompanied by persistent over-valued ideas.
f) Neologisms, breaks or interpolations in the train of thought, resulting in incoherence or irrelevant speech.
g) Catatonic behaviour, such as excitement, posturing or waxy flexibility, negativism, mutism and stupor.
h) 'Negative' symptoms such as marked apathy, paucity of speech, and blunting or incongruity of emotional responses (it must be clear that these are not due to depression or to neuroleptic medication).

These syndromes, symptoms and signs should be present most of the time during a psychotic episode lasting for at least one month.

Looking at the diagnostic criteria in Box 4.3, we can see that someone would receive a diagnosis of schizophrenia if they were to exhibit some combination of positive, negative and disorganised symptoms for at least one month. That all seems reasonable, but the exclusion criteria specified in both *ICD*-10 and *DSM*-5 mean that a person could have many of these psychotic symptoms, but if their symptoms were associated with a mood or a developmental disorder, or could be attributed to the long-term effects of drug use (Barkus & Murray, 2010), then that person would not receive a diagnosis of schizophrenia even though they might be behaving in exactly the same way as someone who did get this diagnosis. For this reason, some researchers and clinicians suggest that it would be better to refer to 'psychosis' as a condition that can be present in a variety of disorders including (what *DSM*-5 and *ICD*-10 refer to as) schizophrenia, bipolar disorder (see Chapter 5), some personality disorders (Chapter 11) and schizoaffective disorder (Bentall, 2003).

There are other problems. If we study large groups of patients with a diagnosis of schizophrenia we will see that on the whole, positive, negative and disorganised symptoms tend to cluster together (Liddle, 1987). However, this doesn't mean that the symptoms always co-occur in each individual patient. It is quite common, for example, to see patients who have delusions, hallucinations and disorganised symptoms, but no negative symptoms at all, particularly when people are first diagnosed with schizophrenia (the first diagnosis is called 'first episode schizophrenia'). However, people with chronic schizophrenia (those who have been hospitalised because of their symptoms, time and time again, over years and even decades) tend to have primarily negative symptoms, but fewer positive or disorganised symptoms (Hulshoff Pol & Kahn, 2008). If we were to interview these people they would seem very different from each other, but each might get a diagnosis of 'schizophrenia' because this covers such a broad range of symptoms. As we will see later in the chapter, it might be more helpful to focus on the various symptoms in isolation, because each symptom is associated with different abnormalities in the brain, and each symptom may have different causes.

Finally, you may be surprised to know that some psychotic experiences, such as auditory hallucinations and delusions, are fairly common even in healthy people. Most of us would accept that it is 'normal' to feel anxious and depressed occasionally, and that Generalised Anxiety Disorder (Chapter 6) and Major Depressive Disorder (see Chapter 5) lie at extreme ends of the spectrum of normal human experience. But we have a tendency to think that hearing voices and having paranoid delusions is a world apart from 'normal' human experience, and therefore people with schizophrenia are qualitatively rather than quantitatively different from 'the rest of us'. Yet this isn't true. 'Schizotypy' refers to a series of personality characteristics, including delusional thinking, hearing voices and social withdrawal, that are fairly common in the general population. For example, Beck and Rector (2003) reported that between 4% and 25% of the general population experience auditory hallucinations at some point in their lifetime, and most of these people do not regard themselves as ill. Therefore many psychotic symptoms are no more distinct from 'normal' or 'healthy' human functioning than are depressed or anxious mood.

Prevalence, course and consequences of schizophrenia

Between 0.3% and 0.66% of the adult population will be diagnosed with schizophrenia at some point in their lives (lifetime prevalence), but this figure rises to 2.3% if all schizophrenia spectrum disorders are included (Van Os & Kapur, 2009). Men tend to be first diagnosed between the ages of 15 and 25 (the average age of onset is 18 years), whereas women are typically diagnosed a few years later (the average age of onset is 25 years) (Saha et al., 2005). A common (mis)conception about schizophrenia is that it has a chronic course and the prospect of a full recovery is poor. However, follow-up studies of patients who received their initial diagnosis of schizophrenia demonstrate a high degree of variability, with about half of patients making a 'good' recovery (e.g. no residual symptoms and no social or intellectual impairment), and about half making a poor recovery characterised by continuous symptoms and repeated re-admission to hospital. Even so, most people who are diagnosed with schizophrenia are able to manage their symptoms and live independent lives, albeit with some support, and if they are re-admitted for treatment they are usually in hospital for only a few weeks at a time (Van Os & Kapur, 2009).

Schizophrenia is associated with marked distress and poor mental health, and it is also associated with adverse effects on physical health. Patients with schizophrenia die on average 10 to 15 years younger than the average population, and this can be attributed to poor diet, obesity, smoking, a lack of exercise and reduced access to healthcare (Van Os & Kapur, 2009).

Section summary

In this section we have discussed how schizophrenia is diagnosed and have distilled its core features: positive, negative and disorganised symptoms. Importantly, the symptoms of schizophrenia are very diverse, and they do not cluster together *for individuals* as neatly as many doctors assume. When we consider the causes of schizophrenia, we need to think carefully about the causes of the 'disorder' (which some people say does not actually exist) versus the causes of the specific *symptoms*, which certainly do exist.

Section 2: How does schizophrenia develop?

Schizophrenia certainly runs in families, and there are clear abnormalities in the brains of schizophrenic patients compared to controls. For years these two observations were explained by fairly simplistic biological accounts of the disease, which led to social and psychological influences being largely ignored. This has changed in recent decades, and there is now growing awareness that the symptoms are strongly influenced by adverse events (particularly during childhood), that they can be maintained by social factors, and that disturbances in psychological processes play an important role.

Heritability and genetics

Schizophrenia is genetically transmitted, at least in part. Gottesman (1991) reported the incidence of schizophrenia in the relatives of people who had the disorder. The incidence in monozygotic twins (who share 100% of their genetic material with the affected proband) is about 50%, compared to around 17% in dizygotic twins (who share, on average, 50% of their genetic material). Looking at other family members, the likelihood of developing schizophrenia decreases in line with the amount of genetic material that someone shares with a schizophrenic individual: the incidence is about 9% for someone who has a schizophrenic brother or sister, or 12% if one of their parents is affected. Siblings and parents are 'first-degree relatives' because you share, on average, 50% of your genetic material with them. The incidence drops to around 5% in the 'second-degree relatives' of schizophrenic individuals, with whom they share, on average, 25% of their genetic material: grandparents, nieces and nephews.

Studies such as this have led to a general consensus that the heritability of schizophrenia ranges between 50% and 80%, which is high compared with most other psychological disorders (Van Os & Kapur, 2009). As with everything, this isn't as simple as it would initially seem. For example, the heritable risk for schizophrenia also confers a risk for other disorders such as bipolar disorder (see Chapter 5) (Craddock et al., 2005). This suggests that we shouldn't hold out too much hope of finding a gene (or genes) that would be specific for schizophrenia. Indeed, an enormous amount of research has been devoted to identifying specific genes that confer an increased risk of schizophrenia. Some individual genes have been identified, but this whole research area is characterised by very small effect sizes, with findings that cannot be replicated (Sanders et al., 2008). Where we *have* found linkages between specific genes and schizophrenia, it seems that those genes are associated with an increased risk of other psychological disorders, such as bipolar disorder, as well (O'Donovan et al., 2008).

So where do we go from here? Many researchers have all but given up the search for the 'schizophrenia gene', and have realised that multiple genetic variations are likely to explain why the disorder runs in families. For example, a recent study involving more than 36,000 patients with schizophrenia and 113,000 controls identified 108 distinct genetic polymorphisms (variations) that were associated with schizophrenia, including genes that are involved in dopamine activity in the brain and immune system function (Ripke et al., 2014). Another promising development is the shift towards identifying genes that are associated with a cognitive 'endophenotype' that is in turn associated with schizophrenia. For example, schizophrenic patients differ from unaffected controls on performance on tasks that measure the control of eye movements (such as the antisaccade task) and on measures of prepulse inhibition of the startle reflex. These characteristics are also seen in unaffected close relatives of schizophrenic patients and they can be detected in schizophrenic patients before they develop any symptoms. Therefore these characteristics may be reliable cognitive markers of the risk for developing schizophrenia (the endophenotype), and they are much easier to identify and measure than a diagnosis of schizophrenia itself! Researchers are optimistic that this may be a more productive way to isolate the genetic risk for schizophrenia (Greenwood et al., 2007; Gur et al., 2007).

Box 4.4   Essential debate

Cannabis and schizophrenia

The relationship between cannabis use and schizophrenia is rarely out of the newspapers, and unfortunately a lot of this coverage is sensationalist and reveals a very poor grasp of statistics by journalists (see www.badscience.net/2007/07/blah-blah-cannabis-blah-blah-blah/#more-476 for an amusing example). There is good evidence that people with schizophrenia are more likely to smoke cannabis than people who do not have schizophrenia, although this doesn't tell us whether cannabis causes schizophrenia, or whether people with schizophrenia use the drug because it makes them feel better.

(Continued)

(Continued)

On one side of the debate, some researchers argue that repeated cannabis intoxication is likely to cause users to lose touch with reality and ultimately develop psychotic symptoms. Opponents of this view point out that the number of people who use cannabis regularly is much higher than the number of people who are diagnosed with schizophrenia, and therefore we shouldn't blame cannabis each time a young person who uses the drug develops schizophrenia.

Findings from several longitudinal studies have gone some way to resolving this debate. These studies reveal that cannabis use does *slightly* increase the risk of having a psychotic episode later on, and this is related to the potency of the cannabis and the amount that is smoked (Di Forti et al., 2009; Moore et al., 2007). But we have to remember that not everyone who smokes cannabis will go on to develop schizophrenia – the vast majority of cannabis users will not – and many people who do develop schizophrenia have never used it at all.

Prenatal trauma

Things that happen before birth (prenatally) are also associated with schizophrenia diagnoses during adulthood. Children of unusually low birth weight, who experience complications during birth, or whose mothers had infections while pregnant, are at increased risk

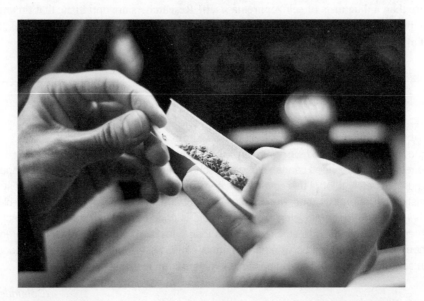

Figure 4.1 Frequent use of high-potency cannabis does increase the risk of developing schizophrenia

of developing schizophrenia later on in life (Rapoport et al., 2012). These prenatal traumas lead to changes in brain structure and function that are characteristic of schizophrenia, but what is interesting is that a child that experiences one of these traumas may appear completely 'normal' until adolescence when the effects become apparent (Meyer & Feldon, 2010). Most researchers agree that schizophrenia is a neurodevelopmental psychiatric disorder, and if any of these traumas occur during 'critical age windows' then the individual is at increased risk of developing schizophrenia later in life (Marco et al., 2011). The effects of prenatal trauma do not seem to become apparent until the brain reaches a critical stage of maturation during adolescence. However, as with genetic factors, there is much debate about whether these effects of prenatal trauma are specific to schizophrenia or whether they confer increased risk to psychological disorders in general.

Adverse events during childhood

Schizophrenic patients are much more likely than unaffected controls to experience adverse events during their childhood. For example, Wicks et al. (2005) investigated the links between socio-economic status during childhood and the incidence of schizophrenia in a sample of two million people, comprising every single person born in Sweden between 1963 and 1983 (impressive!). They found a 'dose–response' relationship between indicators of adversity during childhood (e.g. having parents who were unemployed or were receiving state benefits, or were being raised by a single parent) and the incidence of schizophrenia during adulthood: the higher the level of adversity a person experienced during childhood, the more likely they were to develop schizophrenia later on. Other studies show that a broad range of adverse events during childhood (such as being bullied at school, being neglected by your parents, or the death or divorce of your parents) were all associated with an increased likelihood of developing schizophrenia later on in life (Matheson et al., 2013; Varese et al., 2012). Prolonged separation from the mother during the first two years of life is another risk factor (Anglin et al., 2008).

As discussed in many other chapters of this book, having an unhappy childhood (with severe childhood trauma as an extreme example) is associated with an increased risk of a wide range of psychological disorders. So is there anything special about the relationship between childhood trauma and schizophrenia? Bebbington et al. (2004) showed that experiences of *victimisation* during childhood were particularly closely associated with developing schizophrenia later on. They interviewed over 8,000 adults who suffered from a range of different psychological disorders, including schizophrenia, depression, substance use disorders and generalised anxiety disorder, to identify any adverse events that happened during their childhoods. Their analysis showed that victimisation experiences were selectively linked to schizophrenia rather than other disorders, with childhood sexual abuse being most closely linked to schizophrenia, followed by running away from home, homelessness, and being taken into care. You might have noticed that these adverse events are likely to cluster together, because if a child is sexually abused they are more likely to run away from home, and be homeless for a while, before being taken into care. Bebbington et al. (2004) were able to take all of this into account in their statistical analyses and they found that childhood sexual abuse was closely associated with schizophrenia during adulthood, even after controlling for the other adverse events that tend to occur along with sexual abuse.

Perhaps the apparently close link between childhood sexual abuse and schizophrenia could be explained in other ways. For example, one argument is that parents with schizophrenia are particularly likely to sexually abuse their children. However, when researchers have looked at this they have found no support for this argument (Read et al., 2005). There is overwhelming evidence for a direct link between childhood sexual abuse and schizophrenia, and this is completely independent of the heritable risk of the disorder. A second observation is that most of the available evidence comes from studies that asked schizophrenic and non-schizophrenic adults to recall any adverse events that occurred to them during childhood. Therefore these types of studies are prone to retrospective memory errors, and it is plausible that patients with schizophrenia might fabricate a childhood full of sexual abuse and other unpleasant experiences, particularly if they are currently experiencing paranoid delusions. However, this doesn't seem to be the case. Patients' memories of childhood adverse events are very consistent over time, even when they are asked about them when in the middle of an acute psychotic episode versus when they are in remission (and therefore relatively stable). This suggests that schizophrenic patients aren't simply making up stories about being abused as children because they are in the middle of a psychotic episode (Read et al., 2005).

So why might a history of victimisation experiences during childhood increase the risk of schizophrenia? One suggestion is that they might lead to a dysfunctional style of thinking that places people at risk of developing schizophrenia once they reach a critical stage of maturation. For example, Lataster et al. (2006) reported a strong association between sexual abuse or bullying during childhood, and psychotic experiences (delusional ideation and hallucinations) in adolescents aged between 12 and 16. Importantly, none of these individuals had a diagnosis of schizophrenia at the time. Therefore this study shows a relationship between childhood victimisation and the acquisition of a mental schema in which other people are seen as dangerous, and the person feels that they are constantly under threat. This style of thinking could make the person vulnerable to experiencing paranoid delusions later on, and these could develop into full-blown schizophrenia. However, it is also possible that having psychotic experiences makes individuals vulnerable to victimisation experiences, or that a third factor raises the risk of both victimisation and psychotic experiences. As yet the research has not managed to unpick this relationship.

Social exclusion

Schizophrenia is more common among immigrants (Cantor-Graae, 2007). For example, the incidence is higher among Caribbean immigrants to the United Kingdom compared to the local white population, and to Caribbean islanders who remain at home. You might be thinking that this is because people with schizophrenia are more likely to migrate to a foreign country because they feel persecuted at home, and therefore the increased incidence of schizophrenia in immigrants might simply be an artefact of an increased heritable risk among immigrants. However, some studies suggest that the incidence of schizophrenia is greater in second-generation immigrants (who are born to parents who migrated) compared to first-generation immigrants (the people who actually moved to a different country) (Cantor-Graae, 2007). This fascinating observation is clearly not consistent with the notion that people with schizophrenia are much more likely to emigrate. Cantor-Graae speculates that second generation immigrants are at increased risk because they do not feel that they 'belong' in the country of their birth – which is likely to lead to delusions of persecution. Further evidence comes from the observation that the incidence of schizophrenia is much lower among immigrants if they form a large percentage of the local population than if they are firmly in the minority (Selten & Cantor-Graae, 2005).

Box 4.5   Essential research

Escape to the country

It may surprise you to learn that the incidence of schizophrenia is two to three times higher for city dwellers compared to those who live in the countryside, and this is 'dose-dependent': the longer that children are raised in urban environments, the greater their risk of developing schizophrenia in later life (Meyer-Lindenberg & Tost, 2012). It is possible that this risk factor is related to the increased incidence of schizophrenia in immigrants, who are more likely to live in cramped conditions in big cities. One explanation for this link is that feeling socially excluded is more likely if you belong to an ethnic minority, and/or if you live in a big city, and this feeling of social exclusion leads to delusional thinking, which in turn increases the risk of developing schizophrenia.

Expressed emotion

Families may contribute to the development of schizophrenia in ways other than victimising or abusing their children. Expressed emotion (EE) refers to the tendency of a relative to criticise, be hostile, or demonstrate emotional over-involvement (Miklowitz & Goldstein, 1993) towards a patient. It is commonly measured with the Camberwell Family Interview, which assesses the frequency of critical comments and positive remarks directed from close family members to the schizophrenic patient, and provides global measures of hostility, warmth and emotional over-involvement (Bebbington & Kuipers, 1994).

Many studies have investigated the relationships between the level of expressed emotion in family members, and relapse to psychotic episodes in patients who have received treatment for schizophrenia. For example, in an early study Koenigsberg and Handley (1986) reported that, after initial treatment of schizophrenia, 51% of patients with high EE families had a relapse, as compared to only 22% of patients with low EE families. Bebbington and

Kuipers (1994) suggested that relatives with high levels of expressed emotion are more prone to generate arguments and then escalate them, and they have poor listening skills, which is likely to be very traumatic for patients who are experiencing delusions. Related to this, Hooley (2007) reported that relatives who are high in expressed emotion tend to be less tolerant and flexible, and more likely to believe that affected patients are able to control their symptoms, compared to relatives who are low in expressed emotion.

Some early theoretical models suggested that expressed emotion, together with aspects of 'communication deviance' (unclear or ambiguous communication between family members; see Bateson et al., 1956), were enough to cause schizophrenia because they prevented a child from developing logical thought (leading to delusions) and because they disrupted the normal processing of sensory information (leading to hallucinations). However, evidence suggests that this is not the case. First, although high levels of expressed emotion are associated with relapse in schizophrenia, expressed emotion is actually more closely associated with mood disorders and eating disorders, so it isn't specific to schizophrenia (Butzlaff & Hooley, 1998). Most importantly, prospective studies in which expressed emotion is measured in families *before* a person is diagnosed with schizophrenia show that expressed emotion is not, on its own, sufficient to cause the disorder, although there is little doubt that high levels of expressed emotion can increase the risk of relapse once a patient has been treated for their first psychotic episode (Hooley, 2007). There is some evidence that a child born to schizophrenic parents who is adopted into a non-schizophrenic family where there are high levels of expressed emotion is at increased risk of developing the disorder, and this is a good example of a gene–environment interaction. In this case, the environmental risk factor (high expressed emotion in the immediate family) is not sufficient to cause schizophrenia, but if combined with genetic risk for the disorder it can 'tip a person over the edge' (Hooley, 2007).

We might question why the level of expressed emotion is high in some families of schizophrenic patients but low in others. Perhaps expressed emotion in families increases in response to the behaviour of schizophrenic patients, which becomes increasingly bizarre and difficult to deal with as the symptoms become more severe. The evidence on this is rather mixed, because some studies show that the level of expressed emotion in relatives increases as a patient's symptoms become more severe, whereas other studies show no relationship between the severity of symptoms in patients and the level of expressed emotion in relatives (Hooley, 2007).

Section summary

Schizophrenia is heritable, but the mechanism is unclear and this is far from the whole story. We have shown that adverse events during childhood (and being sexually abused in particular), living in a big city, and belonging to a minority group are all linked to increased risk of developing schizophrenia. All of these things are likely to make people feel threatened and that they do not 'belong'. Furthermore, patients with schizophrenia are much less likely to recover if their family environment is too high in expressed emotion, which may also be a contributing cause of the disorder in combination with other factors.

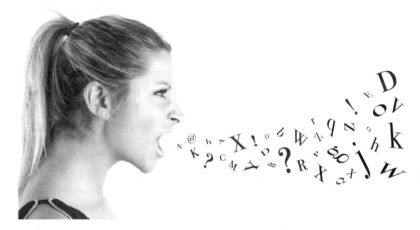

Figure 4.2 High levels of expressed emotion in relatives increase the risk of relapse in patients who have been treated for schizophrenia

Section 3: Brain and cognitive mechanisms in schizophrenia

As we have seen, schizophrenia is likely to be caused by a combination of heritable and environmental factors. However, this doesn't explain *why* and *how* these things lead to schizophrenia. To get a step closer to answering that question, we first need to look at how the brains of schizophrenic people are different from the brains of people who do not have the disorder. These neuropsychological findings can be integrated into general cognitive frameworks, and we will end this section by critically evaluating a few of these theoretical models.

The dopamine hypothesis

A major breakthrough in the treatment of schizophrenia came in the 1950s with the discovery that chlorpromazine had a dramatic effect on many of its symptoms (for an informative history lesson, see Kapur & Mamo, 2003). Chlorpromazine belongs to a class of drugs that are now known as antipsychotics, which are dopamine antagonists that suppress dopamine function in the brain by blocking dopamine receptors. This observation led to 'the dopamine hypothesis': the idea that schizophrenia is the result of increased levels of dopamine in the brain (reviewed by Kapur et al., 2005). The dopamine hypothesis is supported by additional types of evidence. For example, drugs such as amphetamines and L-DOPA, both of which increase dopamine activity, can trigger symptoms that seem very similar to the positive symptoms of schizophrenia when given to healthy volunteers. Finally, patients who are experiencing an acute psychotic episode demonstrate increased synthesis (production) of dopamine, and increased concentrations of dopamine in the brain, relative to healthy control participants (Van Os & Kapur, 2009).

Although the dopamine hypothesis is nice and simple, the reality is a little more complicated. Antipsychotic drugs do not affect the negative symptoms of schizophrenia at all. In addition, dopamine has important roles in motor activity and various psychological functions, including attention, learning and motivation: we cannot simply label it 'the schizophrenia neurotransmitter'. We now know that the effect of antipsychotic drugs on the positive symptoms of schizophrenia is correlated with the degree to which they reduce dopamine activity in the mesolimbic dopamine system, rather than their effects on dopamine function in other parts of the brain (Kapur et al., 2005).

More recent work on the role of dopamine and its dysfunction in schizophrenia was summarised by Kapur et al. (2005). Although dopamine was originally thought to be involved in reward and pleasure, many researchers now believe that its main function is to register novel and salient features of the environment. Kapur's view is that in schizophrenia dopamine is released sporadically and randomly, and the consequence for the patient is that everything in the environment appears 'salient' or important. As a consequence the patient perceives meaning and importance in everything, even things that should be ignored. The patient then attempts to make some sense of these strange feelings that 'everything is important', which leads them to formulate delusions, the content of which is often unique to the individual and their own experiences. If the patient takes antipsychotics, then the patient feels that things in their environment (such as hearing voices) do not seem as significant as they did before they started taking the medication. Kapur makes the point that if antipsychotics block the attribution of salience, this should not eliminate symptoms of schizophrenia but it should make them seem less important. From interviews with patients, Kapur believes that this is in fact the case: patients report that they still hear voices and have strange delusions, but they are less bothered by them. Overall, dopamine seems to play a key role in schizophrenia but its role is not as simple as we initially thought!

Big holes in the brain?

The brain is full of fluid-filled holes called ventricles. If the ventricles are particularly large, they are taking up space that would otherwise be occupied with brain tissue. Post-mortem investigations of the brains of schizophrenic patients reveal enlarged ventricles, particularly in the region that is normally occupied by the temporal lobe, meaning that this part of the brain is generally smaller than it is in controls (Tyrer & Mackay, 1986). Enlarged ventricles, with accompanying reductions in brain tissue volume in this area, have also been demonstrated in living schizophrenic patients using brain scanning techniques (Shenton et al., 2001; Weinberger et al., 1979).

It is unclear whether the ventricles become enlarged to fill the space caused by small brain volumes, or whether the ventricles are responsible for crushing the surrounding brain tissue. Furthermore, enlarged ventricles are not a specific sign of schizophrenia because they are also characteristic of depression and bipolar disorder (see Chapter 5). However, it is interesting to note two things. First, enlarged ventricles are also seen in siblings of schizophrenic patients who do not have the disorder themselves (Staal et al., 2000). Second, enlarged ventricles are seen in 'first episode psychosis', that is, in people who have not yet been taking antipsychotic medication for long periods of time (Staal et al., 2000). These findings suggest that enlarged ventricles are not a consequence of antipsychotic medication, and instead may be one aspect of the genetically-transmitted endophenotype for schizophrenia. In this case, the term 'endophenotype' means the profile of brain function and psychological characteristics that are typical of people who are at increased risk of developing schizophrenia in the future (cognitive features of this endophenotype were discussed in the previous section). The idea that damage to the temporal lobe might have something to do with the onset of psychotic symptoms is discussed in more detail below.

Cognitive deficits in schizophrenia

Schizophrenic patients have marked deficits in cognitive performance, which is unsurprising when we consider that they generally have reduced volumes of brain tissue in the temporal lobes and surrounding areas. These cognitive deficits are very broad (Barch et al., 2009) and include problems with perception, selective attention, working memory, executive control (switching between different task rules and inhibiting inappropriate responses), long-term memory, reinforcement learning, and the processing of social and emotional cues (e.g. judging the emotional state of a person based on their facial expression). In short, schizophrenic patients will perform worse than unaffected controls on almost any cognitive task you can think of. These cognitive deficits are significant for a number of reasons (Mesholam-Gately et al., 2009):

- They can be detected before other symptoms emerge and the patient develops full-blown schizophrenia.
- Mild cognitive deficits are seen in unaffected first-degree relatives of schizophrenic patients.
- Within schizophrenic patients, the cognitive deficits remain even when the other symptoms improve.
- Antipsychotic medication alleviates the positive symptoms but has no effect on cognitive deficits at all.
- Cognitive deficits are not a result of taking antipsychotics for a long period of time because they are seen in patients with first episode psychosis, and they are not noticeably worse in chronic schizophrenia (when patients have taken antipsychotics for many years).

All of these things suggest that cognitive deficits are an important part of the endophenotype for schizophrenia. Clinicians are very interested in cognitive deficits because their severity is an important predictor of 'functional' outcomes in schizophrenia, even more so than positive or negative symptoms (Green, 2006). Functional outcomes relate to how well the sufferer can go back to work, have a social life and look after themselves (e.g. cooking, shopping) without some kind of help. Clinicians who treat schizophrenic patients often assess cognitive impairments in order to work out how much help the patient is likely to need once their symptoms have been stabilised with medication.

The relationship between symptoms and activity in the brain

Other researchers have studied abnormalities of brain function or activity in schizophrenic patients in an attempt to understand how these relate to the severity of positive, negative and disorganised symptoms. A review by Goghari and colleagues (2010) considered a large number of studies that looked at patterns of brain activation in schizophrenic patients, and attempted to relate distinct symptoms to activity in different brain regions while participants completed appropriate tasks. They found that reduced activity in the ventrolateral prefrontal cortex and ventral striatum was related to negative symptoms, including reduced motivation, alogia, anhedonia and flat affect. Positive symptoms, particularly persecutory delusions, were related to increased activity in the medial prefrontal cortex, the amygdala, as well as the hippocampus and surrounding parahippocampal region. It is not possible to say that increased activity in these brain regions reflects increased dopamine activity (fMRI cannot tell us this), but these brain regions are all part of the mesolimbic dopamine circuit and we would expect them to be involved in positive symptoms, so these findings do make sense (Kapur et al., 2005).

Cognitive theories of schizophrenia

We have seen that schizophrenia is caused by genetic factors, adverse events during childhood, and broad social factors such as living in cities and feeling persecuted. We have also seen that the brains of schizophrenic patients are different from the brains of unaffected people, and this brain dysfunction is associated with severe cognitive impairment as well as related to the severity of positive, negative and disorganised symptoms. This moves us closer to an explanation of how schizophrenia develops, but we are not quite there yet. In this section we will consider cognitive theories of schizophrenia. We will also think about a contentious issue among researchers, that is, do we need psychological models that can account for the many symptoms of the *disorder* called 'schizophrenia', or is it more helpful to focus on models of the specific *symptoms* of schizophrenia?

Cognitive theories of schizophrenia as a disorder

In a hugely influential model, Frith (1992) proposed that schizophrenic patients have a deficit in 'self-monitoring', in other words the ability to monitor one's own thoughts and intended actions. For example, our thoughts often take the form of 'inner speech' in which we talk to ourselves without actually speaking. Imagine if you believed that your 'inner speech' was not produced by you: you would then perceive it as an auditory hallucination (an external voice speaking to you). Another example would be if you were to cross the road to look in a shop window but did not realise that you intended to cross the road, you might believe that your behaviour was under the control of a malevolent external force.

Some experimental studies have demonstrated that patients with schizophrenia have deficits in the ability to monitor their own thoughts and actions. For example, McGuire et al. (1995) developed a task that could mimic auditory hallucinations, which required participants to imagine sentences being spoken in another person's voice. When healthy people completed this task, the left inferior frontal cortex and left temporal cortex were activated. By contrast, when patients with schizophrenia who experienced hallucinations completed the task, they had reduced activity in the left temporal cortex but normal levels of activity in the left inferior frontal cortex. This could be the neural substrate of self-monitoring deficits in schizophrenia: a breakdown in connectivity between these parts of the brain means that schizophrenic patients lose awareness of thoughts or actions that they generate themselves, and therefore they perceive these as alien (McGuire & Frith, 1996). Other studies have provided converging evidence for self-monitoring deficits (reviewed by Stephan et al., 2009). For example, patients who have delusions of alien control are not very good at identifying drawings that they have created themselves (Stirling et al., 2001).

Frith's (1992) model can also explain how paranoid delusions develop: patients with schizophrenia are unable to understand the intentions of other people (for the same reason that they cannot properly understand their own intentions), which means they find it difficult to understand what others are thinking or feeling, which then leads to feelings of paranoia. Indeed, some studies show that schizophrenic patients do not 'get' cartoon jokes that require people to understand another person's mental state in order to understand the joke (Marjoram et al., 2005). Finally, Frith argues that negative symptoms develop when patients are overwhelmed by the confusion of being unable to interpret their own intentions and behaviour, as well as those of other people, and this causes them to become withdrawn.

Another model was proposed by Hemsley (1993), who argued that schizophrenia arises when people fail to use their memories and past experiences to make sense of their sensory input (e.g. the things that they see and hear). This causes them to perceive things as unusual and unexpected when in fact they are not (this idea is the basis for Kapur and colleagues' views about abnormal 'salience'; see Kapur et al., 2005). This is likely to result in hallucinations, and then delusions arise when people try to make sense of the barrage of confusing information that they are experiencing. Like Frith, Hemsley also suggested that negative symptoms develop as a coping strategy to escape from this information overload.

Hemsley's theory is supported by the aforementioned source-monitoring studies (e.g. McGuire et al., 1995), as well as by studies which show that schizophrenic patients perform badly on tasks that require them to learn to filter out and ignore irrelevant stimuli (Weiner & Arad, 2009). Both Frith's and Hemsley's models explain schizophrenia as a breakdown in what we might call 'consciousness', and there is evidence for specific instances when consciousness breaks down, as detailed above. One weakness of these models is that they assume that delusions, hallucinations and negative symptoms should be inter-related (e.g. the hallucinations cause the delusions which in turn lead to negative symptoms), and there is some evidence that this simply isn't the case, as we discussed in Section 1. Other theorists think that it is more useful to try to identify the cognitive mechanisms that underlie the different symptoms of schizophrenia, and we turn to these models next.

Cognitive models of specific symptoms

We previously discussed evidence which shows that adverse events during childhood are associated with an increased risk of developing schizophrenia later in life. The reality may actually be a bit more complicated, because it seems that different *kinds* of abuse are associated with specific symptoms. For example, Read et al. (2005) found that childhood abuse and neglect are consistently related to the development of positive symptoms (hallucinations and delusions) but they are completely unrelated to negative or disorganised symptoms. The authors proposed a cognitive model to account for their findings: childhood sexual and physical abuse cause changes in beliefs and attributions (e.g. 'People are dangerous', 'I am vulnerable'), which over time become paranoid delusions. Furthermore, the auditory hallucinations experienced by schizophrenic patients are 'flashbacks' of specific traumatic events experienced during childhood, but the patient does not recognise these as flashbacks, and they cope with the unpleasant emotions by attributing them to an external source.

Other studies suggest that hallucinations and delusions may have distinct causes. For example, Bentall et al. (2012) demonstrated that sexual abuse during childhood was specifically associated with auditory hallucinations in adulthood, whereas disruption of attachment and chronic victimisation (e.g. bullying) during childhood were specifically associated with paranoid delusions during adulthood. For example, rape during childhood was strongly associated with auditory hallucinations, and this association was independent of paranoid delusions. On the other hand, being brought up in institutional care was strongly associated with paranoid delusions, and this association was independent of auditory hallucinations.

Dissociative symptoms might also play a role in the development of auditory hallucinations. Dissociation can be defined as the lack of 'normal' integration of thoughts, emotions and experiences into the stream of consciousness. Schizophrenic patients who have auditory hallucinations report elevated levels of dissociative symptoms compared to patients who do not hallucinate, and studies that use a method known as 'experience sampling' can explain the link between the two. With experience sampling, participants report their symptoms in real-time, in their natural environment, when prompted to do so at random times by alarms delivered on a watch or smartphone. Varese et al. (2011) reported that auditory hallucinations were more likely to occur shortly after people reported an increase in their dissociative symptoms, particularly if they felt stressed at the time. This is consistent with the work on source monitoring (e.g., McGuire et al., 1995). That is, if patients have trouble integrating their thoughts, emotions and experiences into their stream of consciousness (dissociative symptoms), they are more likely to incorrectly attribute internal stimulation (such as the 'inner voice') as having an external source. Other work from this group of researchers suggests that being prone to dissociative experiences fully mediates the relationship between a history of childhood sexual abuse and auditory hallucinations (Varese, Barkus, & Bentall, 2012). Although this research is just beginning, we are starting to form a picture of how environmental triggers can lead to specific psychotic symptoms, and how these can ultimately cascade into other symptoms.

So what about the negative symptoms of schizophrenia? There are conflicting views about whether these develop as a reaction to the positive or disorganised symptoms, or whether they are caused by completely different factors. For example, one view (endorsed by Frith and Hemsley) is that negative symptoms arise because schizophrenic patients gradually disengage from social and other activities because such activities make them feel over-stimulated, or because of their (often paranoid) delusional beliefs, or because they anticipate 'failing' at difficult tasks and social activities. Patients believe that they have very limited psychological resources, and they withdraw because they don't want to waste their effort on social and other activities at which they are likely to 'fail'. Based on this view, negative symptoms seem to be a predictable reaction to the distress caused by positive symptoms and the cognitive and social deficits that are characteristic of schizophrenia. This account is plausible, and indeed some studies do show that the negative symptoms worsen shortly after the positive symptoms have done so. Related to this, antipsychotic medication leads to improvements in positive symptoms, shortly followed by improvements in at least some negative symptoms (Stahl & Buckley, 2007).

There are several pieces of evidence that do not quite fit here (Rector et al., 2005), however. For example, cognitive behaviour therapy (CBT; discussed later) can improve the negative symptoms of schizophrenia even if the positive symptoms do not improve first. The heritable risk for schizophrenia, and obstetric complications, are related to the severity of negative symptoms more so than positive symptoms, and these relationships are mediated (explained) by the extent of ventricular enlargement (Stahl & Buckley, 2007). This suggests that there are fairly clear biological causes for negative symptoms, but these same biological factors are not so closely related to the severity of positive symptoms. These observations are not compatible with the notion that negative symptoms of schizophrenia develop as a response to the positive symptoms of the disorder.

Section summary

Although dopamine function plays a key role in schizophrenia, it is also important to consider the structural and functional changes in the brain that underlie cognitive deficits and specific symptoms. Some cognitive theories of schizophrenia can explain the disorder as a breakdown of self-monitoring (or more broadly, 'consciousness'). This causes the positive symptoms to develop, and negative symptoms develop afterwards as a response. Other theorists suggest that different types of symptoms have distinct causes, and the latest research findings support these theories.

Section 4: How is schizophrenia treated?

Drug therapy

Schizophrenia is primarily treated with medication (antipsychotic drugs), which is unsurprising given the dominance of biological models of the disorder. Dopamine blocking drugs (such as chlorpromazine and haloperidol) and later 'atypical' antipsychotics are widely used today, and are effective in about 70% of patients (Taylor et al., 2012). We will consider the effectiveness of antipsychotic drugs in some detail, and show how clinical trials funded by the pharmaceutical industry have painted a quite misleading picture about the benefits of newer, 'atypical' antipsychotics compared to the older (and less profitable) drugs such as haloperidol.

The majority of patients who receive a diagnosis of schizophrenia will make a significant improvement that will allow them to be discharged from hospital and in many cases lead an independent life, albeit with continued monitoring and support. About a hundred years ago the prognosis was much bleaker, with most patients diagnosed with schizophrenia being committed to asylums for the rest of their lives. A vast improvement in the outlook for schizophrenic patients took place between 1920 and 1970, and it is no coincidence that this overlaps with the widespread introduction of antipsychotics. Widespread prescribing of these drugs has improved the lives of many patients with schizophrenia. However, broad social changes and a move away from the institutionalisation of mentally ill patients also occurred within this period, so we must be cautious before we attribute all of these improvements to antipsychotic medication (Taylor et al., 2012).

The older antipsychotic drugs are effective at blunting the positive and disorganised symptoms of schizophrenia, but they don't seem to improve the negative symptoms, and they may even worsen them. Newer, atypical antipsychotics (such as clozapine and risperidone) were introduced to great acclaim in the 1970s. These drugs affect the serotonin system and have more selective effects on the dopamine system, which means that they can change dopamine activity in some areas of the brain more than other areas (Kapur & Remington, 2001). The initial clinical trials suggested that these drugs were more effective at reducing the positive symptoms, but they ameliorated the negative symptoms as well, compared to the older drugs (Cha & McIntyre, 2012). However, later clinical trials revealed that the atypicals only seemed better than the older antipsychotics in the original trials, because in the early trials atypicals were compared with a very high dose of the older antipsychotics which would have made the negative symptoms worse, and therefore the atypicals would seem much better by comparison (Kapur & Remington, 2001). When better trials were subsequently carried out, comparisons of atypical and typical antipsychotics revealed that the two drugs produced equivalent improvements in positive symptoms, negative symptoms and cognitive deficits. The atypicals have a slight advantage when it comes to affective (negative mood) symptoms, but even then these drugs are no better than a standard antidepressant for those symptoms. There is some evidence that atypicals lead to improved 'quality of life' compared to older antipsychotics, but this difference is very small indeed. Kapur and Remington (2001) state in their review that antipsychotics, even the newer atypicals, work as a 'pharmacological shotgun' because they affect so many different neurotransmitter symptoms. Those authors advocated designing new drugs to specifically target the positive, negative and disorganised symptoms of schizophrenia. Like others, this group of researchers aren't convinced that the 'disorder' exists, and we might be better off trying to treat the individual symptoms instead.

Antipsychotic drugs also have side effects such as body tremors and rigidity, restless leg syndrome, muscular contraction, extrapyramidal side effects (difficulties initiating and controlling movements) and tardive dyskinesia (abnormal movements, especially of the face and tongue). There are several other side effects, such as sedation, weight gain, and (in females) the absence of menstruation and excessive lactation. When the atypical antipsychotics were introduced, the initial studies (which were misleading, as described above) suggested that their side effects were much less severe than those seen with the older drugs. However, we now know that atypicals also produce side effects including weight gain, metabolic and cardiovascular changes and extrapyramidal symptoms. While it is true that extrapyramidal side effects are generally not as severe with atypical antipsychotics, it is also the case that other symptoms such as excessive weight gain are at least as bad (and may be even worse). In addition, more serious symptoms such as agranulocytosis (a decline in white blood cells in the blood that requires careful monitoring) are seen with the atypical drugs, although these are rare (Cha & McIntyre, 2012).

Psychosocial treatments

Cognitive behaviour therapy (CBT)

When CBT and other psychosocial treatments are offered, patients nearly always receive these in addition to (not instead of) antipsychotic medication. The aim of CBT for psychosis is to encourage patients to challenge their dysfunctional beliefs (delusions) through techniques such as 'reality testing' (see Chapter 5) and to think of alternative, more benign explanations for the auditory hallucinations that they experience (Beck & Rector, 2005). Another aim of CBT is to tackle the negative symptoms, for example by encouraging patients to think about the benefits of being more active and engaging with other people. The general idea is that patients who receive CBT should be able to manage their symptoms, and this will reduce their risk of experiencing a relapse into another psychotic episode in the future (see Wykes et al., 2008, for a review).

Patients who take antipsychotic drugs are likely to have some residual positive symptoms, and CBT is effective at reducing their severity, but only if it is delivered by experienced CBT therapists (Wykes et al., 2005; Wykes et al., 2008). One recent study also demonstrated that CBT alleviated symptoms in patients who were not taking any antipsychotic medication (Morrison et al., 2014). It is important to deliver CBT as early as possible after the first psychotic episode, and ideally during the acute phase (Zimmermann et al., 2005). Even if CBT cannot be given during an acute psychotic episode, it is much more effective if given within three years of the initial onset of symptoms (Newton et al., 2005).

As well as reducing symptoms, CBT is effective at reducing the risk of relapse to psychosis in the future (Jones et al., 2000), and a recent meta-analysis revealed that CBT led to symptom

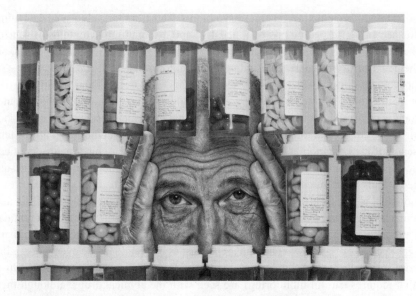

Figure 4.3 While they may be effective, antipsychotic medications affect a broad range of neurotransmitter systems and produce unpleasant side effects

improvement in people who were 'medication resistant', that is, those who did not get better in response to antipsychotic medication (Burns et al., 2014). However, some researchers are more sceptical of the long-term benefits of CBT as compared to other types of psychosocial treatment. For example, the magnitude of the beneficial effect of CBT on symptom severity is approximately halved if the people who are rating the symptoms are blind to group allocation, that is, if they do not know which patients received CBT and which did not. While this type of finding is fairly common in clinical trials (see Chapter 2), it does suggest that at least some of the apparent benefit of CBT can be attributed to wishful thinking on behalf of the researchers who are rating the severity of patients' symptoms (Jauhar et al., 2014; Wykes et al., 2008).

So what about the long-term benefits of CBT? Turkington et al. (2008) studied a group of patients who were receiving antipsychotic medication, and patients also received either CBT, or 'treatment as usual' (no psychosocial treatment), or an alternative non-specific psychosocial intervention ('befriending'). They looked at the symptom severity and overall recovery of their patients five years after they had received therapy. Overall symptom severity was reduced in the CBT group compared to the befriending and treatment as usual groups, as was the severity of negative symptoms of schizophrenia. However, there were no group differences on symptoms of schizophrenia overall. While this study is impressive in terms of the length of its follow-up period (five years), the sample size was small (they were only able to assess 59 out of the original 90 patients at follow-up). Overall, it seems that any benefits of CBT may be short-lived and that in the longer term it is no better or worse than a comparison psychosocial treatment.

For some clinicians, their initial enthusiasm for CBT has been tempered by findings such as these. The general consensus is that for most patients CBT should be delivered alongside medication (not instead of it), and that some may benefit from it in terms of reduced severity of symptoms, acceptance of symptoms, or the effective use of coping skills to live a relatively normal life.

Family therapy

In a previous section we saw that the level of expressed emotion in the families of schizophrenic patients can have a major influence on their prospects of recovery. The aim of Behavioural Family Management (BFM) is to modify expressed emotion in the families of patients with schizophrenia, and there are three broad components:

- educating the family about schizophrenia (this helps to remove attributions of blame from patients);
- communication skills training, in which family members and patients are shown their negative communication patterns and are helped to change them;
- problem-solving skills in which both parties are taught how to approach problematic situations in a collaborative way.

Several studies have shown that patients (and their families) who receive these types of family therapy show less social withdrawal and lower rates of relapse. For example, one study found that only 9% of patients who received a family intervention had suffered a relapse at the nine-month follow-up, as compared to 50% of patients who received a comparison treatment. At a two-year follow-up, even though more patients had relapsed overall, the benefits of family therapy were still apparent (40% vs. 78% had relapsed: see Leff & Vaughn, 1985). Meta-analysis of several studies suggests that in the longer term family therapy reduces the risk of relapse by about 20% in comparison to standard care (i.e. medication only; see Pitschel-Walz et al., 2001). It is particularly effective for the amelioration of negative symptoms and the improvement of social functioning, and a further benefit is that patients who receive family therapy are more likely to take their medication as instructed (Pharoah et al., 2010). However, one big disadvantage of family therapy is that it (obviously) cannot be used on individuals who live alone, and this rules out about half of those patients with schizophrenia.

Social skills training

The many symptoms of schizophrenia mean that sufferers often have difficulty interacting with others. Even if the 'primary' symptoms can be treated with medication and CBT, many patients struggle to engage in normal social interaction once they have recovered from the acute psychotic episode. The aim of social skills training is to remedy this inability to interact with others and modify some of the socially awkward behaviour exhibited by patients with the disorder (e.g. talking too loudly, standing too close to others). Although research on this type of treatment is limited, it does seem to be a useful adjunct (add-on) to other types of treatment: it improves the social functioning of patients, even those with chronic schizophrenia (Bellack, 2004). A meta-analysis of the available evidence revealed medium-sized effects on functioning and independent living, psychosocial functioning and negative symptoms, but no reliable effects on positive and disorganised symptoms, or the risk of relapse (Kurtz & Mueser, 2008).

Cognitive remediation

We saw previously that schizophrenia is characterised by severe and wide-ranging cognitive deficits, and their severity is a good predictor of the long-term course of schizophrenia. The goal of cognitive remediation is to improve cognitive functions such as attention, memory and executive function in the hope that this 'brain training' will produce benefits that lead to knock-on improvements in the other symptoms of schizophrenia. Demily and Franck (2008) suggest that we should view cognitive remediation as a therapy that sits somewhere in between antipsychotic drugs (which target a brain dysfunction) and CBT (which targets specific symptoms). The idea is that a cognitive process such as attention cannot be reduced to the level of dopamine dysfunction, but if we can improve attention this might lead to benefits in specific symptoms such as auditory hallucinations and apathy.

So does it work? McGurk et al. (2007) conducted a meta-analysis of the available studies and found that cognitive remediation had reliable effects on cognitive functioning, and smaller (but statistically significant) effects on symptoms and social functioning, particularly if patients were receiving psychiatric rehabilitation at the same time as cognitive remediation. However a subsequent meta-analysis (Wykes et al., 2011), which included more studies, reported that any effects on symptoms were very small, and they tended to disappear at follow-up.

Which treatment is best?

The short answer is that each of these treatments has a role to play, and in an ideal world patients would be able to receive all of them. They should not have to choose one over the other. The more complicated answer is that these treatments work in different ways, for example by 'damping down' symptoms (antipsychotic medication), teaching patients skills to manage their symptoms (CBT), or improving their general social functioning (social skills training). Another way to look at it is that improvements in symptoms can ultimately be gained either by intervening at the cellular level (antipsychotics) – an intermediate level based on strengthening cognitive processes (cognitive remediation) – or by directly targeting the symptoms themselves (CBT). There is no reason why different psychosocial treatments cannot be combined, as Drury and colleagues (2000) did in their treatment combining elements of CBT, family education and an activity programme that included the teaching of 'life skills'. After receiving this therapy patients had fewer symptoms compared to a control group at a nine-month follow-up, although unfortunately these benefits had disappeared at a five-year follow-up.

Finally, studies of psychosocial treatments demonstrate that they produce meaningful improvements in the symptoms of schizophrenia in the short term, but these benefits tend to disappear in the longer term, after people stop receiving treatment. This is also the case for antipsychotic medication (which is why patients are constantly reminded to take their medication), but for some reason it is not widely appreciated for psychosocial interventions. If healthcare budgets allowed it, patients might show long-lasting improvements in symptoms of schizophrenia if they received psychosocial treatments over a long period of time, perhaps for years or even decades. A priority for future research is to investigate the effectiveness of very long-term psychosocial treatment, in addition to investigating new types of treatments that make use of the latest technology (see Box 4.6).

Box 4.6   Essential research

Transcranial magnetic stimulation (Aleman & Larøi, 2011)

Around 30% of patients who are treated with antipsychotics do not report any improvement in their auditory hallucinations, so alternative treatments are needed. With repetitive transcranial magnetic stimulation (rTMS), regions of the brain that are overactive during auditory hallucinations are targeted by repeatedly activating a magnetic field that is placed on the scalp, directly above the cortical region of interest (it doesn't hurt!). If the magnetic field pulses on and off fairly slowly, this has the effect of reducing brain activity in that part of the cortex. Several recent studies found that rTMS directed at speech production areas of the brain, such as the temperoparietal junction, led to reductions in the severity of auditory hallucinations. In some of these studies the improvements were maintained for follow-up periods of several months. For future research we need to know if any therapeutic gains are maintained in the longer term as well as which regions of the brain we should target, and we need to refine technical aspects of the procedure (e.g. the optimal frequency of stimulation). Most crucially, we need to understand how rTMS works in the longer term: does it 're-wire' the brain?

Section summary

Antipsychotic drugs give rise to symptom improvement in the majority of patients with schizophrenia, although they are certainly not a panacea! Psychological treatments such as CBT, cognitive remediation, social-skills training and family therapy all have a role to play, although the research on these is limited. Ideally, patients would receive a combination of different treatments that was tailored to their individual needs.

Essential questions

Some possible exam questions that stem from this chapter are:

- Is schizophrenia a disorder, or a cluster of unrelated symptoms?
- To what extent is schizophrenia a heritable biological disorder?
- What role do families play in the development of schizophrenia?
- To what extent is schizophrenia caused by adverse events during childhood?
- How well do cognitive models explain the symptoms of schizophrenia?
- What is the best way to treat schizophrenia?

Further reading

Kapur, S., Mizrahi, R., & Li, M. (2005). From dopamine to salience to psychosis – Linking biology, pharmacology and phenomenology of psychosis. *Schizophrenia Research*, 79(1): 59–68. (A very readable, critical and thought-provoking overview of biological accounts of schizophrenia.)

van Os, J., & Kapur, S. (2009). Schizophrenia. *The Lancet*, 374(9690): 635–645. (A broad summary that is aimed at clinicians so is mainly useful for understanding diagnosis and treatment.)

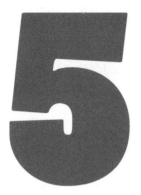 **MOOD DISORDERS**

General introduction

In this chapter we describe the diagnostic criteria for major depressive and bipolar disorders in *ICD*-10 and *DSM*-5, and we discuss some controversial changes to the diagnostic criteria that occurred between *DSM-IV* and *DSM*-5. We then also discuss the causes of these disorders, including heritable and environmental factors, and gene × environment interactions. The largest section of the chapter is devoted to the cognitive distortions that underlie mood disorders, their relationship to abnormalities of brain function, and a critical evaluation of cognitive theories which posit that negative thoughts and cognitive biases are the most important causes of mood disorders. Finally, in the last section we take a look at how mood disorders are treated, with a consideration of the psychological mechanisms of the action of 'talking therapies', and a critical look at the effectiveness and mechanism of the action of medications.

Assessment targets

At the end of the chapter, you should ask yourself the following questions:

- Can I explain how major depression and bipolar disorder are diagnosed?
- Do I understand the key psychological processes that characterise major depression and bipolar disorder?
- Are mood disorders heritable and can I explain their biological basis?
- Can I explain how distorted cognitive processes might play a role in the initial development of mood disorders, and in the maintenance of those disorders?
- Do I understand how mood disorders are treated, and can I relate those treatments back to theoretical models?

Section 1: What are depression and mania?

This section will look at how we diagnose the two major types of mood disorder. These are *depression*, which is known as 'recurrent depressive disorder' in *ICD*-10 and 'major depressive disorder' in *DSM*-5, and *manic depression*, the official name for which is 'bipolar disorder' (*DSM*-5) or 'bipolar affective disorder' (*ICD*-10). We will refer to them as major depression and bipolar disorder for the remainder of this chapter. The disorders are characterised by extreme mood states (deep sadness and manic over-excitability, respectively), and these extreme moods correspond to distinct patterns of behaviour and cognition. You can probably remember a time when you felt sadness, ruminated on bad things that had happened, and felt pessimistic about the future. You can probably also remember times when you felt full of energy, very confident, and optimistic about your future. These are normal human characteristics, but they are taken to the extreme in people who suffer from mood disorders.

The *ICD*-10 diagnostic criteria for recurrent depressive disorder are shown in Box 5.1. Bipolar disorder is diagnosed if a person has experienced at least one manic episode (Box 5.2) and at least one depressive episode (Box 5.1). The experience of living with a close family member who has bipolar disorder is depicted in Box 5.3.

Box 5.1   Essential diagnosis

For major depression

According to *ICD*-10 (World Health Organisation, 1992), Recurrent Depressive Disorder is characterised by recurrent *depressive episodes*, but there must be no history of manic episodes (see Box 5.2). Typical symptoms of depressive episodes, which should be present for at least two weeks to warrant diagnosis, are as follows:

- Depressed mood to a degree that is definitely abnormal for the individual, present for most of the day and almost every day, and largely uninfluenced by circumstances.
- Loss of interest or pleasure in activities that are normally enjoyable.
- Decreased energy or increased fatiguability.
- Loss of confidence and self-esteem.
- Unreasonable feelings of self-reproach or excessive and inappropriate guilt.
- Recurrent thoughts of death or suicide, or any suicidal behaviour.
- Diminished ability to think or concentrate.
- Change in psychomotor activity, with agitation or retardation.
- Sleep disturbance of any type.
- Change in appetite (decrease or increase) with corresponding weight change.

The *ICD* also distinguishes between mild, moderate and severe depressive episodes, depending on the number and severity of the above symptoms that are present during the episode.

The *DSM*-5 (American Psychiatric Association, 2013) applies a different label (Major Depressive Disorder) but the diagnostic criteria are similar to those described by *ICD*-10. As with other disorders, both *ICD*-10 and *DSM*-5 require the symptoms to be associated with clinically significant distress and/or impairment in social and occupational functioning.

Box 5.2   Essential diagnosis

ICD-10 diagnostic criteria for a manic episode (World Health Organisation, 1992)

ICD-10 distinguishes between three degrees of severity of manic episode, which are hypomania (least severe), mania without psychotic symptoms and mania with psychotic symptoms (most severe). The criteria for *mania without psychotic symptoms* are:

A. A mood which is predominantly elevated, expansive or irritable and definitively abnormal for the individual. The mood change must be prominent and sustained for at least a week.
B. At least three of the following must be present (four if the mood is merely irritable), leading to severe interference with personal functioning in daily living:

- Increased activity or physical restlessness.
- Increased talkativeness ('pressure of speech').
- Flight of ideas or the subjective experience of thoughts racing.
- Loss of normal social inhibitions resulting in behaviour which is inappropriate to the circumstances.
- Decreased need for sleep.
- Inflated self-esteem or grandiosity.
- Distractibility or constant changes in activities or plans.
- Behaviour which is foolhardy or reckless and whose risks the subject does not recognize e.g. spending sprees, foolish enterprises, reckless driving.
- Marked sexual energy or sexual indiscretions.

The *DSM*-5 criteria for a manic episode (American Psychiatric Association, 2013) are similar, and both *ICD*-10 and *DSM*-5 require symptoms to be present for at least one week and to be associated with social or occupational impairment in order to warrant diagnosis.

Both *ICD*-10 and *DSM*-5 recognise subcategories and specifiers of major depression and bipolar disorder. For example, one specifier of major depressive disorder in *DSM*-5 is 'with seasonal pattern', which is more commonly known as 'seasonal affective disorder' or the 'winter blues'. Subtypes of bipolar disorder distinguish the severity of manic episodes. For example, manic symptoms can be 'hypomanic' (less severe) or 'with psychotic symptoms' (more severe). In the latter case, inflated self-esteem and grandiose ideas develop into grandiose delusions, or irritability and suspiciousness can develop into paranoid delusions. At this point the distinction between a severe manic episode and other psychotic disorders such as schizophrenia (Chapter 4, see Box 4.3) becomes very blurred indeed!

The diagnostic criteria for major depressive disorder in the previous version of the *DSM* (*DSM-IV*) contained a 'bereavement exclusion' criterion, which meant that a person could not be diagnosed with major depression if they were recently bereaved (a similar exclusion criterion applies in *ICD*-10). However, this exclusion criterion was removed from *DSM*-5. This has divided opinion among the scientific community. On the one hand, it seems reasonable because although it is normal to feel depressed when suffering a bereavement, why shouldn't it be possible to develop major depression after such a traumatic life event? On the other hand, critics argue that this change to the criteria will lead to a massive over-diagnosis of major depression among people who are having a normal and predictable reaction to an unpleasant life event, but who are likely to recover by themselves in time (Wakefield & First, 2012). We saw in Chapter 1 that this general widening of diagnostic criteria is likely to result in much 'normal' human experience being sufficient to warrant a diagnosis of a psychological disorder, and this is one of the main criticisms of categorical approaches to psychological disorders in general, and *DSM*-5 in particular.

Box 5.3   Essential experience

Living with bipolar disorder (Eyers & Parker, 2008)

Depression has the Black Dog. In our home, bipolar has the Polar Bear. A code word created between my sister and me when she was first diagnosed as bipolar aptly describes the illness and our experience of living with this 'animal'.

Polar bears look cute and cuddly, and most of the time my sister is open, funny and playful. Polar bears enjoy company, and my sister has a wide circle of friends, enjoys sport, movies and going out. Polar bears are also versatile, living on land and in deep waters, and my sister is managing her illness extremely well, aged 21, having had the illness since she was 14, attending university and singing in a local church group.

However polar bears also have a predatory side, and this is when we see the illness emerge and my sister goes from gorgeous to grizzly.

The early warning signs for us are over-reaction, over-emotion and extreme irritability. My sister is aggressive with my parents and myself and favours her friends over us. This is brought about by a lack of sleep and racing thoughts. The racing thoughts are ones of anxiety and worries such as being late, organising her room, meeting people, failing in her studies – all mixed up in her mind. As a result she stays up late and cannot relax.

My sister's illness is quite brittle. Within a couple of days she is in a full bipolar episode, and a few days after the inevitable hospital admission she is back home and in recovery. She has experienced far more manic episodes than depressive episodes. Seeing other friends with depression the manic episode is actually easier to handle, believe it or not. Although it requires a higher level of prowess and fitness (like when her thoughts become too overwhelming and she decides to leave home regardless of the time of night, with the result that my family and I have had some stealthy midnight strides across the local shire where we live!), the mania is highly transparent. Depression is hidden and darker: we can't tell what she is thinking or feeling, and it is far harder to help and takes far longer to resolve.

As the episode progresses we also see a change in clothing: haphazard dressing where she tries to wear everything that she likes … all at once, regardless of the weather and venue, like a haute couture model! The final indicator for my family and me is the episode's 'theme tune'. My sister listens to her iPod constantly throughout her illness, and chooses one song that she will play repeatedly: J-Lo, Eminem, Dido, have made up our 'bipolar soundtrack' over the years.

Prevalence, course, comorbidity and the financial burden of mood disorders

The lifetime prevalence of major depression has been estimated at between 7% and 17%, although there is much debate about the true figure which could be even higher (Richards, 2011). The incidence of major depression is about twice as common in women as it is in men. The lifetime prevalence of bipolar disorder is much lower, at approximately 1% (Merikangas & Pato, 2009), and the prevalence of the most severe subtype of bipolar disorder is equal in men and women. However, female bipolar sufferers may have more depressive episodes than males.

Symptoms of both major depression and bipolar disorder first appear in late adolescence and early adulthood (Merikangas & Pato, 2009; Richards, 2011). Depressive episodes last for around six months on average, and most people will make a full recovery after experiencing a depressive episode. Unfortunately, and in common with the chronic nature of other psychological disorders, the majority of people will have at least one additional major depressive or manic episode at some point after recovering from the first one, although they could be symptom-free for many years before experiencing a recurrence of symptoms (Richards, 2011).

Both major depression and bipolar disorder are often comorbid with anxiety disorders and substance use disorders. For example, 70% of people with a diagnosis of bipolar disorder also have panic disorder, and 50% will also have social anxiety disorder (see Chapter 8) (Merikangas & Pato, 2009). With regard to substance use disorder, chronic substance use lowers brain 'reward thresholds', and this leads to a syndrome that looks very similar to major depression (see Chapter 9).

The disabling effects of chronic mood disorders cannot be overstated: the global burden of disability attributable to major depression is second only to that which can be attributed to heart disease (Murray & Lopez, 1996). The economic burden of major depression (attributed to healthcare costs, work absenteeism and reduced productivity) was estimated at 118 billion euros in 2004 (Richards, 2011).

Section summary

We have seen that both *ICD*-10 and *DSM*-5 recognise two broad types of mood disorders, characterised by extreme sad mood (major depression), or alternations between extremely sad and manic states (bipolar disorder). Bipolar disorder is relatively rare and in its extreme form it can be difficult to distinguish this from other psychotic disorders such as schizophrenia. On the other hand, major depression has been called 'the common cold of psychiatry' because it is one of the psychological disorders that psychologists will see most often.

Section 2: How do mood disorders develop?

Do mood disorders run in families?

Both major depression and bipolar disorder run in families, although the heritability of bipolar disorder (estimated at around 70%) is much greater than that for major depression (about 30% to 40%). This issue is complicated because there is shared heritability for the two disorders. This means that a child born to a parent with bipolar disorder is at increased risk of developing both major depression and bipolar disorder, and the same is true for a child who has one or more parents with major depression (Lau & Eley, 2010; Merikangas & Pato, 2009).

Specific genetic variants associated with bipolar disorder have not yet been identified (Merikangas & Pato, 2009). However, polymorphisms (variations) in genes that are involved in serotonin function have been linked to the heritable risk for major depression. For example, genes that code for serotonin transporters seem to differ in people with major depression and unaffected controls, and these genetic variants are associated with personality traits such as neuroticism that are in turn related to major depression (Lau & Eley, 2010). Unfortunately, as with much of the research on psychiatric genetics, many findings in this area cannot be replicated across different studies. Even when we consider the findings that do seem to be reliable, closer examination of individual studies reveals that there is little consistency between different studies (Lau & Eley, 2010; see Box 5.4). Other researchers have identified a relationship between major depression and genes associated with Brain Derived Neurotrophic Factor

(BDNF), which is involved in the regeneration of neurons that are damaged during exposure to stressors (Lau & Eley, 2010). There is undoubtedly a heritable risk for both major depression and bipolar disorder, but our search for the specific gene variants that are involved seems unlikely to succeed until we have a better understanding of how genetic polymorphisms are related to the structure and function of the brain.

Environmental influences

It is easy to think of life events that can cause us to feel sad (e.g. the break-up of a relationship) or ecstatically happy (e.g. passing your exams). However, one-off life events such as these are probably insufficient causes for the development of major depression or bipolar disorder by themselves, because the majority of people will return to 'normal' in time. The risk of developing major depression is increased if people experience a series of negative life events in quick succession (e.g. losing their job, then getting divorced, then being diagnosed with cancer), probably because it is difficult to cope when faced with multiple stressors at the same time (Bender & Alloy, 2011). Similarly, chronic stress associated with poverty, unemployment and low social

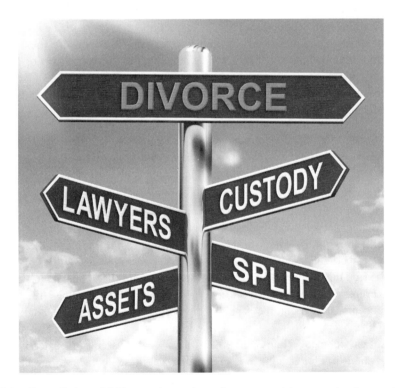

Figure 5.1 One-off stressful life events, such as divorce, can trigger major depressive episodes but they are unlikely to lead to major depressive disorder unless experienced as part of a sequence of negative life events

status is associated with increased risk for major depression, and this has also been attributed to psychological coping resources being overwhelmed (see Bender & Alloy, 2011).

Another explanation for why multiple stressful events can lead to chronic major depression or bipolar disorder is the kindling hypothesis, proposed by Post (1992). 'Kindling' is a biological term, which refers to a progressive decline in the strength of the electrical current that is needed to trigger a seizure in mice. At first a high voltage would be needed to cause a seizure, but a second seizure could be triggered by a slightly lower voltage than that needed to cause the first one. The threshold continues to drop until eventually the animal can experience seizures in the absence of any electrical stimulation at all.

The basic idea of the kindling hypothesis of mood disorders is that a major life stressor is needed to trigger the initial depressive or manic episode. However, once the person has recovered from this episode, their threshold for experiencing a subsequent episode is lowered. This kindling process continues until at some point a very minor stressor (e.g. having a minor argument) is sufficient to cause a major depressive or manic episode. After that episodes might occur spontaneously without any environmental trigger at all. Although this idea was originally inspired by a biological process (kindling), we should note that cognitive theories can also account for kindling effects in terms of a progressive strengthening of depressogenic cognitions over time (see Section 3).

In support of the model, there is a declining relationship between life stress and major depressive episodes over time: the first episode is almost always linked to a major stressor, but recurrences can occur independent of life stress (Monroe & Harkness, 2005). However, the model has been less well-supported when applied to bipolar disorder, because there are many inconsistent findings in the literature (Bender & Alloy, 2011).

Gene–environment interactions

In Chapter 1 (Box 1.9) we introduced the many ways in which genes and environment can interact (commonly termed 'G×E' interactions). As reviewed by Lau and Eley (2010) there are many examples of G×E interactions in relation to mood disorders. For example, individuals with a heritable risk for mood disorders are more likely to report symptoms of depression, but only after a stressful life event. In the absence of a stressful life event, there is no relationship between heritable risk for depression and experiencing the symptoms of depression. Attempts to extend this work by identifying the specific genes that moderate the influence of stressful life events on depression have so far yielded inconclusive findings (see Box 5.4). It has also been demonstrated that the gene and environment cannot be disentangled as easily as we would like, because people at increased heritable risk for depression also tend to have more stressful environments (Lau & Eley, 2010), as we discussed in Chapter 1. The study of G×E interactions is a burgeoning area of research, but these interactions are likely to take many forms. In the future major advances are likely to come from the study of epigenetics (how gene expression is influenced by environmental factors; see Chapter 1) and attempts to identify the depressed endophenotype, that is, the characteristics of people who are at increased familial risk for mood disorder, but have not yet developed a disorder.

Box 5.4   Essential research

When an apparently reliable finding isn't so reliable after all

A landmark study by Caspi et al. (2003) has pride of place in many psychology textbooks, because it demonstrates a very clear GxE interaction that seems to play a major causal role in depression. The authors studied a genetic polymorphism of a serotonin transporter gene, and explored how individuals who differed on this genetic polymorphism reacted to stressful life events. They reported that the number of stressful life events that people experienced was directly related to the number of depressive symptoms that they reported (and the severity of those symptoms), but this was only seen amongst people who possessed a certain polymorphism of this serotonin transporter gene. People who had a different genetic polymorphism seemed to be 'immune' to depression, in other words no matter what life threw at them, they just didn't get depressed.

In the years that followed, other reports were published which seemed to directly replicate these findings. Had we found the gene which determined who would be vulnerable (or resilient) to depression? Unfortunately not. When Munafò and colleagues (2009) conducted a meta-analysis of all of the studies that had investigated this issue, they found no reliable evidence for the GxE interaction reported by Caspi et al. (2003). To make matters worse, some of the studies that claimed to directly replicate the findings from the original study had actually shown a completely different pattern of results, but they had interpreted those results incorrectly. This example illustrates the dangers of over-interpreting results from a single study, and the problems that arise when we are too quick to interpret an apparent replication of a novel finding. Perhaps most crucially, it demonstrates the power of meta-analysis to provide the bigger picture on a given topic (see Chapter 1).

Section summary

We have seen that both major depression and bipolar disorder are influenced by stressful life events and that both have a heritable basis, although the heritable basis of bipolar disorder is likely to be more substantial than that for major depression. The roles of nature and nurture are less important than the interaction between the two, and we are beginning to recognise how gene × environment interactions have the potential to explain why people develop mood disorders.

Section 3: Biological and psychological mechanisms in mood disorders

Neurotransmitters

According to the monoamine hypothesis (for an historical overview, see Heninger et al., 1996) depression is caused by reduced levels of serotonin, noradrenalin and dopamine (the monoamines) in the limbic system. Several pieces of evidence support the theory. First, the most commonly prescribed antidepressants are selective serotonin reuptake inhibitors (SSRIs) and noradrenalin reuptake inhibitors (NRIs). These drugs work by increasing activity in serotonin and noradrenalin systems, respectively, and both are effective at alleviating the symptoms of major depression (see Section 4). Neuroimaging and post-mortem studies of depressed patients' brains show that they have fewer serotonin receptors, and their receptors tend to be less sensitive compared to healthy controls (Drevets et al., 2008). Second, other studies have investigated the effects of depleting tryptophan, a biological precursor of serotonin. If we give an amino acid drink that depletes levels of tryptophan (and therefore levels of serotonin in the brain) to formerly depressed patients who have recovered, this can trigger a recurrence of their depressive symptoms (Drevets et al., 2008). Finally, the recreational drug ecstasy increases monoamine activity, and when people take it they report strong feelings of euphoria. On the basis of all of these observations, it can be argued that reduced levels of these neurotransmitters play a causal role in major depression, and that increased levels might cause mania.

However, some evidence is not consistent with a simplistic monoamine hypothesis. First, the SSRIs alter serotonin function immediately, but people need to take them for several weeks before they see an improvement in symptoms. Second, the observed deficits in serotonin function might reflect changes in the brain that occur as a consequence of chronic depression, rather than being a cause of it. Finally, and more fundamentally, we know that neurotransmitters do not function in isolation, and we have to consider the interactions between different neurotransmitters (including glutamate, GABA and acetylcholine) in order to understand mood disorders properly (Drevets et al., 2008). This is why current biological theories of mood disorders focus on abnormal function in different regions of the brain, rather than the activity levels of different neurotransmitters.

Abnormal brain function in depression

Drevets et al. (2008) proposed that a network of brain structures was implicated in major depression and bipolar disorder. These are regions included within the medial prefrontal cortex (MPFC), the limbic system, and the connections between the two. In mood disordered patients we can see reduced grey matter volume (a structural deficit) and glucose metabolism (a marker of brain activity, i.e. a functional deficit) in specific regions of the MPFC, particularly the left anterior cingulate cortex (ACC). This is important because the MPFC normally inhibits activity in the limbic system, so one indirect consequence of reduced activity in the MPFC would be increased activity in the limbic system. This is exactly what we see in mood disorders: activity in the limbic system (particularly the amygdala) is increased in major depression and bipolar disorder patients when they are in the middle of a major depressive episode, and the level of increased activity in these regions is associated with the magnitude of emotional processing biases in depressed patients (Drevets et al., 2008; emotional processing biases are discussed later in this chapter). Furthermore, antidepressants normalise activity in these regions (Goldapple et al., 2004). Cognitive behaviour therapy (CBT) may work in a different way, by increasing activity in the MPFC and therefore indirectly increasing inhibition of the limbic system. In essence, both antidepressants and CBT can normalise an overactive limbic system, but their mechanism of action is very different: a 'top-down' action for CBT (the MPFC changes first, and then influences activity in the limbic system) versus a 'bottom-up' action for antidepressants (the limbic system changes first, and then activity in the MPFC changes afterwards) (Goldapple et al., 2004).

Drevets et al.'s (2008) model represents a notable advance on simplistic monoaminergic theories of mood disorders: it acknowledges that serotonin plays a key role, but it also shows how it is important to investigate the function of different networks in the brain, and the interplay between many different neurotransmitter systems within these networks.

Cognitive factors: Learned helplessness

Martin Seligman and colleagues undertook several experiments in the 1960s to demonstrate how the lack of control of aversive outcomes was linked to helplessness in dogs. An overview of these experiments is shown in Box 5.5.

Box 5.5   Essential research

Classic studies of 'learned helplessness' (e.g. Seligman et al., 1968)

Seligman's basic paradigm used chambers that had two compartments separated by a barrier. Both sides of the chamber had a metal floor through which a strong electrical current could be passed – thus shocking anything that happened to be in that compartment. They studied two groups of dogs. The first group could escape the electric shocks by jumping across the barrier to the opposite compartment, in which the shock was not activated. This group could escape the shocks by jumping, so they had some control over what happened to them. For the second group, however, both compartments were electrified, so this group of dogs received a shock no matter what they did – they had no control over negative events.

In the second stage of the experiment, both groups of dogs could escape the shock by jumping the barrier and entering the opposite compartment. However, the dogs that had no control in the first part of the experiment didn't do this; instead they cowered passively in a corner and whimpered. Even when the experimenters dragged them across the barrier into the safe chamber, they did not learn that they could escape the shock. These dogs had learned to be helpless.

Subsequent studies replicated the basic learned helplessness effect in animals and demonstrated that this also occurs in humans (for a review and some discussion, see Forgeard et al., 2011). For example, Hiroto and Seligman (1975) demonstrated that if participants were exposed to an aversive noise that they could not turn off, they were slow to learn to press a button in order to terminate the noise in a second phase of the experiment. The learned helplessness theory of depression (Seligman, 1975) evolved from these experiments: it suggests that depression arises from a perception that environmental events cannot be controlled. For example, loss of a loved one or repeated abuse may lead to passivity and a belief that the person is unable to prevent negative things that might happen to them in the future.

When people learn to be helpless, this can be seen in cognitive changes (they believe that whatever they do, bad things will happen), motivational deficits (they have no motivation to try to change things) and emotional changes (depressed mood). Seligman's subsequent studies with dogs showed that helpless animals showed other biological changes that were associated with depression: reduced aggression, a loss of appetite and reduced serotonin function (Maier & Seligman, 1976). Therefore, learned helplessness was a plausible explanation for why uncontrollable negative life events could lead to the development of major depression.

Unfortunately, the original formulation of learned helplessness theory struggles to explain the importance of 'dependent' versus 'independent' life events on the development of major depression. Think of someone who loses their job. This might happen because their employer went bankrupt, in which case this would be 'independent' of how the person behaved. Alternatively, the person might have been a bully and they were sacked when their employer had finally had enough of them. This would be a 'dependent' life event, because the person's behaviour was directly responsible for the outcome (i.e. losing their job). Based on learned helplessness theory, we would expect people to be more likely to become depressed after experiencing independent rather than dependent negative life events. But this is not generally the case: people are more likely to become depressed if they experience a negative life event that they had some influence on (a dependent event) rather than if they experienced an independent negative life event (Hammen, 2005).

Learned helplessness theory had a cognitive makeover when it was revised by Abramson, Seligman, and Teasdale in 1978. According to reformulated helplessness theory, the experience of helplessness is not enough to cause depression. Instead, 'when a person finds that he is helpless, he asks *why* he is helpless. The causal attribution he makes then determines the generality and chronicity of his helplessness deficits as well as his later self-esteem' (Abramson et al., 1978: 50).

Reformulated helplessness theory posits that people with major depression make causal attributions about negative life events that have the following characteristics:

- Events are attributed to *internal* (rather than external) factors, for example: 'It's my fault that I fell out with my friend, because I behaved badly.'
- Events are attributed to things that are *stable over time* (rather than something that was specific to that particular time), for example: 'I fell out with my friend because I am a bad person, and I will always be a bad person.'

- Attributions are *global* (rather than something that was specific to that occurrence), for example: 'I am a bad person and not only does this make my friends dislike me, it also makes me perform badly at work.'

Abramson et al. (1978) suggested that people who make these types of causal attributions are more likely to blame themselves for negative events and to expect to experience negative events in the future. The resulting expectations lead to increased helplessness, a loss of self-esteem and feelings of hopelessness. There is good evidence that depressed people think in this way, which has been called a 'depressogenic' attributional style. For example, Quiggle et al. (1992) reported that depressed children were more likely than nondepressed controls to attribute negative life events to internal, stable and global causes. Furthermore, prospective studies show that a depressogenic attributional style predicts the onset of depressive symptoms in response to a negative life event (Metalsky et al., 1993). A large longitudinal study from Alloy et al. (2006) found that a depressogenic attributional style predicted depressed mood at later time points, and similar findings have been reported in children (Abela, 2001) and adolescents (Auerbach et al., 2014)

Reformulated helplessness theory may describe the way that depressed patients think, but it doesn't explain why they think in this way (and non-depressed patients do not). What we need to know is why some people acquire this depressogenic cognitive style in the first place. Alloy et al. (1999) extended the theory by proposing that attributions have a developmental origin. Given that depression tends to run in families, they proposed that depressed parents have a depressogenic cognitive style and their own children acquire this attributional style as they are growing up, which ultimately causes them to develop depression themselves. After reviewing the evidence, Alloy et al. identified four pathways by which children could acquire attributional styles from their parents:

- *Modelling*: children might learn to explain environmental events simply by copying their parents' attributions. The evidence for this was mixed, with some studies finding an effect and others failing to do so.
- *Parental feedback*: depressed parents provide depressogenic feedback to their children about the causes of negative life events ('You fell off your bike because bad things always happen to our family'). There was some evidence for this happening in interactions between depressed parents and their children.
- *Parenting style*: parents who suffer from depression are likely to adopt a critical, commanding and threatening style of parenting, and this can lead their children to develop depressogenic cognitions.
- *Childhood maltreatment*: neglect and emotional, physical and sexual abuse during childhood are associated with a depressogenic cognitive style during adulthood. This relationship may be particularly strong for emotional abuse, for example being told 'Of course you didn't get invited to the prom. You're ugly'. Alloy et al. (1999) speculate that comments such as this could be internalised, leading to the formation of depressogenic cognitions.

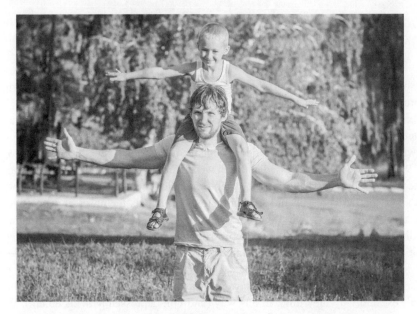

Figure 5.2   Children may learn to explain life events by copying their parents' attributions for them

Beck's cognitive model of depression

Beck's (1967) theoretical model of depression and his formulation of cognitive therapy (Beck, 1976) are based on the idea that during childhood we acquire a set of schemata, a 'world view', based on our early experiences and/or by modelling the world view held by our parents (as discussed in the previous section). If children have negative experiences such as major trauma (e.g. the death of a parent, parental divorce), rejection or criticism from friends, parents or teachers, or if their parents have a negative view of the world, then they are likely to acquire dysfunctional beliefs about the world. These negative schemata will usually lie dormant but can be 'reactivated' by negative life events in the future. So, for example, failing your psychology exam might trigger a set of beliefs that were formed during childhood, such as 'I am stupid' and 'I always disappoint the people who love me'. Once these negative schemata are (re)activated, this leads to a stream of what Beck called negative automatic thoughts (NATs), which are negatively valenced intrusive thoughts that the person cannot control. Other symptoms of depression such as negative mood and reduced motivation, together with automatic cognitive biases for negative information (see below), follow on from this barrage of negative thoughts. This depressogenic cognitive style is then maintained by a number of cognitive distortions or logical errors that influence how the person will interpret life events (see Box 5.6).

Box 5.6 Essential experience

Examples of cognitive distortions ('logical errors')
proposed by Beck (from Field, 2003)

- *Arbitrary inference*: if you visit your friend but they do not answer the door, you assume that they are ignoring you.
- *Selective abstraction*: in the early days of a new romantic relationship, the person tells you they would really like to see you again and that they really like you but that they're busy for a few days. You interpret their unavailability as a signal of their 'true' feelings, that is, that they don't really like you.
- *Overgeneralisation*: you have an argument with an acquaintance and this causes you to think that all of your friends dislike you.
- *Magnification and minimisation*: magnification would be taking a relatively minor incident and blowing it out of proportion; for example, if you are late to meet someone this makes you think 'All of my friends will think I'm always late'. Minimisation would be playing down positive feedback; for example, if someone tells you that 'You look good', you take it to mean 'They are telling me that I look slightly less disgusting than normal'.
- *Personalisation*: this is the 'world revolving around me' syndrome. For example, if nobody seems to be having fun at a party you assume that it must be your fault.
- *Absolutistic dichotomous thinking*: for example, 'If I fail my exams, my life is ruined', or 'Without my girlfriend, I am nothing'.
- *'Should' and 'must' statements*: for example, 'I must be best at everything' and 'I must be liked by everyone'. Even for the most high achieving and popular person, these statements are unlikely to be true *all* of the time.

There is a great deal of overlap between Beck's model and reformulated helplessness theory (Abramson et al., 1978; remember that Beck's theory was published first!). Beck's theory can incorporate Abramson et al.'s ideas about attributional style, but arguably the additional cognitive distortions specified by Beck (e.g. those in Box 5.6) make it a more complete cognitive theory of depression. Many clinical reports suggest that depressed patients do think in the way described by Beck (Haaga et al., 1991). There is also good evidence that depressed patients have automatic cognitive biases for negative information, as predicted by the theory. For example, people with major depression have a memory bias: they preferentially remember negative information. They also have an interpretive bias: they are more likely to infer negative information from ambiguous scenarios. Finally, they have an attentional bias for negative information, in the sense that they struggle to disengage their attention from such information once they have focused on it (Gotlib & Joormann, 2010). However, while this evidence suggests that Beck's model is a useful way of *describing* the depressive thinking style, it doesn't tell us whether depressogenic cognitions are the *cause* of depressive episodes.

If depressogenic cognitions have a causal influence on depression rather than being an irrelevant by-product of negative mood, then the onset of depressive episodes should be explained by an interaction between depressogenic cognitions and the occurrence of stressful life events. Results from several longitudinal studies support this prediction, and many of these were discussed in the previous section as support for the reformulated helplessness model. For example, Brown et al. (1995) looked at depressive symptoms in students who didn't do as well as they expected to in their exams. As they predicted, they found that depressogenic cognitions (which were measured before the students got their results) interacted with the extent to which the students underperformed in their exams to predict the severity of depressive symptoms shortly after the students got their results. In another study, Kwon and Oei (1992) found that the interaction between depressogenic cognitions and negative life events predicted symptoms of depression three months later. Alloy et al.'s (2006) cognitive vulnerability to depression (CVD) project studied a large sample of undergraduates over a five-year period. They found that people with high levels of depressogenic cognitions at the start of the study were much more likely to be diagnosed with major depression at the end of the study than participants with low levels of depressogenic symptoms. Furthermore, any participants who were cognitive 'high risk' and had a history of major depressive episodes in the past were much more likely to experience a recurrence of depressive symptoms (i.e. another major depressive episode) than participants who also had a history of major depressive episodes but were cognitive 'low risk'. However, one review of the evidence concluded that the effects from these longitudinal studies were small and many of the methods used were inadequate (Lakdawalla et al., 2007).

Mood priming experiments are another way to test Beck's theory. In these experiments, researchers compare the effects of a laboratory mood induction (e.g. listening to sad music or watching a sad film) on depressogenic cognitions in remitted-depressed and control participants. According to Beck's theory, all participants should report depressed mood after negative mood induction, but only people who have a cognitive vulnerability to depression should show an increase in depressogenic cognitions. Several studies have demonstrated such findings, and therefore this is strong support for Beck's theory (reviewed by Scher et al., 2005). For example, Miranda and colleagues (1998) reported a study in which healthy controls and remitted depressed patients initially completed the Dysfunctional Attitudes Scale (DAS), a questionnaire that measures many of the negative thinking styles that are central to Beck's theory. Participants then watched either a depressing or a neutral film before completing the DAS again. DAS scores increased in the remitted depressed patients who had seen the depressing film (but not those who had seen the neutral film), while DAS scores did not change in the group of healthy controls regardless of which film they had watched. Therefore, depressogenic cognitions can be 'reactivated' by a depressing life event in patients who have experienced major depressive episodes in the past. Importantly, other studies have shown that the extent to which depressogenic cognitions reappear after negative mood induction in remitted depressed patients predicts the recurrence of major depressive episodes in the future (Segal et al., 1999). These studies support Beck's theory because they show that depressogenic cognitions are 'latent' in patients with a history of major depression, just waiting to be activated by a negative life event.

More recently, Beck (2008) showed how his model could be integrated with genetic influences on depression (see Section 2) and abnormalities of brain function (earlier in this section). For example, variations in serotonin transporter genes have been linked to hyperactivity of the amygdala, which in turn is related to negative cognitive biases. Finally, the clear evidence that CBT is an effective treatment for major depression strongly suggests that depressogenic cognitions play a role in maintaining depression, because changes in these depressogenic cognitions that occur during a course of CBT are what cause a patient's mood to improve during treatment (see Section 4).

Cognitive processes in mania and bipolar disorder

While the cognitive processes involved in major depressive disorder have been well researched and are fairly well understood, we cannot say the same for manic episodes and bipolar disorder. During depressive episodes, patients with bipolar disorder display the same types of depressogenic cognitions as those with major depression (Scott et al., 2000), and much of the evidence discussed above applies here. One influential theoretical model of cognitions in bipolar disorder (Winters & Neale, 1985) proposes that when patients experience a negative event this would normally trigger a major depressive episode. Alternatively, in some (not clearly specified) circumstances, bipolar disorder patients may have a defensive reaction to these negative cognitions that takes the form of a manic episode. Evidence in support of this theory comes from a study (Lyon et al., 1999) which showed that bipolar disorder patients had implicit negative beliefs about themselves regardless of whether they were experiencing a depressive or manic episode at the time. However, patients who were in the middle of a manic episode reported positive beliefs about themselves, whereas patients who were in the middle of a depressive episode reported negative beliefs about themselves. Therefore, both manic and depressive episodes are associated with negative automatic thoughts, but bipolar disorder patients during manic episodes may try to compensate for this by reporting that they feel positively about themselves ('manic defence'). Other theories have focused on the behavioural approach system (BAS), which is implicated in motivational responses to rewarding stimuli. BAS activity is elevated during manic episodes, and therefore it may be useful to consider this individual difference in order to understand the root causes of manic episodes. However, while the model can explain mania, it cannot account for the cycling between manic and depressive episodes that is seen in bipolar disorder (Johnson et al., 2012).

Section summary

In this section we have shown that we can investigate brain dysfunction in mood disorders at two different levels: individual neurotransmitters, and different regions of the brain. Whilst serotonin and noradrenalin function seem to be disrupted in major depression and bipolar disorder, this does not provide a complete picture. It is more useful to think about different regions of the brain, and interconnections between different brain networks, in order to understand what goes wrong in the brain in mood disorders. This doesn't mean that we can ignore neurotransmitters – this is how different brain regions communicate with each other, after all – but it does mean that neurotransmitters are only one part of the overall picture.

Cognitive theories of major depression are able to explain the core symptoms of the disorder, and they provide a convincing explanation of how the disorder develops and how the symptoms are maintained. There is overwhelming evidence that depressogenic cognitions can be triggered by negative life events, and that once activated they play a causal role in vulnerability to depression. These theories are beginning to be integrated with biological models of mood disorders. Cognitive distortions can also explain why bipolar disorder patients experience major depressive episodes, although our understanding of why bipolar disorder patients cycle between manic and depressive episodes is limited.

Section 4: How are mood disorders treated?

Pharmacotherapy (drug treatments)

Antidepressant medications for major depression increase the activity of the monoamines, particularly serotonin and noradrenalin. The various types are monoamine oxidase inhibitors (MAOIs, e.g. phenelzine), tricyclics (e.g. amitryptiline) and selective serotonin reuptake inhibitors (SSRIs, e.g. fluoxetine; the best known brand of this is Prozac) and noradrenalin reuptake inhibitors (NRIs, e.g. venlafaxine). Although different types of drugs have different mechanisms of action (and MAOIs are now rarely used because of their side effects), they all ultimately work because they prevent the reuptake or breakdown of serotonin or noradrenalin from the synapse. This means that these drugs increase the amount of serotonin or noradrenalin activity in the brain. When taken for long periods of time, they enhance transmission within these neurotransmitter systems.

There is little doubt that antidepressants are effective in the sense that people who take them are more likely to get better: around 50% of those who take them report significant improvements in mood (Anderson et al., 2008). Furthermore, antidepressants reduce the risk that patients will experience a recurrence of symptoms (i.e. another major depressive episode) by about 70%, compared to receiving no treatment at all (Anderson et al., 2008). There is also an emerging body of evidence showing that patients treated with antidepressants show improvements in cognitive biases, for example improvements in memory biases such that tendencies to recall more negative rather than positive material are reduced in people who have received antidepressants (Harmer et al., 2004). Harmer and Cowen (2013) showed that antidepressant-induced improvements in cognitive biases were seen slightly before the drugs led to an improvement in depressed mood. They suggested that improvements in cognitive biases might ultimately explain why antidepressants work: the drugs alleviate automatic cognitive biases, and this takes a while to filter through and influence subjective mood.

However, all types of antidepressants have side effects, although these are less severe with the SSRIs. In Box 5.7 we discuss the controversial topic of the role of the placebo effect in the response to antidepressant drugs. Another important point to note about antidepressants is that people are very likely to relapse (i.e. experience another major depressive episode) when they stop taking them, whereas patients who receive CBT seem to be more resilient to depression after they have finished the treatment (see Box 5.8 later).

Box 5.7   Essential debate

The drugs don't work … or do they?

A meta-analysis of clinical trials of antidepressants hit the headlines in 2008 (Kirsch et al., 2008). Unlike previous meta-analyses, this one was based not just on published trials but also on unpublished trials from pharmaceutical companies. Their results were startling: compared to a placebo, antidepressants were only minimally effective at alleviating the symptoms of depression, and the effects were moderated by the severity of depression. In severely depressed patients, antidepressant drugs had a modest effect on symptoms. But in mildly and moderately depressed patients, the drugs were not effective at all! This isn't to say that patients who receive an antidepressant in the real world will not get better (many of them will). Instead most people will improve if they receive a placebo, and only a minority will show an additional improvement if they receive an antidepressant drug.

The implications were clear. To begin with, the majority of depressed patients (who are not classed as 'severely' depressed) may as well take a sugar pill, and added to this, the apparent effectiveness of antidepressants could be explained by pharmaceutical companies hiding the results from trials that did not show a benefit for their drugs over a placebo.

However, other researchers – most of them not connected to the pharmaceutical industry – have been very critical of this study. A subsequent meta-analysis from Horder and colleagues (2011) argued that Kirsch et al. (2008) had used inappropriate data analyses, and when more appropriate analyses were used (on the same data) the benefits of antidepressants over a placebo were much larger. Horder et al. (2011) were also very critical of many of the assumptions made by Kirsch et al. (2008), and the way in which they interpreted their results. Both papers are an entertaining read (and not too technical) and come highly recommended.

One thing that researchers can agree on is that there is a big placebo response to antidepressants, in other words many depressed patients who take part in drug trials will get better even if they receive a placebo. It is also clear that patients who receive an antidepressant drug will show a bigger improvement than patients who receive a placebo. The ongoing debate is how large, and how clinically significant, that difference between antidepressants and a placebo actually is.

Lithium and other medications for bipolar disorder

As with many psychiatric medications, the psychological effects of Lithium (a common salt which used to be an ingredient in 7-Up!) were discovered by accident. The drug is effective at stabilising mood in about 60% of patients, and it prevents bipolar disorder patients from oscillating between depressive and manic episodes (Geddes et al., 2004). Its mechanism of action is unclear, but it may ultimately work because of a general effect on neurotransmission throughout the brain. Given its effectiveness, it is currently recommended as a first-line treatment for bipolar disorder. However, it is more effective at blunting manic episodes than alleviating depressive episodes, and for this reason many bipolar disorder patients may be prescribed other medications at the same time. Importantly, the side effects of lithium (which can be toxic) mean that patients require careful monitoring when they are maintained on the drug, and many patients stop taking the drug because of the side effects. Other medications, such as Valproate (an anti-seizure medication originally developed for the treatment of epilepsy) and some antipsychotic drugs, are also effective for the treatment of manic episodes (Goodwin, 2009).

Cognitive behaviour therapy (CBT) for major depression

The primary aims of CBT are to educate clients about the role of negative cognitions in mood disorders, and to teach strategies that will help them to think in a more positive (or optimistic) way (Beck, 1976). There is also a behavioural element to this: given that depression is associated with anhedonia and a reluctance to engage in activities that might otherwise be viewed as pleasurable, behavioural activation and event scheduling are used to increase activity and engagement in activities, such as going to the shops or socialising (Kanter et al., 2010). Clients usually receive between 6 and 20 one-to-one sessions with a qualified CBT therapist, although the homework that clients do between sessions and afterwards is recognised as a vital component of therapy.

In order to challenge depressogenic cognitions, a client is taught exercises that can help them evaluate their pessimistic attributions for negative life events rather than accepting them uncritically. Some of the techniques that a therapist might use are as follows:

- *Thought catching*: the client recalls a recent incident that led to depression and then lists their thoughts and feelings at the time. The therapist and client then determine which thoughts were reasonable reflections of reality, and which were negative automatic thoughts (NATs) brought on by the incident.
- *Task assignment*: the client thinks of activities that they are avoiding (e.g. they don't go to social events) and then makes predictions about the bad things that would happen if they were to engage in these (e.g. being ignored by others). After the therapy session, the client completes the activity, and at the next session the client and therapist discuss the extent to which the client's predictions were accurate. The client will usually have overestimated the negative consequences of engaging in the activity.

- *Reality testing*: this is similar to the above but is focused on disproving specific beliefs. The client generates tasks to test the reality of a given belief (e.g. phoning a friend to disprove the belief that the friend does not want to speak to them). The client completes the activity and at the next session the client and therapist discuss the outcome; again, the idea is that the client will realise that their expectations were unrealistically negative.
- *Cognitive rehearsal*: once the client has performed some of these tasks, they move on to using cognitive rehearsal. For this they think of potentially negative situations that are likely to arise in the future, and plan for how they will apply task assignment and reality testing to a situation. The general idea is that the client starts to use these cognitive techniques in their everyday life, in a range of situations. Eventually, they will get better at identifying and challenging their negative automatic thoughts, and thinking in a more positive and optimistic way during challenging situations.

CBT for depression is undoubtedly effective. In a meta-analysis of previous meta-analyses (serious amounts of data!) Butler et al. (2006) reported overall large effect sizes for CBT in comparison to other treatments, including other psychological therapies (also see Tolin, 2010). There is some evidence that CBT may be more effective for patients with less severe depression, that patients with severe depression may respond better to antidepressants first, and that they may be more receptive to CBT once their mood has stabilised.

Direct comparisons of CBT with antidepressants generally reveal that the treatments are equally effective in the short term, but CBT has a more enduring effect. In a now-classic study, Hollon et al. (2005) followed up remitted depressed patients for two years after they had finished a course of either antidepressants or CBT. Of those who were symptom-free one year after treatment had finished, 80% of patients who had received CBT remained symptom-free one year later, in contrast to 50% of patients who had received antidepressants. Studies such as this have led to suggestions that CBT might work because it offers a kind of cognitive 'vaccine' against future episodes of depression (see Box 5.8).

Box 5.8   Essential treatment

Is CBT a cognitive vaccine?

Clients who receive CBT are at reduced risk of experiencing a relapse (i.e. another major depressive episode) in the future (Hollon et al., 2005). This might mean that CBT works as a cognitive 'vaccine', because it stops NATs from re-emerging whenever clients experience a negative life event. A study by Segal et al. (1999) suggests that this might be the case. Remitted depressed patients who had previously been treated with either CBT

(Continued)

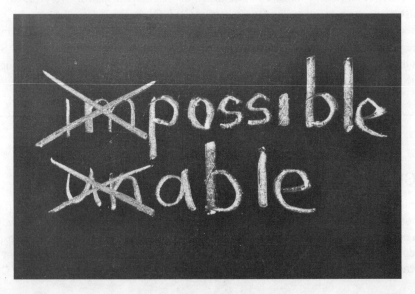

(Continued)

or antidepressants completed measures of depressogenic cognitions before and after exposure to a negative mood induction procedure. They found that the negative mood induction caused depressogenic cognitions to increase in both groups, but to a much smaller extent in the group that had previously received CBT. Perhaps most notably, individual differences in cognitive reactivity to the mood induction procedure predicted a recurrence of depressive symptoms later on. Taking these findings together, it seems that CBT can reduce the activation of depressogenic cognitions in response to negative events, and this in turn is associated with a reduced risk of recurrence of symptoms.

Other studies of CBT have shown that improvements in depressive symptoms only happen after depressogenic cognitions have changed, and that for patients who receive CBT, cognitive change mediates the subsequent change in negative mood (see Garratt et al., 2007). By contrast, patients who receive other types of treatment (including antidepressants and other psychological treatments) also show improvements in depressogenic cognitions, but these changes occur after improvements in negative mood in these patients (Garratt et al., 2007). In other words, different types of treatment might ultimately result in improved mood and a more optimistic way of thinking. The important difference is that the cognitive change is what causes the improvement in mood among patients who receive CBT, but patients who receive other types of treatment show improvement in mood first, and changes in cognition follow on afterwards.

Figure 5.3   Adopting a more positive, optimistic cognitive style may explain why CBT leads to improved mood in depressed patients

Other treatments for major depression

You have probably heard about electro-convulsive therapy (ECT), which involves the application of a high voltage electrical current to the dominant brain hemisphere, usually over repeated sessions. It is not a first-line treatment for major depression (because of its side effects), but may be offered to patients with severe depression who have not responded to antidepressants or are at high risk of suicide. It is considered effective for such patients, and its beneficial effects are seen more quickly than with antidepressants (McCall, 2001). Other types of psychological treatment, including mindfulness (Piet & Hougaard, 2011), are also effective, although CBT usually emerges as the most effective treatment when compared with others.

Psychological treatments for bipolar disorder

CBT for bipolar disorder utilises many of the same approaches as those used in regular CBT for depression (see above), but with additional components aimed at challenging cognition and behaviour during manic episodes. A meta-analysis from Szentagotai and David (2010) concluded that this approach had small but reliable effects on reducing symptoms of bipolar disorder, although the effects at follow-up (and prevention of recurrence of manic or major depressive episodes) were not impressive. As a consequence, CBT (and other psychological therapies) may be recommended as well as medication, but there is no convincing evidence that they should replace medication as the primary treatment for bipolar disorder.

Section summary

In this section we have shown that both antidepressant medication and cognitive behaviour therapy are effective treatments for major depression. Although both are equally effective in the short term, CBT has the edge in the longer term, perhaps because it has more enduring effects on depressogenic cognitions. Drug therapy remains the first-choice treatment for bipolar disorder because it improves symptoms in the majority of clients who take it.

Essential questions

Some possible exam questions that stem from this chapter are:

- Why do negative life events cause depression to develop?
- Critically evaluate the role of gene × environment interactions in the development of depression.
- Do depressogenic (pessimistic) cognitions play a role in the development of major depressive disorder, and in the recurrence of major depressive episodes after recovery?
- Do antidepressants work?
- Does cognitive behaviour therapy improve the symptoms of major depressive disorder, and if so how does it work?

Further reading

Beck, A. T. (2008). The evolution of the cognitive model of depression and its neurobiological correlates. *American Journal of Psychiatry*, 165(8): 969–977. (An excellent overview of the cognitive model of depression from the guru of this topic, with some accessible explanations of how the theory relates to brain dysfunction in mood disorders.)

Garratt, G., Ingram, R. E., Rand, K. L., & Sawalani, G. (2007). Cognitive processes in cognitive therapy: Evaluation of the mechanisms of change in the treatment of depression. *Clinical Psychology: Science and Practice*, 14(3): 224–239. (Engaging discussion on the role of cognitive change in the mechanism of the action of different treatments for major depression, with a focus on CBT.)

Scher, C. D., Ingram, R. E., & Segal, Z. V. (2005). Cognitive reactivity and vulnerability: Empirical evaluation of construct activation and construct diatheses in unipolar depression. *Clinical Psychology Review*, 25(4): 487–510. (Very readable dissection of the evidence on the causal influence of depressogenic cognitions on depressed mood.)

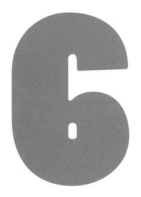

GENERALISED ANXIETY DISORDER

General introduction

In this chapter we introduce the diagnostic criteria for generalised anxiety disorder, before considering its overlap with other mood and anxiety disorders. We then discuss how heritable and environmental factors, particularly parenting, may cause children to develop into anxious adults. The largest part of this chapter is devoted to a discussion of cognitive mechanisms in anxiety, particularly the roles of excessive worry and cognitive biases for threatening information. In the final part of the chapter, we consider how generalised anxiety disorder can be treated, and we evaluate whether treatments need to influence cognitive processes if they are to have a beneficial effect on anxiety.

Assessment targets

At the end of the chapter, you should ask yourself the following questions:

- Can I explain the diagnostic criteria for generalised anxiety disorder?
- Do I understand the roles of genetic and biological factors in generalised anxiety disorder?
- Can I explain how distorted cognitive processes might play a role in the initial development of generalised anxiety, and in the maintenance of the disorder?
- What can people do to help reduce their worrying?
- Do I understand how generalised anxiety disorder is treated, and can I relate treatments (particularly cognitive treatments) back to their theoretical models?
- Is cognitive bias modification likely to prove superior to existing treatments for generalised anxiety disorder?

Section 1: What is generalised anxiety disorder?

Diagnosis of generalised anxiety disorder

The primary feature of generalised anxiety disorder (GAD) is excessive worry that interferes with everyday functioning. This worry is associated with high levels of distress, and with concentration problems, sleep disruption and restlessness. Box 6.1 contains the diagnostic criteria for generalised anxiety disorder in *ICD*-10. The *ICD*-10 diagnostic criteria are similar to those provided in *DSM*-5, which are themselves largely unchanged from those in the previous version (*DSM-IV*) and the one before that (*DSM*-III). Unlike other disorders considered in this book, the way in which we conceptualise GAD has not changed much over time.

Box 6.1   Essential diagnosis

Generalised anxiety disorder

The *ICD*-10 (World Health Organisation, 1992) criteria for generalized anxiety disorder are:

A. A period of at least six months with prominent tension, worry, and feelings of apprehension, about every-day events and problems.
B. At least four of the following symptoms are present, one of which must be from (1):

   1. Palpitations or pounding heart; sweating; trembling or shaking; dry mouth.
   2. Difficulty breathing; feeling of choking; chest pain or discomfort; nausea or abdominal distress; feeling dizzy, faint or light-headed; feeling that objects are unreal ('derealisation') or that one's self is distant or 'not really here' (depersonalization); fear of losing control, going crazy, or passing out.

The *DSM*-5 criteria (American Psychiatric Association, 2013a) are similar to those described in *ICD*-10, although *DSM*-5 is more vague on the physical symptoms of anxiety. In both *DSM*-5 and *ICD*-10, *worry* or apprehension is assigned a key role.

The key features of these diagnostic criteria are that the worry and apprehension must happen most days and persist over a long period of time. The worry should also be associated with various physical symptoms (restlessness, sleep disturbance, etc.) and impairment of general functioning. A typical experience of GAD is shown in Box 6.2. As with most disorders, it is important to rule out a better diagnosis. This is particularly important in GAD because of a potential overlap with the other anxiety disorders. Therefore, the focus of the anxiety and worry should not be confined to features of another psychological disorder: the anxiety or worry should not be about having a panic attack (as in panic disorder; see Chapter 8), being embarrassed in public (as in social phobia; see Chapter 8), intrusive thoughts (as in obsessive-compulsive disorder), being away from home or close relatives (as in separation anxiety disorder; see Chapter 3), gaining weight (as in anorexia nervosa; see Chapter 10), having multiple physical complaints (as in somatisation disorder), or having a serious illness (as in hypochondriasis).

Anxiety disorders in general are closely associated with mood disorders (most notably depression; see Chapter 5) and substance-use disorders (see Chapter 9). It is estimated that up to 90% of people with GAD will suffer from a different psychological disorder as well (Grant et al., 2005), and in many cases GAD will precede the onset of the other disorder (Ruscio et al., 2007). The interaction with tobacco smoking is interesting: GAD sufferers are more likely to smoke, often because they believe that it helps them to relax, whereas the evidence suggests that anxiety can make nicotine withdrawal worse and that smoking can increase the risk of developing anxiety disorders later on in life (Morissette and colleagues, 2007). Anxiety, mood and substance-use disorders have some shared heritable influences and environmental risk factors, and this goes back to our general point about the diagnostic boundaries between different psychological disorders being very blurred. However, there are also distinctive environmental risk factors for GAD that are not shared with other disorders (Newman et al., 2013).

Box 6.2   Experience of generalised anxiety disorder

(National Institute of Mental Health, 2014)

I always thought I was just a worrier. I'd feel keyed up and unable to relax. At times it would come and go, and other times it would be constant. It could go on for days. I'd worry about what I was going to fix for a dinner party, or what would be a great present for somebody. I just couldn't let something go.

When my problems were at their worst, I'd miss work and feel just terrible about it. Then I worried that I'd lose my job. My life was miserable until I got treatment.

I'd have terrible sleeping problems. There were times I'd wake up wired in the middle of the night. I had trouble concentrating, even reading the newspaper or a novel. Sometimes I'd feel a little lightheaded. My heart would race or pound. And that would make me worry more. I was always imagining things were worse than they really were. When I got a stomach ache, I'd think it was an ulcer.

Prevalence and consequences of generalised anxiety disorder

The lifetime prevalence rate of GAD is about 6%, and the 12-month prevalence rate is 3% (Kessler & Wang, 2008), although these are likely to be underestimates due to their reliance on retrospective reports. As with most psychological disorders there is considerable variation in the prevalence of GAD in different countries. For example, the point prevalence estimate for the whole of Europe is about 2%, but there is a lot of variation between countries, a situation that is not helped by patchy data for some countries (Lieb et al., 2005). The lifetime prevalence rate across Europe has been estimated at 2.8%, but around double that (at 5.7%) in the USA, which might reflect different attitudes to diagnosis rather than national differences in prevalence (Michael et al., 2007). The ratio of female to male sufferers is approximately 2:1 (i.e. it is twice as common in females). In addition, the disorder is more common in people who are unemployed, on a low income, living alone or who have fewer years of education (Grant et al., 2005; Michael et al., 2007). The average age of onset is 21 years (although getting reliable estimates of this is very difficult), which is considerably later than that for other anxiety and mood disorders. However, once established, GAD tends to follow a chronic course, with many patients recovering but later experiencing a recurrence of symptoms (Newman et al., 2013)

Newman et al. (2013) argue that GAD is often perceived as a disorder that afflicts the 'worried well', which implies that it is not particularly debilitating. They demonstrate that this is not the case: the disability associated with a GAD diagnosis is comparable to that associated with chronic health conditions such as arthritis, is similar to the disability associated with major depression, and is higher than that seen in patients with personality disorders and substance use disorders. GAD sufferers are more likely to be unemployed and to suffer from a number of health conditions such as heart disease. While these complications are very unpleasant for the individual with GAD, they mean that the disorder also has financial consequences for society, in the form of a loss of productivity, incapacity benefits and medical costs.

Section summary

In this section, we have shown how GAD is diagnosed and we have identified chronic, uncontrollable and unrealistic 'worry' as its central feature. We have demonstrated that it is fairly common in the general population, although when we think of the estimated lifetime prevalence rate of 6% in relation to the proportion of people who occasionally worry about things (arguably this is close to 100%), then GAD starts to seem rare!

Section 2: How does GAD develop?

Heritable influences

GAD does seem to run in families, although its heritability is low compared to other disorders. Hettema and colleagues (2001) conducted a twin study and found that concordance rates for GAD were relatively low. The heritability estimate for GAD was 15% to 20%, and heritability did not differ for men and women. A more recent meta-analysis from Bienvenu et al. (2011) reported a heritability estimate for GAD of 28%, which you may think is high but it was much lower than the heritability estimates for bipolar disorder (81%), schizophrenia (81%), alcohol use disorder (56%) and major depressive disorder (37%), reported in the same paper.

Any heritable risk for GAD does not seem to be specific to that disorder: several twin studies suggest that the heritable risk for GAD is shared with that for other anxiety disorders and major depressive disorder. This might mean that what is actually inherited is a personality trait, such as neuroticism, that predisposes to all of these disorders (Schienle et al., 2011).

If GAD is heritable, have we found the gene (or genes) that lead to the development of the disorder? Schienle et al. (2011) reviewed the available studies and concluded that, despite some studies showing associations between GAD and variations in genes that code for dopamine and serotonin function in the brain, the overall picture is clouded by studies with small sample sizes and a lack of consistency across different studies (as is the case for other psychological disorders). The search for the GAD gene(s) has not really got off the ground, and given the shared heritability between GAD and many other disorders, most researchers are sceptical that we will ever find these.

Trauma, childhood attachment and parenting

You will not be surprised to learn that unpredictable, negative life events (e.g. the death of a family member, divorce, unemployment) can increase the risk of developing GAD, in much the same way that they increase the likelihood of developing many other psychological disorders, including schizophrenia, major depression and substance use disorders (see Chapters 4, 5 and 9). In the case of GAD, Newman et al. (2013) suggest that this occurs because such events, particularly if they occur unpredictably, can make people question the stability and predictability of their world, which causes them to become continuously anxious so that they can prepare for other potentially unpredictable events. One obvious problem with such an account is that it does not explain why many (in fact, most) people who experience these kinds of trauma do *not* go on to develop GAD, or indeed any other kind of psychological disorder. Many of the issues that we discussed in Chapter 5 on the relationship between traumatic life events and depression are equally applicable here.

We know that severely traumatic events experienced during childhood, such as the death of a parent or sexual abuse, can massively increase the risk of developing schizophrenia (Chapter 4) and substance use disorders (Chapter 9) during adulthood. This is also true for GAD, as sexual abuse during childhood increases the likelihood that a person will develop GAD later on in life (Bulik et al., 2001). However, we have to remember that childhood sexual abuse is fortunately very rare whereas GAD is not. Therefore, sexual abuse during childhood cannot explain the majority of cases of GAD in adults.

In Chapter 3 we asked whether parents were responsible for the development of anxiety disorders in their children, and the answer was, as it often is, 'maybe' (see Box 3.11 in particular). Therefore it is reasonable to ask whether the attachments that people form with their parents, and their parents' style of parenting, are associated with individual differences in anxiety *during adulthood* (Newman et al., 2013). Different 'attachment styles' can be distinguished, and this important topic is covered elsewhere in this book in detail (see Chapters 3 and 11 in particular). For example, infants who feel rejected by their parents might form an 'anxious/avoidant' attachment, whereas infants whose parents are inconsistent or intrusive (very affectionate one moment, but disinterested or angry the next) might form an 'ambivalent/resistant' attachment. Newman et al. (2013) reviewed evidence which demonstrates that compared to infants who formed healthy attachments with their parents, the formation of anxious, insecure attachments during infancy is associated with anxiety later in life. For example, teenagers who reported that they formed insecure, anxious attachments with their parents were more likely to have GAD, or to worry more, than teenagers who reported forming healthy attachments with their parents (see Newman et al., 2013). The conclusions from these retrospective studies, which are obviously prone to bias, are supported by longitudinal studies which show that infants who are ambivalently attached at 12 months old are more likely to be diagnosed with GAD or social anxiety disorder during adolescence (e.g. Warren et al., 1997).

As discussed in Chapter 3, no one has been able to exclude the possibility that children with an early predisposition to anxiety (which could be heritable) might develop insecure attachments because of this predisposition, rather than vice versa. Another issue that seems to be significant is parenting style, which was also discussed in Chapter 3. There is evidence for a direct link between parenting styles and GAD symptoms during adulthood. Adolescents and adults with a GAD diagnosis are more likely to report that they felt rejected by their parents, that their parents were over-controlling, or that they seemed emotionally cold (Newman et al., 2013). One suggestion is that children who are over-controlled in this way might start to form the belief that they cannot handle difficult situations without their parents' help, leading to anxiety, which is why these kinds of parenting styles might cause GAD to develop and then persist during adulthood (Newman et al., 2013). In summary, if parenting style can increase the risk of anxiety disorders in children (and that is quite a big 'if'), these effects could be quite long-lasting.

Kertz and Woodruff-Borden (2011) identified modelling as another way in which parents can influence anxiety levels in their offspring. They argued that if children see their parents reacting in an anxious way in response to things that happen, this will influence a child's interpretation of threat and the ways in which they will cope with that threat, and some modelling of the parents' behaviour is likely to occur (similar mechanisms could explain the familial transmission of depression; see Chapter 5). There is good evidence that this is the case for anxiety: experimental studies show that children will avoid a particular toy if their parents had a negative emotional reaction to it (Gerull & Rapee, 2002). In a clever naturalistic study, Greenbaum and colleagues (1988) observed mothers and their children in a paediatric hospital waiting room, and found that anxious behaviours in the mother tended to precede anxious behaviour in the child, with some evidence for the reverse pattern of influence as well (i.e. anxious children made their mothers more anxious), depending on the mother's level of trait anxiety. This issue was discussed in more detail in Chapter 3.

In summary, there is evidence that parenting plays a key role in the development of GAD. However, before we 'blame the parents' for every instance of GAD in adults, we need to consider the many ways in which children interact with their parents, all of which make it difficult to confidently conclude that bad parenting leads to GAD in adults.

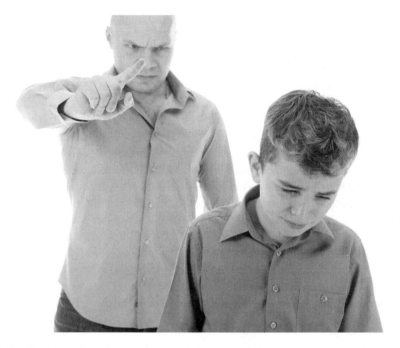

Figure 6.1   Certain styles of parenting can increase the risk that children will develop anxiety disorders when they reach adulthood

Section summary

In this section we have shown that GAD is a heritable disorder but the degree of heritability is low. This suggests that environmental influences play an important role in the development of GAD. It is clear that the type of parenting children receive, and the attachments they form with their parents, are likely to play a part in the development of GAD later in life.

Section 3: Brain and cognitive mechanisms in GAD

Are anxious brains different?

GAD sufferers show hyper-responsivity in the amygdala, a part of the brain that is clearly implicated in negative emotional reactions to stimuli, particularly fear (Schienle et al., 2011). For example, the amygdala is activated when people see unpleasant images, and the degree of activation is greater in people with GAD than matched controls. There are also structural differences: the amygdala is larger in GAD patients than controls, and this may explain why the degree of amygdala activation is enhanced when GAD sufferers view unpleasant images (Newman et al., 2013). Other research has identified functional abnormalities in a network of brain regions, including the amygdala and the anterior cingulate and dorsolateral prefrontal cortices, which suggests that the brain abnormality in GAD might reflect changes in a broad network of brain regions, rather than abnormalities in one region alone (Schienle et al., 2011).

However, when we consider this research we should remember that these types of studies tell us what is going on in the brains of patients with GAD, so they clarify how activity in the brain is associated with the psychological symptoms we can see. But these studies don't offer any kind of explanation as to 'why' or 'how' people develop GAD in the first place.

Another way to study brain abnormalities in GAD is to look at different neurotransmitters instead of different parts of the brain. For example, benzodiazepines (which increase GABA activity) and selective serotonin reuptake inhibitors (SSRIs; these increase activity in serotonin systems) are widely prescribed to treat GAD, and both seem to be effective (see Section 4 of this chapter). Further evidence for the role of these neurotransmitters can be found in studies that give people different drugs that reduce GABA or serotonin activity; these drugs tend to make people feel more anxious (Schienle et al., 2011). But while this information is very informative regarding the role of neurotransmitters in anxious states, you should think critically about what these studies tell us about the biological *causes* of the disorder that we call GAD. For example, if you drink alcohol (a drug that affects the GABA system in similar ways to benzodiazepine drugs) you will feel more relaxed and less anxious. But does this mean that you had an abnormality in the first place, one that was 'corrected' by drinking alcohol?

Cognitive mechanisms in GAD

Worry

Arguably, excessive 'worry' is the defining feature of GAD. Worry is a word that we intuitively understand and most of us know what it feels like to worry. Nevertheless, it is important for researchers and clinicians to define the term so that it can be distinguished from other negative emotions. Also, if worrying is an everyday activity for people who are otherwise healthy, then we need to know how the process differs in people with GAD: Is there a qualitative difference in the way that GAD sufferers worry? This section looks first at how worry is defined and then considers the ways in which worry in GAD is different from normal experience.

Worry has been described as a 'chain of thoughts and images, negatively affect-laden and relatively uncontrollable' (Borkovec et al., 1983). Worry appears to have some similarities with rumination, a central feature of major depression (Chapter 5). Both worry and rumination are repetitive, iterative and somewhat uncontrollable thought processes. However, worries are focused on future events whose outcomes are uncertain but there is a possibility that a negative outcome could occur, whereas rumination typically focuses on past events and experiences (Hirsch & Mathews, 2012).

Differences between normal and pathological worry

Craske et al. (1989) classified the worries of 19 GAD patients and 26 non-anxious controls and found that these fell into five categories:

- family, home and interpersonal relationships;
- finances;
- work or school;
- illness, injury and health;
- miscellaneous.

There were no reliable differences between GAD patients and controls in the content of their worries or the anxiety they produced. However, one factor that did significantly distinguish the groups was the controllability of the worries: patients with GAD felt that they could not stop worrying! This finding has been replicated in other studies (e.g. Ruscio & Borkovec, 2004). There are several reasons why worry might become uncontrollable, and this leads us on to look at psychological theories of uncontrollable worry.

Why worry?

Behar et al. (2009) and Newman et al. (2013) reviewed several cognitive theories of worry in GAD. It is notable that whilst some of these theories make predictions that directly compete with each other (and we flag up when this occurs), other theories talk about psychological processes that can explain different aspects of worrying, so they are not necessarily inconsistent with each other, and each of them might be 'true' to an extent. For example, the Cognitive Avoidance Model (Borkovec et al., 2004) proposes that the function of worry is to suppress the emotional processing of fear. People engage in worry in an attempt to control their negative emotions, and also because they superstitiously believe that it will prevent bad things from happening to them. The main idea is that worry is a verbal-linguistic, thought-based activity (the 'inner voice') that inhibits vivid mental imagery (picturing the bad things that might happen in the 'mind's eye') and the physiological arousal and emotional distress that are associated with imagery. In order for fear to be extinguished, people need to experience this emotional distress (see Chapter 7). Therefore worry is a form of cognitive avoidance, and worry is reinforced precisely because it reduces emotional distress. As predicted by the theory, worry does seem to be a verbal-linguistic process rather than an imagery-based process (Behar et al., 2009). Other support for the theory comes from accounts from GAD sufferers themselves, who claim that they worry because it prevents them from engaging in deeper, more upsetting thoughts about the events they fear (Borkovec, 1994). Supportive evidence can also be found from experiments which show that worry leads to reduced physiological arousal (Behar et al., 2009).

Newman and Llera (2011) proposed the Contrast Avoidance Model. The main idea is that GAD sufferers engage in chronic worry because it makes them distressed, and they like it that way because it means that they are always prepared for the worst possible thing to happen to them! It might seem strange that anyone would want to feel distressed all of the time, so to explain this we have to consider a phenomenon known as affective contrast. This refers to the observation that the impact of an emotional experience will be moderated by the emotional state we are in before we experience it. To give an example: if you find out that you have won the lottery, that's wonderful and you will feel very happy, but you will be more elated if you were previously feeling a bit miserable rather than if you were previously feeling quite happy. According to Newman and Liera (2011), affective contrast is relevant to GAD because individuals with GAD report feeling more distraught than controls when they experience this affective contrast (a rapid shift from a positive mood state to a negative mood state). Because of this, people with GAD may worry all the time because it minimises their affective contrast when bad things do happen to them.

The Contrast Avoidance Model was only proposed fairly recently, so it hasn't been thoroughly tested yet. There is some debate as to whether worry actually alleviates negative emotional states (as predicted by Borkovec et al.'s (2004) Cognitive Avoidance Model) or increases them (as predicted by the Contrast Avoidance Model). Different types of studies seem to support different theories (a level of complexity we won't get into here). However, compelling evidence comes from prospective studies which show that engaging in worrying causes an increase in the physiological markers of negative mood, an effect that persists for several hours (Zoccola et al., 2011). This evidence is consistent with the Contrast Avoidance Model, but not the Cognitive Avoidance Model.

Regardless of the *actual* effect of worrying on a person's emotional state, it could be that worrying becomes uncontrollable because GAD sufferers *believe* that worrying serves this purpose. In other words, worry might be *superstitiously reinforced* because, in general, people (including those with GAD) don't have as many negative emotional experiences as they expect to, and this means they might perceive a causal relationship between the relative lack of bad things happening to them and their excessive worrying ('It didn't happen because I worried about it'). Anecdotal reports from GAD patients suggest that worrying does serve this purpose (Newman & Llera, 2011), and this function of worry is consistent with both the Cognitive Avoidance and Contrast Avoidance models of worry.

Wells (1995) proposed the Metacognitive Model of worry, which has some shared features with the models described above, but also makes some unique predictions. Wells distinguishes between type 1 and type 2 worries. Type 1 worries are the kinds of worries that we all have, about our relationships, work, finances and so on. The cognitive and emotional processes that determine the uncontrollability of these types of worries are similar to those proposed in the Cognitive Avoidance and Contrast Avoidance Models, discussed above. Wells' unique prediction is that GAD sufferers begin to worry about their worrying, a process that he calls 'meta-worry' (or type 2 worrying). The important distinction here is that healthy people (those who do not have GAD) experience type 1 but not type 2 worries. Only GAD sufferers have type 2 worries, and these serve to maintain the cycle of constant worrying. When GAD sufferers experience meta-worry (type 2 worry) they fear that their worrying has become uncontrollable and may be very harmful for them, which sets off a psychological cascade that in turn makes the worry even more uncontrollable. This includes strategies to manage and cope with worry including thought suppression, distraction, and avoiding negative situations. Each of these strategies is unsuccessful (and indeed often counter-productive), which reinforces the belief that the worry is uncontrollable, and this makes the whole situation worse. Wells argues that negative attitudes about worrying are likely to develop from, amongst other places, the media, family and other social and cultural domains. Once negative attitudes to worrying develop, they may be exacerbated if people compare their own worrying behaviour to that of others, or by the fact that any increased propensity to worry will lead to a greater probability that worrying will, by chance, become associated with something negative. This all builds up to increase the amount of time that a GAD sufferer spends worrying about the fact that they worry. There is evidence that 'meta-worry' is related to, and has a causal influence on, the controllability of worries. However, it seems that meta-worry is not specific to GAD, and does in fact occur in a range of psychological disorders (Behar et al., 2009).

Another cognitive process that has been linked with worry is intolerance of uncertainty, which is a negative emotional response to situations that are ambiguous or uncertain. The Intolerance of Uncertainty Model (IUM; see Freeston et al., 1994) proposes that people with GAD get particularly distressed in such situations, and they engage in worry in an attempt to prepare for ambiguous or uncertain events or to prevent them from happening at all. The problem is that worrying in this way does not actually help to 'solve the problem'; all it does is maintain and exacerbate the worry (there is some overlap with this function of worry and the 'superstitious reinforcement' function, as discussed previously). This model is not inconsistent with the other cognitive models of worry we have looked at: its main novel prediction is that GAD sufferers are more prone to uncontrollable worry because they are so intolerant

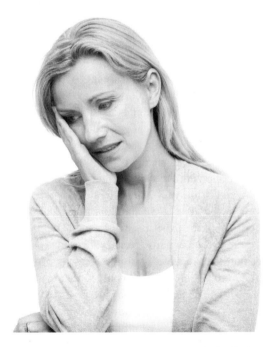

Figure 6.2 Worrying about things is normal, so many psychological models of GAD attempt to explain what is abnormal about worry in GAD

of uncertainty, and therefore any treatment should try to target the intolerance of uncertainty rather than the worry itself. There is some supportive evidence for the model: intolerance of uncertainty is more closely associated with a GAD diagnosis than other measures of worry cognitions (Behar et al., 2009).

Other cognitive distortions in anxiety

Attentional biases

Many experimental studies have used a task called the 'Emotional Stroop' and have demonstrated that anxious individuals, including individuals with GAD, are relatively slow to name the colour in which words are printed when those words are threatening, even when those words are presented too quickly to consciously read them (Mathews & MacLeod, 1994; Mogg et al., 1993). Other studies have used the visual probe task (see Box 6.3) combined with eye movement monitoring to demonstrate that patients with anxiety disorders will preferentially focus their attention on anxiety-provoking words and pictures presented on a computer screen, compared to control words (Cisler & Koster, 2010). Research conducted over the past two decades has revealed that attentional biases for threatening information are a reliable feature of anxiety disorders (including GAD), and they are also related to trait anxiety levels in healthy people: people who feel more anxious are more likely to attend to threatening stimuli. Cisler and Koster (2010) reviewed this evidence and concluded that attentional biases could be broken down into the following:

1. biases in the detection of threat, which can be related back to the hyperactive functioning of the amygdala (see Section 2);
2. difficulty disengaging attention from a threat, which may be linked to disrupted function in regions of the prefrontal cortex;
3. attentional avoidance, that is, something that anxious people might deliberately do in order to reduce how anxious they feel when they encounter something threatening.

A number of recent studies have investigated whether attentional biases have a causal influence on subjective anxiety. Following the seminal study by MacLeod et al. (2002, described in Box 6.4) See, MacLeod, and Bridle (2009) investigated the effects of attentional bias modification on anxiety levels in response to a natural stressor. They tested college students in Singapore who were shortly about to experience a stressful situation: moving to Australia to begin a university degree. One group of participants were trained to direct their attention away from threatening words, and they received multiple sessions of this training shortly before they left for Australia. A control group received no attentional bias modification training. As would be expected, both groups experienced an increase in anxiety at around the time that they moved to Australia. What was most significant, however, was that the group that had received the 'avoid threat' attentional training showed a blunted stress response when they moved to Australia, which provides further evidence that the attentional bias for threat seems to have a causal influence on the anxiety experienced during a stressful situation. These studies (and others like them) have led to interest in the use of attentional bias modification as a treatment for GAD and other anxiety disorders, and we discuss this in Section 4.

Box 6.3 Essential research

The effects of attentional bias modification (ABM) on emotional vulnerability

In a now-classic study, MacLeod et al. (2002) used a modified visual probe task to train participants to direct their attention either towards or away from negative words. On each trial of this task, a pair of words (one negative and one neutral) was presented slightly above and below a fixation point in the centre of the screen for either 20 or 480 milliseconds before those words disappeared and were replaced by a 'visual probe' (a pair of dots). Participants had to respond to this probe as quickly as possible.

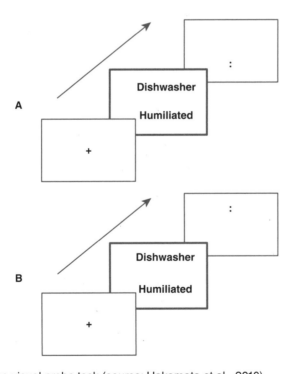

Figure 6.3   The visual probe task (source: Hakamata et al., 2010)

(Continued)

(Continued)

Normally, this task is used to measure attentional biases for threat: the probes replace the 'threat' words ('Death' in this example) and the neutral words ('Model' in this example) equally frequently, and if participants are faster to respond to probes that replace threat words than probes that replace neutral words, this indicates that they have an attentional bias for threat.

In the MacLeod et al. study, the position of probes was varied by experimental group. Participants were randomly allocated to either the 'Attend Negative' group, for whom the probes usually replaced the threat pictures, or the 'Attend Neutral' group, for whom the probes usually replaced the neutral pictures. After 576 trials of this attentional bias modification, additional trials were introduced in which the probes could appear in either location. The reaction time data for those trials are shown below.

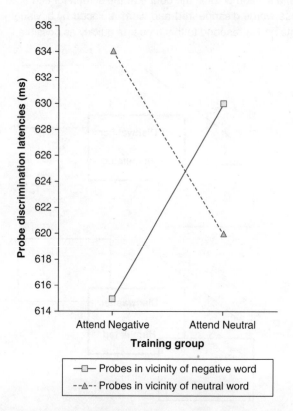

Figure 6.4 The attentional bias data from MacLeod et al. (2002)

What these results show is that the ABM manipulation was effective: participants in the 'attend negative' group were much faster to respond to visual probes that replaced negative words versus probes that replaced neutral words, which means that they had an attentional bias for the negative words, whereas in the 'attend neutral' group the reverse was true: this group had an attentional bias for the neutral words, or a bias *away* from the threat words. This part of the experiment revealed that attentional biases for threatening words could be experimentally manipulated.

The really interesting part of the experiment came next. To begin with, the participants rated how anxious and depressed they felt. All of them were then exposed to a stressful task, in which they had to solve difficult anagrams while being recorded on a video camera, but after they had finished they were told that they had performed very badly on the task and the video of their performance would be shown to psychology students for teaching purposes (how embarrassing!). Finally, all the participants rated their mood once more.

Their mood ratings (the average of anxiety and depression ratings) are shown below. As we can see, the ABM procedure did not influence mood before the stressful task, but the stressful task caused all the participants to feel much more anxious and depressed. Most importantly, this increase in negative mood after the stressful task was much larger in the group who had been trained to focus their attention on threat words compared to the group who had been trained to look away from the threat words.

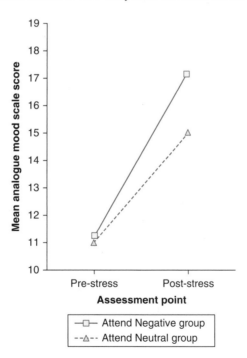

Figure 6.5 The mood data from MacLeod et al. (2002)

This study suggests that although attentional bias does not have an immediate effect on subjective anxiety, an attentional bias for threat can increase the negative emotional response to a stressful situation.

Interpretive biases

Eysenck et al. (1991) presented 32 different ambiguous sentences to groups of anxious, recovered anxious and non-anxious individuals. Two examples are: 'The two men watched as the chest was opened' and 'The doctor examined little Emma's growth.' Later on, the same individuals were presented with both a positive and negative interpretation of each sentence and they had to identify which sentence they had read earlier on. For example, they were shown a negative sentence such as 'The doctor looked at little Emma's cancer' and a positive one such as 'The doctor measured little Emma's height'. Even though the participants had seen none of the test sentences before, anxious individuals reported having previously seen many more negative statements than non-anxious individuals: they had a bias to interpret ambiguous scenarios as threatening.

In order to investigate the influence of this interpretive bias on symptoms of anxiety, more recent studies have attempted to 'train' that bias so that people are more likely to perceive a benign, non-threatening meaning in ambiguous scenarios of this sort. Wilson and colleagues (2006) reported that training people in this way led to a blunted (reduced) emotional response to stressful situations, that is, much the same effects that we see with attentional bias modification (described above). Studies such as this suggest that a negative interpretive bias, like attentional bias, plays a causal role in subjective anxiety. People are more likely to feel anxious in stressful situations if they have attentional or interpretive biases for threatening information.

An integrative model of cognitive distortions in anxiety

The cognitive biases described above imply that people suffering from GAD perceive more threat in their environment than people without anxiety disorders. Therefore it is fair to say that these people live in a more anxiety-inducing world than people without these biases: it isn't surprising they are more anxious! Hirsch and Mathews (2012) combined theories of cognitive bias and worry into an integrated cognitive theory of pathological worry, which is illustrated in Figure 6.6. This theory predicts that threat-related biases in selective attention and the interpretation of ambiguous information mean that threat information is more likely to intrude on conscious awareness, and this will be experienced as a negative thought. Once the negative thought intrudes on their consciousness, the GAD sufferer engages conscious attempts to resolve the source of threat by thinking of solutions to avoid it (i.e. worrying). However, automatic cognitive biases continue to exert a (pessimistic and catastrophic) effect on this reasoning process, and anxiety-induced impairments in attentional control mean that people find it difficult to 'break off' from worrying when in this anxious state.

Section summary

We discussed the brain mechanisms involved in anxiety before evaluating various theories that can account for the cognitive processes that underlie uncontrollable worry, the defining feature

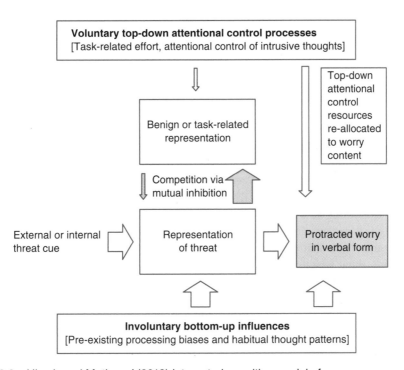

Figure 6.6   Hirsch and Mathews' (2012) integrated cognitive model of worry

of GAD. We have also seen how cognitive biases such as attentional bias and interpretive bias are implicated in GAD, and how these might play a role in maintaining anxiety. Finally, we showed how it is possible to integrate worry and cognitive biases into a unified cognitive model of worry in GAD.

Section 4: How is GAD treated?

Cognitive theories dominate our understanding of GAD. Therefore it should come as no surprise that one of the most effective treatments is cognitive behaviour therapy (CBT), which aims to directly target distorted cognitions. You may also be aware that waiting lists for CBT tend to be very long (although a recent government initiative called 'Increasing Access to Psychological Therapies' (IAPT) is attempting to remedy this), and if you are ever unfortunate enough to be diagnosed with GAD you might be offered medication, which is also effective. Finally, a different type of cognitive treatment aims to directly target cognitive biases (attentional bias and interpretive bias), and this type of therapy, called cognitive bias modification (CBM), has been heavily researched in recent years with some promising findings. In this section we will explain how all of these treatments work and show how they relate to theories of GAD, before evaluating their effectiveness.

CBT

The overarching goals of CBT are to:

> teach coping skills that encourage an active, problem-solving approach to stressful events, and a greater tolerance and acceptance of anxiety symptoms (Durham, 2007: 185)

Exposure to a feared stimulus is an essential component of cognitive behavior therapy for other anxiety disorders, including simple phobias (Chapter 7) and social phobia and panic disorder (Chapter 8). However, exposure, in the traditional sense, plays a less vital role in GAD because there are no specific triggers for the anxiety: the patient is constantly anxious about everything so what on earth should you expose them to? What happens in CBT for GAD is that patients are exposed to their cognitions. This may sound a little odd, but essentially the idea is that they are encouraged to imagine the worst possible consequence of something about which they have been worrying for a prolonged period, until they feel more relaxed, and then to consider other possible explanations or possible outcomes for the thing they are worried about. For example, if they are worried that they are not doing very well at work then they imagine a horrible situation (e.g. the boss being angry with them), and after that, when they are calm, generate benign reasons for why he might be angry (he's having a bad day). This, first and foremost, helps them get used to their cognitions (so this is a form of exposure therapy), but it also helps them practise not misinterpreting ambiguous information (this is called 'cognitive restructuring'). So it treats both the anxious response and the cognitive distortion (interpretive bias in this case). CBT is commonly delivered one-to-one with a therapist in the form of 6 to 20 hour-long sessions over a period of three to six months, although it can also be delivered in groups, over the telephone, and more recently over the internet (Durham, 2007).

CBT does seem to be effective, and while the table in Box 6.4 only shows recovery rates for people who received CBT, many studies have compared CBT with 'no treatment', or with different psychological therapies, and it consistently comes out as more effective than the alternatives. Its overall effectiveness, including newer variations (see below), was confirmed in a recent meta-analysis (Hanrahan et al., 2013). To give an example of an individual study, Butler and colleagues (1991) reported that CBT produced greater and more stable cognitive changes than behaviour therapy, and these gains were maintained at a six-month follow-up. Durham et al. (1994) also reported similar success for CBT compared to psychoanalytical therapy: six months after the end of treatment, 76% of those who had received CBT were better as compared to 42% of those who had received the psychoanalytical therapy.

Although CBT is effective (in comparison to other psychological treatments), we cannot exactly call it a 'cure' for GAD, because only 38% of patients who receive it are completely recovered at a six-month follow-up, with another 38% showing no improvement or getting worse, and the remainder showing a slight improvement (see Box 6.4). In addition, studies with even longer follow-up periods (10 to 14 years in one study) show that most patients relapse in the longer term, even after receiving CBT (Durham, 2007). On a more positive note, CBT does lead to reductions in attentional biases for threat in anxious patients (Mathews et al., 1995), which suggests that it produces (at least temporary) improvements in the core cognitive distortions that characterise GAD.

The cognitive models of worry that we discussed in the previous section have given rise to the development of some variations of CBT (see Behar et al., 2009, for a detailed review). For example, therapy based on Wells' Metacognitive Model targets meta-worry (worrying about worry) by focusing on patients' unrealistic beliefs about the uncontrollability of their worrying, and the benefits and consequences of worrying. Wells (2006) argued that dysfunctional beliefs about worry have to be specifically addressed through behavioural experiments (which we discussed in the context of CBT for depression in Chapter 5) and cognitive techniques that target the negative beliefs that drive the meta-worry. So if someone is worried that they will lose control, they could be encouraged to try to lose control of their worrying: the patient should discover that even if they try they cannot lose control. Likewise, if they believe that worrying will result in bad things happening, they should be encouraged to worry more or less to see that their level of worry doesn't change the number of bad things that happen to them. One trial of this type of CBT found that 75% of patients had completely recovered when assessed 12 months after the end of treatment (Wells & King, 2006).

Box 6.4   Essential treatment

Overall outcome of treatment aggregated across six clinical trials of CBT for GAD (Fisher & Durham, 1999; cited in Durham, 2007)

	Worse (%)	No change (%)	Improved (%)	Recovered (%)
Post-treatment	3	45	20	32
Six-month follow-up	2	36	24	38

Drug treatments

Patients with GAD may be prescribed a class of drugs called benzodiazepines (Xanax and Valium are well-known versions of these). These drugs are known as anxiolytics for their anxiety-relieving properties, and they work by stimulating GABA receptors in the brain. Their mechanism of action in the brain is similar to that of alcohol, which is interesting because many anxious patients choose to 'self-medicate' their anxiety by drinking alcohol, which can lead to alcohol problems (Grant et al., 2004), and this partly explains the high co-morbidity between anxiety disorders and alcohol use disorders (covered in Chapter 9). Therefore it is much safer to prescribe a drug that has a similar action in the brain, but is less harmful to bodily organs than alcohol is (in case you were wondering why we don't tell anxious patients to just go out and get drunk all the time!).

Benzodiazepines are an extremely effective treatment for GAD: about 35% of patients who take them experience a complete remission, and another 40% of people see some improvement (Davidson et al., 2001). The problem is that benzodiazepines are addictive: many people find it difficult to stop taking them, and when they do they experience unpleasant withdrawal symptoms including rebound anxiety. Because of this doctors in the USA and some European countries try to minimise prescriptions of benzodiazepines, and if they must be given to patients they are prescribed for only a minimal period of time (two to four weeks), which is long enough to stabilise debilitating anxiety but brief enough to make it unlikely that addiction will develop (Durham, 2007).

Other treatments for GAD are the selective serotonin reuptake inhibitors (SSRIs), for example escitalopram, and other antidepressants including tricyclics. Although these drugs were initially used to treat major depressive disorder (see Chapter 5), they are now the first-choice drug treatment for GAD. They are more effective than anxiolytics, and the rates of improvement are similar with SSRIs and tricyclic antidepressants, although SSRIs are preferred because they have fewer side effects (Rocca et al., 1997).

If the drugs that target the GABA and serotonin systems are effective at alleviating the symptoms of GAD, at least in the short term, does this tell us anything about the biological causes of the disorder? As we discussed in Section 3, the effectiveness of these drugs does not necessarily mean that GAD is caused by some kind of abnormality in these neurotransmitter systems. So we cannot say that these medications work because they correct an underlying 'chemical imbalance' in the brain. However, some studies suggest SSRIs reduce interpretive bias as well as improving symptoms (self-reported anxiety) in GAD patients (Mogg et al., 2004), which also suggests that these drugs may work because they change dysfunctional cognitions, at least in the short term.

Are psychological and drug treatments equally effective?

Some studies have directly compared improvements in GAD symptoms in patients who received benzodiazepines versus those who received cognitive therapy. A meta-analysis revealed that both types of treatment were more effective than a control treatment (a drug placebo) in the short term. However, the medium- and long-term improvements were more pronounced in people who receive cognitive therapy (Gould et al., 1997). It is becoming clear that the benefits of cognitive therapy are maintained in the medium term, but the benefits of benzodiazepines are not maintained once people stop taking the drugs.

SSRIs fare a little better than benzodiazepines: here, the medium-term effects are comparable with those seen after cognitive therapy, with about 50% of patients achieving a complete recovery three to six months after the end of treatment. But the longer-term pattern is the same, with clearly superior effects for cognitive therapy compared to SSRIs at longer-term follow-ups (Durham, 2007).

A plausible explanation for this pattern of results is that cognitive therapy teaches people how to reverse the maladaptive thinking patterns that caused them to feel anxious, whereas anxiolytics relieve the anxiety but don't make any difference to the maladaptive thinking processes. So once people stop taking the drugs, the maladaptive thinking processes are able to generate anxiety, and the whole cycle starts again. You might be thinking that it should be a good idea to combine SSRIs and cognitive therapy in order to gain the maximum possible benefit, that is, an immediate improvement that is maintained long term. However, few clinical trials have made such a comparison, and those that have combined the two have shown no clear benefit compared to either treatment delivered on its own (see Newman et al., 2013). Furthermore, some therapists believe that cognitive therapy is likely to work best on unmedicated patients, so that they can see how the cognitive changes that they practise have a direct effect on their anxiety levels (Durham, 2007). We discussed this issue more generally in Chapter 2.

Cognitive bias modification

Psychological therapies such as CBT aim to rectify the dysfunctional thinking processes that underlie uncontrollable worry. However, research on cognitive biases (such as attentional bias and interpretive bias) shows that faulty cognitions in GAD may also operate at a more automatic level. Indeed, Hirsch and Mathews' (2012) theoretical model suggests that these cognitive biases for threat are what trigger the worry cognitions in the first place. Therefore, there is a good theoretical reason to believe that directly targeting cognitive biases might be an effective way to treat GAD (and other anxiety disorders). In Section 3 we talked about some of the earlier research that used cognitive bias modification (CBM) to demonstrate that cognitive biases can have a causal effect on anxiety. In more recent years, the effectiveness of CBM in clinical populations of anxious patients has been studied.

In their review of the literature, MacLeod and Mathews (2012) concluded that multiple sessions of attentional bias modification could improve the symptoms of GAD (particularly uncontrollable worry), although they also noted that there were very few randomised controlled trials of its effectiveness. Similarly, positive findings have been reported for interpretive bias modification. Hallion and Ruscio's (2011) meta-analysis offered cautious support for both types of CBM, although they concluded that the effects of interpretive bias modification on anxiety symptoms were larger than those for attentional bias modification.

While these results are encouraging, there are many challenges. Most of the studies that evaluated CBM compared it to a 'no treatment' control condition, but what we really need are studies that compare it to the current 'gold-standard' treatment for GAD (which is CBT), or integrate it with conventional CBT to see if this combined therapy is better than conventional CBT by itself. It is important to compare the effectiveness of CBM with that of CBT, because this will inform clinical decisions about which type of treatment patients should get first. Even if CBM proves to be *less* effective than conventional CBT in absolute terms (as many believe it will), it could still be useful because it can be offered to patients if they do not respond to conventional CBT. In addition, we need to ensure that any changes in cognitive bias which occur as a result of CBM reflect a broad change in the way that GAD sufferers process threat, rather than a change in reactivity that is limited to the particular words or pictures that were used during training, although the available evidence does suggest that multiple sessions of CBM do lead to generalisable effects (MacLeod & Mathews, 2012). There are also several promising features of CBM: the potential to deliver the treatment over the internet means that it presents an opportunity to reach people who might be unable or unwilling to seek one-to-one treatment with a therapist, and it can be combined with conventional CBT (Rapee et al., 2013) which should, in theory at least, lead to a treatment that is able to target all aspects of dysfunctional cognitions in GAD simultaneously (Hirsch & Mathews, 2012). However, meta-analyses of published trials of CBM have reached quite different conclusions about its effectiveness in the 'real world', and we discuss this debate in Box 6.5.

Box 6.5   Essential debate

How effective is cognitive bias modification?

A number of meta-analyses of the CBM literature have been published in recent years, and despite including many of the same studies they reached some quite different conclusions. The first meta-analysis (Hakamata et al., 2010) only included trials that investigated the effects of attentional bias modification on anxiety symptoms and reported a medium effect size ($d = .61$). In subsequent meta-analyses, some of which included both attentional and interpretive bias modification for both anxiety and depression, the overall effect size was statistically significant but also noticeably smaller than that reported in the earlier meta-analysis (Beard et al., 2012; Hallion & Ruscio, 2011; Mogoaşe et al., 2014).

It is clear that CBM has potential as a treatment for anxiety disorders as well as mood disorders (see Chapter 5) and substance use disorders (see Chapter 9), because in principle it can be delivered via the internet and even via mobile phones (Enock et al., 2014). Therefore it could be accessible to patients who may be reluctant to take medication or engage with conventional psychological therapies. However, rather disappointing results from some meta-analyses, combined with the observation that it may work better in the laboratory with healthy participants rather than in the 'real world' with anxious patients, led one clinician to disparage cognitive bias modification and argue that conventional psychological treatments are more effective, at least for some disorders (Emmelkamp, 2012). Other researchers have strongly disagreed, and have pointed out that many of the existing studies that investigated CBM were not able to change cognitive biases after extended CBM training, so we should focus on tinkering with CBM so that it produces robust changes in cognitive biases before judging its effects on symptoms (Clarke et al., 2014). The next few years should yield research findings that can settle this debate once and for all, and tell us whether CBM is a 'flash in the pan' that cannot improve on conventional treatments, or whether it represents a revolution in the treatment of psychological disorders as its proponents claim.

Section summary

In this section, we have shown that GAD can be treated with cognitive behaviour therapy (CBT) or with drugs that target GABA or serotonin neurotransmitters in the brain. Both types of treatment are effective, although the beneficial effects of CBT are maintained for a much longer period of time than those for drugs. Both CBT and drug treatments change cognitive biases, and recent studies suggest that directly targeting cognitive biases with cognitive bias modification (CBM) might also be an effective way to treat GAD.

Essential questions

Some possible exam questions that stem from this chapter are:

- Compare and contrast psychological theories of uncontrollable worry.
- Evaluate psychological and drug treatments for generalised anxiety disorder.
- Does Cognitive Bias Modification have the potential to be a useful treatment for generalised anxiety disorder?

Further reading

Durham, R. C. (2007). Treatment of generalized anxiety disorder. *Psychiatry*, 6(5): 183–187. (A very readable and concise overview of the effectiveness of CBT and drug treatments of GAD, with a comparison between the two.)

Mogoaşe, C., David, D., & Koster, E. H. W. (2014). Clinical efficacy of attentional bias modification procedures: An updated meta-analysis. *Journal of Clinical Psychology*, in press.

(Continued)

(Continued)

(A recent meta-analysis of research on attentional bias modification, with some good balanced discussions of why different meta-analyses have yielded different findings.)

Newman, M. G., Llera, S. J., Erickson, T. M., Przeworksi, A., & Castonguay, L. G. (2013). Worry and generalized anxiety disorder: A review and theoretical synthesis of evidence on nature, etiology, mechanisms, and treatment. *Annual Review of Clinical Psychology*, 9: 275–297. (Comprehensive and engagingly written summary of pretty much everything to do with GAD.)

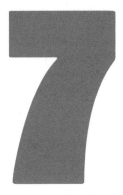

SPECIFIC PHOBIAS

General introduction

In this chapter, you will learn what it is like to have a specific phobia, how these are diagnosed and how common they are. We will discuss two of the main theories of how phobias develop, namely learning theory and cognitive theory, and consider the relevant evidence for some criticisms of these theories. We will then look at how psychologists treat phobias, and how successful this is.

Assessment targets

At the end of the chapter, you should ask yourself the following questions:

- Can I explain the key diagnostic criteria for specific phobia?
- Can I explain how phobias are learnt, and do I know the limitations of these explanations?
- Can I explain preparedness theory, and am I aware of its limitations?
- Do I understand how specific phobias are treated and can I relate the therapy back to the theories on which it is based?

Section 1: What is a specific phobia?

In this section we will start by looking at what a phobia is by exploring some of the common phobias that you might have already come across. We will then describe the *ICD*-10 criteria for specific phobias, consider some of the problems with the diagnostic criteria, and briefly consider the prevalence of phobias.

Diagnosis of specific phobias

There are actually three forms of phobia: specific phobia (sometimes called 'simple phobia'), agoraphobia and social phobia (see Chapter 8). Specific phobias are unique within this group because they are confined to a specific object or situation. Most of us will have come across some form of phobia in our lives: for example, lots of us might have, or know people with, mild forms of arachnophobia (a fear of spiders), ophidiophobia (snakes) or acrophobia (heights). However, it's possible to acquire a phobia of virtually anything and we would encourage you to look at www.phobialist.com/ which is an excellent website about phobias: amongst other things, it lists a staggering array of recognised phobias. There are some relatively common phobias such as nosophobia (injury/illness) and thanatophobia (death), but there are more unusual ones too. Some of our favourites are pogonophobia (a fear of beards) and melanophobia (not the fear of large yellow fruits, but fear of the colour black).

Box 7.1   Essential diagnosis

ICD-10 diagnosis of specific phobias (World Health Organisation, 1992)

A. Either (1) or (2):

   (1) marked fear of a specific object or situation not included in agoraphobia or social phobia;
   (2) marked avoidance of such objects or situations.

B. Symptoms of anxiety in the feared situation at some time since the onset of the disorder, with at least two symptoms present together, on at least one occasion, from the list below, one of which must have been from items (1) to (4):

Autonomic arousal symptoms

   (1) Palpitations or pounding heart, or accelerated heart rate.
   (2) Sweating.
   (3) Trembling or shaking.
   (4) Dry mouth (not due to medication or dehydration).

Symptoms concerning chest and abdomen

   (5) Difficulty breathing.
   (6) Feeling of choking.
   (7) Chest pain or discomfort.
   (8) Nausea or abdominal distress (e.g. churning in stomach).

Symptoms concerning brain and mind

   (9) Feeling dizzy, unsteady, faint or light-headed.
  (10) Feelings that objects are unreal (derealization), or that one's self is distant or "not really here" (depersonalization).
  (11) Fear of losing control, going crazy, or passing out.
  (12) Fear of dying.

General symptoms

  (13) Hot flushes or cold chills.
  (14) Numbness or tingling sensations.

C. Significant emotional distress due to the symptoms or the avoidance, and a recognition that these are excessive or unreasonable.
D. Symptoms are restricted to the feared situation, or when thinking about it.

If desired, the specific phobias may be subdivided as follows:

- animal type (e.g. insects, dogs)
- nature-forces type (e.g. storms, water)
- blood, injection and injury type
- situational type (e.g. elevators, tunnels)
- other type

Looking at Box 7.1 you will notice that you can only get a diagnosis of a specific phobia if your symptoms cannot be explained better by another diagnosis (e.g. agoraphobia or social phobia). This is a safeguard that most disorders have, in order to ensure that a clinician seeks alternative explanations for the symptoms and only makes a firm diagnosis when they are convinced it is the one that best fits the symptoms. For instance, someone who has an intense fear of parties probably doesn't have 'party phobia'; instead Social Anxiety Disorder (also known as 'Social Phobia' in *ICD*-10) may better explain their symptoms.

Diagnosis controversies

Diagnostic criteria can be useful. They can help a time-pressed clinician to decide where they should focus their treatment, and nowadays countries will often issue guidelines about how the different disorders should be treated. In the UK we have the National Institute for Clinical Excellence (NICE) which produces guidelines on how diseases should be treated, and increasingly guidelines are being written for psychological disorders: in order to follow such guidelines, a therapist needs to diagnose clients' conditions correctly. Diagnostic criteria are also important for researchers who need to be able to describe their participants clearly and reliably, and establish that they are researching exactly the same condition as everyone else. However, there are some controversies surrounding the use of diagnostic criteria. Many psychologists think that you cannot and should not reduce a complex individual down to a simple label, and that the best therapies are 'formulation-based', that is, they draw up an idio-syncratic picture of what is causing their patient's specific difficulties and base their treatment on that (see Chapter 2 for more details). You will notice that some of the criteria for specific phobia are very vague in the terms that they use. For example, what constitutes 'excessive or unreasonable'? Most of us might agree that running away screaming from a peanut is an excessive response, because even while to someone with a nut allergy the peanut may pose a lethal threat, most peanuts don't jump up into people's mouths of their own free will. However, is a fear of spiders out of proportion to the threat that they present, given that some of them can actually kill you? Box 7.2 describes what a severe phobia can look like.

Box 7.2   Essential experience

Phobia

Keith is a middle-aged man who is extremely scared of crane flies (those sort of flying daddy-long-legs that appear everywhere in the UK in August and September). He knows that crane flies can't hurt him, but they scare him anyway. During the crane fly season Keith keeps all of the windows in his house closed for fear that one may find its way in. When leaving the house he traps himself in the porch and his wife then has to check outside for crane flies. Once she has given the all-clear, he runs, flapping a fly swatter around his head, to the waiting car (the door of which is opened with clinical precision so as to stop any particularly cunning crane flies from entering the car when no one is looking). Think of the diagnostic criteria in Box 7.1: do you think Keith has a specific phobia?

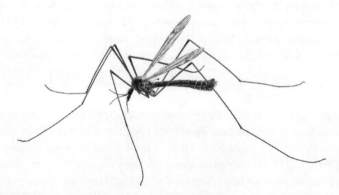

Figure 7.1   Keith had a specific phobia of crane flies

Prevalence of phobias

It is safe to assume that phobias are pretty common. In one large and well-conducted British study, 18% of adults had a diagnosis of a phobia (Jenkins et al., 1997). In children the reported prevalence rates for phobias vary dramatically, but surprisingly seem rather lower than the prevalence rates reported for adults. For instance, the most recent large and well-conducted British epidemiological survey reported that only about 1% of children had a phobia (Ford et al., 1999), and a number of other studies have reported rates than were not much higher (Bergeron et al., 1992; Briggs-Gowan et al., 2000). However, this discrepancy between the child and adult prevalence rates should not be taken to indicate that adults have more phobias than children. On the contrary, most phobias develop during childhood, and (in the absence of treatment) are often resistant to the passage of time, meaning that the true prevalence rates are probably very similar in adults and children. It may be that the research shows lower figures for children because they are more reluctant to own up to their phobias than adults are. Alternatively, it could be that the adults measuring anxiety in childhood are less willing to assign a diagnosis of a phobia to a fearful child, as fears are, to some extent, a normal part of growing up. And finally, what about students … ? According to one (admittedly rather small) study (Davis et al., 2007), they are the most frightened of the lot. The study showed that 34% of respondents had a spider phobia, 22% had a snake phobia, 18% a height phobia and 16% an injection phobia. If you like a challenge have a look at this study, and see if you can work out the reasons why these figures have come out so high.

Is there a gender bias in specific phobias?

As with other anxiety disorders, research shows that adult women are consistently more likely to suffer from phobias than men. For instance, in the study described above (Jenkins et al., 1997) 25% of women reported phobias compared to 18% of men. Can you think why there is such a gender bias? It is held that it could, in part, be due to a reporting bias (men may be more likely to think that admitting to being scared of something makes them look like a wimp). Alternatively, it might be that this concern about being seen as a wimp means that men are more likely to grit their teeth and face up to minor fears, meaning that these are less likely to develop into phobias. For a review of this area, see McLean and Anderson (2009).

Which phobias are the most common?

Using *DSM-IV* criteria for specific phobias, Fredrikson et al. (1996) went about diagnosing a range of common phobias in a large sample of randomly selected adults. Their top three phobias were heights (7.5%), snakes (5.5%) and closed spaces (4.0%). Surprisingly, spider phobia only scraped in at fourth place, with a paltry 3.5%.

Section summary

This section has taught us how clinicians diagnose specific phobias and how common they are. We've seen that specific phobias are excessive fears of identifiable objects or situations. In the next section we explain how phobias develop.

Section 2: How do we acquire phobias?

There are several possible ways in which people could acquire phobias. As with the other psychological disorders that are covered in this book, we can examine nearly any clinical disorder in terms of nature or nurture: Are we born with a disorder, or do we learn this by interacting with our environment?

It is clear that some people are predisposed to developing anxiety even before they are born. We know that genetics has a big part to play in anxiety disorders (Eley et al., 2003). It is also clear that stress during pregnancy predisposes the unborn child to a range of mental health difficulties, including anxiety (O'Connor et al., 2003). There is a theory that at this very sensitive stage of development, unborn children are being primed as to what to expect of the world. If their mother is very stressed, for any reason, the baby develops in a way that maximises its chances of survival after birth, and it is born prepared for a dangerous world. In a truly dangerous world it is quite useful to be very attuned to threat, and very quick to respond with the fight-flight response (see below for more detail on the fight-flight response). In other words, if the world is very dangerous it pays to be born very anxious. However, if the world is really not that dangerous (and for most children born in the developed world in the twenty-first century, childhood is the safest it has ever been), then having a hair-trigger fight-flight response will cause far more trouble than it will save.

In fact all anxiety disorders arise as a combination of factors, including genes *and* environment. And as we are now discovering, these are not separate things. Our genes fundamentally manipulate the environment we grow up in. So, for example, a very shy, nervous child, who gets upset easily and is very difficult to console, will shape the care that they receive from adults. Those adults will often, quite unconsciously, become more protective of this child, reducing their exposure to potentially frightening situations, and stepping in very quickly once the child gets upset. As we saw in Chapter 3, overprotective parenting such as this has been linked with anxiety disorders, but in this case it is really difficult to attribute the disorder to heritable or environmental causes, or the interaction between the two (see Wermter et al., 2010).

Clearly, the nature/nurture debate is not a simple one, but this section will now focus on what happens after birth, and then examine the evidence that fears and phobias are heritable, before turning its attention to the role of learning processes.

Heritability of phobias: Are we born to fear?

So is there a genetic component to phobias? Van Houtem et al. (2013) carried out a meta-analysis of twin studies that looked at the heritability of fears and phobias, and found really quite large differences between studies. For instance, the range of heritability found for blood/injury/injection fears ranged from just 2% up to 71% in the studies they included. However, broadly speaking, when all the studies were combined, all the fears and phobias appeared to have a substantial genetic component, with the means for the heritability of different fears and phobias ranging from 25% to 45%.

This should not be taken to mean that we are born with our fears and phobias, however. The heritability figures reported by Van Houtem et al. (2013) leave a substantial role for environmental factors. And then, of course, there are gene–environment interactions to consider, as nicely demonstrated in a study by Hettema et al. (2003). Here, the authors rounded up a large sample of twin pairs, and attempted to condition them to have fears, and to then get rid of those fears (i.e. extinguish them). In order to do this they gave the twins mild electric shocks whilst showing them pictures of 'fear-relevant' stimuli (snakes and spiders) and 'fear-irrelevant' stimuli (geometric shapes). They found that both the propensity to learn to be afraid of stimuli that were paired with a shock and the ease with which this fear could then be extinguished (by showing the stimulus many times without giving a shock) were heritable, with 35% to 45% of the variance attributable to genetic transmission. Tellingly, heritability was higher for ease of conditioning towards the fear-relevant stimuli (snakes, spiders) than the fear-irrelevant stimuli (geometric shapes), which suggests that we may be genetically predisposed to acquire some fears more easily than others.

Observations that phobias of spiders, snakes, dogs, heights, water, death, thunder and fire are much more prevalent than phobias of modern threats to safety such as hammers, guns, knives and electrical outlets, and that fears of these stimuli are more easily acquired in the laboratory (see above), suggest that humans might be hard-wired to easily acquire a fear of these objects. This idea is known as the 'preparedness theory'.

Preparedness

Preparedness is the idea that we are born to acquire fears of certain stimuli more easily than others, because these stimuli were a threat to our ancient ancestors. If we are born with a 'hard-wired' fear of certain stimuli or situations then we might expect two things: that children would be scared of certain things from birth, and that there should be common themes in what people fear. We saw in the previous section that such common themes exist, and we also saw that children go through a fairly fixed developmental pattern of normal fears. In addition, Menzies and Clarke (1993a, 1993b) suggest that water and height phobics do indeed report having been scared for as long as they can remember. One explanation of these findings is Seligman's (1971) preparedness theory. Seligman suggested that people are born with a tendency to *learn to fear* certain stimuli that were in some way dangerous or lethal to our ancient ancestors. Therefore, because our 'caveman' ancestors were under threat from certain animals (e.g. snakes) or situations (e.g. heights, water, fire), we have evolved a predisposition to be wary of these stimuli (and so these stimuli are known as fear-relevant). The rationale is that if someone fears a stimulus then they are likely to avoid it, so the scared caveman would have avoided potentially lethal situations and survived to pass on his 'scared' genes.

Many students incorrectly think that preparedness theory means that people are born with phobias. However, Seligman only suggested that we are born with *a predisposition to learn to fear* these stimuli more quickly. So if we have a negative experience with a snake say, we are more likely to learn a phobic response than if we have a negative experience with a knife, for example.

Preparedness provides a very elegant explanation for why it is that certain phobias are more common (i.e. snakes, spiders, insects, heights, water, fire, thunder, open spaces). It also doesn't exclude the possibility that people can develop unusual phobias (e.g. a phobia of cardboard) because the theory merely says that we learn to fear certain stimuli more quickly. Finally, preparedness can also explain some irrational fears. For example, spider phobia is very common in the UK and yet there is not one species of spider in the UK that can do us even the slightest amount of harm.[1] Preparedness would explain this by suggesting that although spiders in the UK are not currently a threat, there might have been threatening spiders lurking around in our ancestral past. Box 7.3 discusses whether preparedness is a useful theory.

Box 7.3   Essential debate

Is preparedness a useful theory?

For one thing, did these stimuli really threaten our caveman ancestors? Although it's certainly true that our ancestors came from far and wide, there are remarkably few spiders on the planet that can actually kill humans. On a daily basis, the average caveman probably had more to fear from the ancestors of cats, woolly mammoths and the tribe next door than they did from the average spider. So why did we acquire a predisposition to spiders and not to other animals such as tigers and elephants (elephant and woolly mammoth phobias are rare!)? One answer is that we do have a predisposition to fear tigers and the like, but because we have little or no contact with them, that predisposition is never put to use. However, equally true is that our contact with spiders is usually non-threatening (unless you live in Sydney and annoy a Funnelweb!), so why haven't we learnt not to fear them? There is also a theoretical problem with making statements about evolutionary processes: in the absence of a time machine, we can never know the specific threats our ancestors faced. Although it's appealing to think that a natural disposition to fear would have helped them to survive and pass on their genes, we will never be certain as to whether this actually happened. The key point here is that the theory is *unfalsifiable* (i.e. we will never be able to prove that it is incorrect, even if it is), and thus breaks a fundamental principle of the scientific method.

---

[1] Useless trivia to scare people with: lots of spiders in the UK are extremely poisonous; however, they pose no threat to humans because their fangs are not strong enough to pierce our skin and inject their venom. Comforting thought, eh?

The Learning Model of Fear

So it is clear that, although we have some genetic propensity to develop fears and phobias, environmental processes have an important role to play. In this section, we will show how fears and phobias can be learnt.

Children experience general patterns of normative fear throughout their development (see Field & Davey, 2001). These fears often appear and disappear spontaneously and follow a predictable course. A wealth of research (e.g. Bauer, 1976; Campbell, 1986; Muris, Merckelbach, & Collaris, 1997; Muris, Merckelbach, Meesters, & Van Lier, 1997; Ollendick & King, 1991; Silverman & Nelles, 1989) suggests that normal fears follow a distinctive developmental course: during infancy children tend to fear stimuli within their immediate environment (e.g. loud noises, objects and separation from a caretaker); as they get older (four to eight years old) they typically start to fear ghosts and animals; just before adolescence they become more likely to fear physical injury; and in early adolescence they fear social situations and criticism. These fears are not usually phobias though, and are just a normal part of development. However, this developmental pattern does correspond to the retrospectively reported age for the onset of related adult phobias (see Field & Davey, 2001). For example, people with height and water phobias usually claim to have always had their fear (Menzies & Clarke, 1993a, 1993b) while the mean ages for the onset of animal, blood/injection and social phobias are 7, 9 and 15 to 20 years respectively (Öst, 1987). Yet this correspondence between the developmental pattern of normal fears and the onset ages of adult phobias does not mean that normative fears will necessarily develop into phobias. Experience is a key determinant of specific fears and phobias, and the role of basic associative learning mechanisms is discussed in Box 7.4.

Box 7.4   Essential research

Learning to be afraid

Almost a hundred years ago, Watson and Rayner (1920) conducted a now legendary experiment that showed how a nine-month old child, Albert B (or 'Little Albert' as he became known) could be conditioned to fear a white rat. Albert was pre-tested to ensure that he was not initially fearful of the rat, and that he was naturally fearful of a loud noise made by banging a claw hammer on an iron bar. Albert was placed in a room with the rat and every time he approached or touched the rat, Watson scared Albert by hitting the iron bar. After several pairings of the rat with the loud noise, Albert began to cry whenever he saw the rat (remember that initially he had not been scared of the rat). The implication from this experiment was that an excessive and persistent fear could be acquired by experiencing any innocuous stimulus in temporal proximity to some fear-inducing or traumatic event.

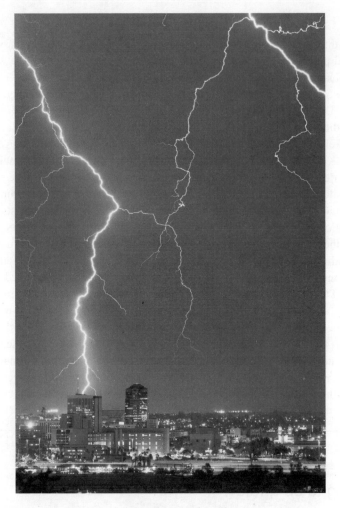

Figure 7.2 Can a single traumatic event cause a phobia?

Can you learn to fear something just from one bad experience? Dollinger et al. (1984) found that children surviving a severe lightning strike showed more numerous and intense fears of thunderstorms, lightning and tornadoes than control children. Similarly, Yule et al. (1990) found that teenage survivors of a sinking cruise ship showed an excess of fears relating to ships, water travel, swimming and water, and even other modes of transport than their peers did. Both of these studies suggest that a single event, if traumatic enough, can lead to intense fears of stimuli related to that trauma. However, it is vital to note that many people who experience very frightening events do not develop related phobias. Also, arguably, many of the examples given above describe other anxiety disorders such as post-traumatic stress disorder rather than phobias.

Mowrer's Two Factor Theory

The Learning Model of Fear suggests that people acquire their fear of a stimulus simply because they have come to associate this with a negative or traumatic outcome. Mowrer's (1960) influential paper extended this idea to a two-stage theory. In the first stage a person learns to associate a stimulus (an object or situation) with an unpleasant, aversive outcome, resulting in a learnt fear response. In the second stage that person learns that by avoiding the now scary stimulus they can reduce their fear. The relief they feel from this avoidance is very powerful, and acts as an incentive for further avoidance, thus causing a vicious cycle of avoidance and perpetuation of the fear (see Box 7.5). So, for instance, someone who has been bitten by a dog might start to feel afraid whenever they see a dog, and when this happens might run away, which then makes them feel much better. The relief they get from running away means that doing so is powerfully reinforced, and they are even more likely to run away next time they see a dog.

Box 7.5   The problem with avoidance

- When we avoid things we are scared of, we deny ourselves the chance of finding out that the object/situation won't really hurt us.
- When we avoid scary things, we will never find out that those nasty feelings we get in our body are perfectly safe, and that we are very unlikely to throw up, go mad, or die of fright.
- Avoidance feels good! Every time we avoid something we are scared of, we get a rush of relief. This relief rewards the avoidance and means that we are even more likely to run away next time, causing a vicious cycle of fear and avoidance that is difficult to break free from.

The Learning Model updated

The learning model is useful because it demonstrates how any stimulus could come to be fear-evoking (if you happen to be eating cabbage when a tornado hits your house you could develop an irrational fear of cabbage ...). However, Rachman (1977) pointed out that there are several important things that the simple learning model can't explain. First, not all people who have phobias can remember experiencing a traumatic experience at the onset of their phobia (we mentioned earlier that height and water phobics, for example, often claim to have always had their fear). Second, not all people who experience a traumatic event go on to develop a phobia. For example, not everyone who experiences pain or a traumatic event whilst at the dentist goes on to acquire a phobia (Lautch, 1971), and not all people who experience a traumatic flying accident develop a fear of flying (Aitken et al., 1981). Finally, based on learning, we would expect that all stimuli are equally likely to acquire fear-evoking properties, and yet there is an uneven distribution of phobias. Phobias of spiders, snakes, dogs, heights, water, death, thunder and fire are much more prevalent than phobias of hammers, guns, knives and electrical outlets, even though the latter group of stimuli seem to have a high likelihood of being associated with pain and trauma (see Field & Davey, 2001 for more details of the criticisms of the Learning Model).

However, the model can be saved through advances in our understanding of human conditioning processes. The construct of preparedness (discussed previously) can explain why we are more likely to fear some objects than others. To give another example, Davey (1997) has suggested that the likelihood of an association being made between a stimulus and a traumatic outcome depends upon a person's expectations prior to the learning episode. So, for example, if we expect something bad to happen when we see a spider, and something bad does indeed happen, then we're more likely to make the connection between spiders and trauma than if we'd previously expected something good to happen when we see a spider. These are called *outcome expectancies*.

Rachman's Model

So what is likely to influence our expectancies? According to Rachman's (1977, 1991) model, there are two types of experience, other than direct learning, that contribute to phobias: learning through observing others (vicarious learning) and the transmission of fearful information.

Vicarious learning (also known as *observational learning* or *modelling*) is learning something by watching someone else. So because of this we might learn that mice are scary because we've seen our parent standing on a chair screaming as a mouse runs around the floor! And indeed, it does appear that you can learn fear by watching someone else's fear. For instance, Gerull and Rapee (2002) showed that parents' faked reactions to a toy snake influenced the likelihood of their children developing a fear of it. If a parent pretended to be scared of the snake, the child was significantly more likely to show fear towards it too. Similarly, lab-reared rhesus monkeys learn to fear snakes just by watching videos of wild monkeys responding anxiously towards a snake (Mineka et al., 1984).

Fear information, for example hearing from someone else that a stimulus is scary, is another way in which learning can occur. This also seems to have some effect on fear beliefs: Field and colleagues (2001) demonstrated that fearful information (especially from adults) about unknown animals increased children's fear of those animals.

We also know that events in the past, and in particular the consequences of an event, can subsequently be revalued and come to be viewed as traumatic, even if they did not feel frightening at the time (see Box 7.6 below) (Davey, 1997).

Box 7.6 Essential experience

Revaluing of experiences (from Davey et al., 1993)

H.B. was severely spider phobic. She had lived in Rio de Janeiro in Brazil during her childhood and once, at the age of 10 years, when she woke during the night, a large tropical spider walked over her face. Although calm at the time (she did not have a traumatic experience), when she told her parents about what had happened the next morning they expressed extreme concern. From that moment on H.B. was extremely frightened of spiders and exhibited severe phobic behaviour. This example demonstrates how an initially non-traumatic event came to evoke anxiety because its consequences were revalued (in this case by the parents expressing concern at how dangerous the spider might have been).

Section summary

This section has looked at how preparedness can explain why certain fears are more prevalent than others, but we have also seen that this theory has some limitations. We have seen how learning processes can contribute to the learning of fears and looked at both the traditional Learning Model and some later developments of this. The next section looks at the ways in which individuals with phobias might think differently from people without phobias.

Section 3: Do we think ourselves into being scared?

The learning and preparedness models largely ignore the thoughts of the person with the phobia. However, it seems that some people actually think differently about threats in their environment. As a result, they become scared of certain stimuli or situations partly because they perceive the world in a different way. This section looks at some of what we know about cognitive processing biases in people who have specific phobias. There is an accumulation of evidence for the role of cognitive factors in anxiety generally, and so when reading this section you should also look at corresponding sections in the chapters on GAD (Chapter 6) and panic disorder and social phobia (Chapter 8).

Cognitive theories of specific phobias

Cognitive theories are based on the idea that phobias are caused by cognitive biases or mal-adaptive thinking. The learning explanations earlier in this chapter pretty much ignored thoughts and relied instead on fear responses being learnt at a relatively reflexive level. Therefore, these theories give rise to the prediction that to treat the phobia you simply need to treat the learnt behaviour. Cognitive theories instead assume that cognitive biases drive the phobia and cause the fear response. These theories then lead to a different prediction about how to treat phobias: if you treat the cognitions, the behaviour should vanish.

People with phobias do seem to attend to threat-relevant material more than non-phobic people: they show an *attentional bias* towards material related to their fear (attentional biases were discussed in detail in Chapter 6). Öhman and colleagues (2001) found that spider- and snake-fearful students took longer to name the colour of pictures of spiders and snakes than they did of neutral objects, suggesting that their attention was being caught by these frightening images. This experiment used a version of the Emotional Stroop Task, in which participants have to name the colour of words or pictures when some are threat-relevant (e.g. 'fangs', 'hairy' and 'spider' to a spider phobic) and others are threat irrelevant (e.g. 'chair', 'spoon'). Williams et al. (1996) reviewed the evidence from this kind of task and found that anxious people (and not just people with specific phobias) take longer to process threat-relevant words than non-threatening words, whereas for non-fearful controls there was no difference. This suggests that anxious people's attention is captured by threatening words and pictures.

People with phobias may also have reasoning biases that come into play when they are faced with the stimulus they are afraid of. For instance, in one study 15 people with spider phobias (and a group of people who were not scared of spiders) were told that they were about to interact with a spider. The participants with a spider phobia rated the spider as more likely to bite them than the non-fearful participants did. They also rated the injuries they would receive from such bites as more serious than the non-fearful participants did. Finally, when asked how reasonable and rational their fears were, the phobic participants rated their (highly unrealistic) fears as *more* reasonable than the non-fearful participants did (Jones & Menzies, 2000).

There are a couple of problems with the cognitive approach, however. First, it doesn't convincingly explain that these cognitive biases *cause* the fear. It's a chicken and egg situation: Does the phobia come from the thoughts or do the thoughts come as a result of the phobia? One possibility is that psychological disorders are learnt independent of cognition, but that cognitive biases act to *maintain* or *exacerbate* the feelings of anxiety. Second, all effective treatments for phobias contain a behavioural component, in other words they include some form of exposure to the feared object. It is very unlikely that cognitive therapy on its own would be effective, and to our knowledge, no researcher has ever tried this.

Section summary

In this section we have looked at how people with phobias might have cognitive biases or distortions in the way in which they think. Such people may selectively attend to threatening stimuli in their environment, and be prone to reasoning or thinking in a biased fashion about the thing they are scared of. However, purely addressing these cognitive biases would be unlikely to solve the problem, and 'behavioural' components are always used in effective treatments. The next section looks in more detail at how phobias are treated and how successful that treatment is.

Section 4: How are specific phobias treated?

We've had a look at various theories of how phobias develop. The final part of this chapter examines how these are put into practice in therapeutic settings. In reality, modern therapy typically tries to change both people's learnt behavioural responses (as described in Section 2) and cognitive biases (as described in Section 3). Cognitive behaviour therapy (CBT) for phobias blends exposure to the fear-evoking situation with cognitive techniques to help to reduce the fear.

How therapy for specific phobias works

As we explained in Chapter 2, therapy is usually made up of two overlapping phases: assessment and intervention.

Assessment

During assessment, the first aim of the clinical psychologist will be to take a baseline measure of a client's difficulties. An initial assessment can be done using validated measures such as the Fear Survey Schedule (Wolpe & Lang, 1974, reprinted 2008). Usually, however, idiosyncratic measures will also be taken, which ask the patient how afraid they feel in the particular situations that upset them. The therapist may also use Behavioural Approach Tests (BATs) to try to get an objective measure of the client's fear. In a BAT, the psychologist will ask the client to approach a situation or object that they are afraid of (e.g. a dog) and will measure how far they can get. These baseline measures are then recorded in the client's notes, and their progress throughout therapy is measured against them.

A second aim of the assessment is to develop a formulation of the client's difficulties. In order to draw up this formulation, the psychologist will want to find out several things. How did the phobia start? What triggers the phobia now? What does the client think and feel when they encounter the feared object/situation? What do they do when they feel afraid? Does anyone else do anything that helps or hinders?

A simple formulation of a client presenting with a phobia of spiders is reproduced in Box 7.7.

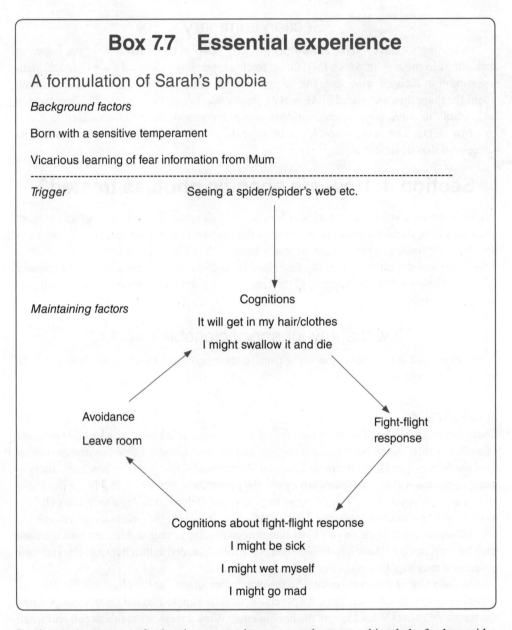

Box 7.7 Essential experience

A formulation of Sarah's phobia

Background factors

Born with a sensitive temperament

Vicarious learning of fear information from Mum

Trigger   Seeing a spider/spider's web etc.

Maintaining factors

Cognitions

It will get in my hair/clothes

I might swallow it and die

Avoidance

Leave room

Fight-flight
response

Cognitions about fight-flight response

I might be sick

I might wet myself

I might go mad

Sarah was a young, professional woman who came to therapy seeking help for her spider phobia. She had always managed to keep her severe fear of spiders covered up, but had recently got a new job in an old building that had vast numbers of spiders. This was causing her real distress, and she had considered giving up the job. Her phobia probably started when she was very small. Her mother had a phobia of insects, and Sarah remembered that whenever her mother encountered a spider she would scream and try to get out of the room as quickly as possible. Therefore, the psychologist hypothesised that Sarah had learnt part of her phobia from her mother via a process of 'vicarious learning'. However, she also reported that she had been a shy, quiet child, who got upset easily, and the psychologist suspected that she had been born with a sensitive temperament. It is thought that people born with these sorts of sensitive temperaments are at increased risk of developing anxiety disorders (e.g. see Van Ameringen et al., 1998).

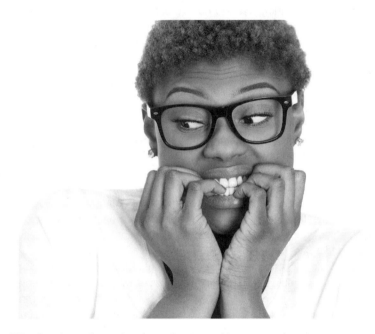

Figure 7.3   Sarah confronts her fears (portrayed by an actor)

The trigger for Sarah's fear was, not surprisingly, seeing a spider. However, because phobias *generalise* over time, Sarah now finds that she feels edgy and scared when she is in any room that is a bit dusty and has dark corners where spiders could lurk. The psychologist, James, assessed whether she had any distorted beliefs about spiders; he asked Sarah what she thought would happen if she came across a spider, and could not get away from it. Sarah was a bit embarrassed, but admitted that she had strong images of the spider running into her clothes, and getting into her mouth or tangled in her hair. She was also afraid that if she swallowed a spider perhaps she would die.

As a result of thinking all of these thoughts when in the presence of a spider, Sarah recognised that she would then begin to feel very tense and edgy, and an important process called the fight-flight response would begin (see Box 7.8).

Box 7.8   The fight-flight response

Think about the last time you felt really scared. What feelings did you get in your body? Just guessing here, but did you feel shaky, sweaty, sick? Did you have palpitations, want to go to the loo, have a tight chest or a lump in your throat? By any chance did your head or your eyes feel funny or fuzzy?

Now try to imagine something. You are a caveman, wandering the ancient forests, in search of your lunch. Unfortunately, you are not the only thing that is hungry. You turn a corner, and ahead of you you see an enormous sabre toothed tiger. He licks his lips. What do you do? Well if you are anything like the authors of this book you would turn tail and run. If you have your spear on you, and are slightly less of a coward, you might decide to fight the tiger to the death. But in order to run this fast, or to put up a decent fight, what does your body need to do? A quick biology lesson is perhaps necessary here. First, the sympathetic nervous system is activated and large quantities of stress hormones, particularly *adrenalin*, are secreted. These hormones act as chemical messengers, which instruct the body to prepare to *fight* or *fly*. The heart begins the powerful pumping of oxygen-rich blood to your muscles so that they can run fast or fight hard. In order to get the oxygen into your blood your lungs must start working overtime, pulling large quantities of air in through your nose and mouth. All of this blood has to come from somewhere, and so your body takes the blood away from parts of your body that don't have quite such an urgent need for it, such as your stomach and intestines. At the same time your brain will be working overtime, and may well be heightening your senses, such as your vision, so that you are well prepared to find a hiding place and detect further threats.

Okay, so how do you think our caveman's body feels right now? His heart will be racing, his chest will be aching, his mouth will be dry, and his muscles will feel weird. His head might feel funny, and his abdomen will be feeling the effects of having all that blood drawn away. Do you notice anything here? Well done if you spotted that the feelings we get as our body prepares to fight or fly are exactly the same feelings that we get when as modern twenty-first century humans we are scared of something. This is known as the *fight-flight response* and it is key to understanding anxiety disorders. Although as social and cultural beings we have moved on immeasurably since our days in caves, our bodies and brains have not, and we still respond to fearful stimuli as if we need to fight them or fly away from them.

All of the physical feelings that were caused by the fight-flight response were very unpleasant for Sarah. Increased arousal levels made her feel shaky and sick, and also made her abdomen feel tight, as if she badly needed to go to the loo. She interpreted these as signs that she might be sick, or even wet herself, although she had never done so. Sometimes the thoughts racing around her head felt so bad that she thought she was on the verge of going mad.

All of these frightening thoughts about being sick/wetting herself/going mad, made Sarah want to escape the scary situation. So whenever she saw a spider, or even thought that she might, she would move to a different room as quickly as she could. James explained to Sarah why avoidance is a problem when we are suffering from anxiety disorders (see Box 7.5 for more information on this). In short, the avoidance was stopping her from getting over her phobia, and meant that the next time she saw a spider she felt just as bad, and the whole vicious cycle started up again.

In addition there was another factor that Sarah and her psychologist, James, decided might be worth putting into the formulation. Sarah had a very sympathetic boyfriend. Whenever she saw a spider and got upset, Steve would go and remove the spider (allowing Sarah to engage in even more avoidance) and would give her lots of sympathy and attention which she found very pleasant. Although neither of them realised it at the time, Steve's behaviour may have been reinforcing Sarah's distress. This process, whereby a patient gets some positive consequences as a result of their symptoms, is known as 'secondary gain'.

A final aim of assessment is to establish the goals of therapy. The psychologist and the client need to work these out together. In this case the goals were fairly simple. By the end of the intervention, Sarah and James hoped that she would be able to handle a spider confidently and without distress.

At the end of an assessment the psychologist and the client should have a pretty good idea of what is causing the problem, and what they are going to do about it. However, a good psychologist will not leave it there: they will carry on gathering information as long as they are seeing that client, and will use this to update the formulation and then modify the treatment that flows from it.

The intervention

By the end of the assessment, the intervention has usually already begun. In Sarah's case, during the assessment sessions, James had been working hard to explain to her what was causing her anxiety, so by the start of the intervention she was already aware of where her problems lay, and also had a good idea of what she needed to do to sort those problems out.

At the start of the intervention, the psychologist will have a plan of action. This is never set in stone, and will evolve along with the formulation. For Sarah, the psychologist's initial plan was as follows:

- Use cognitive techniques to loosen some of Sarah's beliefs about spiders.
- Draw up a fear hierarchy for Sarah, and get her doing some exposure to spiders. Include behavioural experiments to further loosen her beliefs about spiders.
- If Sarah agrees, get Steve involved, and talk to him about not helping her to engage in avoidance as well as the secondary gain aspect.

1 Cognitive techniques
James began by talking to Sarah about what would happen if she met a spider. At the start of the conversation, Sarah's beliefs were as shown in Table 7.1.

Sarah could see that some of her beliefs were a bit outlandish, but because she got so upset about it she had never spent much time thinking logically about these. After a bit of time talking about her beliefs, and looking at the evidence she had for them, Sarah believed the thoughts about spiders much less. Also, James taught her about the fight-flight response, and

Table 7.1 Sarah's beliefs about spiders at the start and end of the first treatment session

Belief	Rating (0–100%) at start of session	Rating (0–100%) at end of session
The spider will get in my clothes	90	80
The spider will get in my hair	90	75
The spider will get in my mouth, and if I swallow it I could die	70	20
If I touch a spider, I will be so scared I will be sick	95	70
If I touch a spider, I will be so scared I will go mad	75	15
If I touch a spider, I will be so scared I will wet myself	65	25

explained that this was why she felt sick and as if she needed to go the loo. James explained that no one had ever gone mad as a result of a phobia, and that the spaced-out feelings she experienced were just all to do with the fight-flight response. Sarah's ratings at the end of the first treatment session are also shown in Table 7.1.

2 Fear hierarchy and behavioural experiments

Although the first session had gone very well, James knew that the only way to really crack Sarah's beliefs about the effects of meeting a spider was to get her to face her fears and test them out. This is called 'exposure'. So together, Sarah and James drew up a fear hierarchy. This hierarchy had, at the very top, the most scary thing that she could imagine, which was handling a large live spider. In the early days of behaviour therapy Sarah's treatment would have simply involved making her dive straight in and hold a big hairy spider. This was called 'flooding'. Fortunately psychologists have seen the error of their ways and are now much gentler. Instead of asking so much of clients in one go we realise that it is usually much better to do exposure by taking things step by step and working up gently to the scariest thing. So Sarah and James drew up a list of steps, starting with something that she thought she could manage fairly easily. These steps are shown in Box 7.9.

Box 7.9   Sarah's fear hierarchy

Step 8	Handling a large live spider
Step 7	Handling a small live spider
Step 6	Looking at a live spider
Step 5	Handling a dead spider

Step 4	Looking at a dead spider
Step 3	Looking at photos of spiders
Step 2	Looking at lifelike drawings of spiders
Step 1	Looking at rubbish cartoon drawings of spiders

Sarah and James agreed to start her 'exposure' to spiders by working their way up the hierarchy. For the first step James drew some very bad drawings of spiders and gave them to Sarah to look at. As she did this James asked her to rate her *subjective units of distress* (SUDs). This is a score (usually out of 10) rating how anxious someone feels at that precise moment. At first Sarah felt terrible and rated her SUD as 10 out of 10. James encouraged her to just accept the feeling, and keep looking at the drawings until her her score had come down to 0. This will usually take anywhere between a few minutes and an hour. After about 20 minutes, Sarah was so relaxed with the cartoon drawings that she was laughing, and reported that her SUD was down to 0. The psychologist also did some behavioural experiments, that is, he got Sarah to test out some of her beliefs about what would happen when she looked at the spider pictures. After she had done her exposure to the drawings, Sarah said that her belief that she would be sick with the fear, or that she would go mad or wet herself, had been fairly well tested out, and that she now believed these just 10%.

Clinical psychologists generally try to give homework to their clients. This is meant to consolidate what has been achieved in the treatment session, to prepare for the next one, and to ensure that the results of therapy generalise to the outside world. For homework James asked Sarah to look at the drawings for 15 minutes every day, and longer if she started to feel scared of them again.

At the next session Sarah was completely relaxed with the drawings of the spider, and she agreed with James that it was time to move on to step 2, in other words, more lifelike drawings of spiders. Therapy continued in this vein for several weeks, with Sarah gradually working up her fear hierarchy in exactly the same way. Each time, she stayed with the feared object until her SUDs had fallen to 0. Each time, she re-rated her beliefs about the effects that fear and/or spiders could have on her. By the eighth session of treatment she had triumphantly handled a large spider for the first time. She didn't even find it that scary. She was no longer scared of spiders, and was much more confident in general. As well as discovering that spiders couldn't harm her, she had realised that her anxiety could not harm her either.

3 Secondary gain

Sarah did very well in therapy on her own, and decided that she was not keen to have her boyfriend involved, even though the formulation had included a small role for him. The psychologist respected her decision, and instead they thought about ways that Sarah could get Steve to help her with her phobia. They decided that she would explain the formulation to Steve, and ask him not to collude with her avoidance by always getting spiders out of the bath. Instead he would give her loads of encouragement when she handled spiders on her own.

4 Maintenance and generalisation

Although Sarah had done very well in treatment, James was well aware that many clients relapse after successful treatment. This happens for two main reasons:

- Therapy is too restricted, and although the patient is fine in the psychologist's office or in their own home, when they meet their feared stimulus in a new situation they panic and don't cope very well.
- The client forgets to keep practising their confident new behaviour, and the old phobia gradually creeps back.

To minimise the chances of this happening, James asked Sarah to keep handling spiders as often as possible, and in as many different situations as possible.

Finally, James carried out a last assessment to do a formal check on how Sarah was doing. The questionnaires and the BAT all showed that her fear had reduced dramatically.

How successful is therapy?

Therapies for simple phobias have changed relatively little since the exposure-based therapies of the 1960s. This is because the evidence suggests that they are very effective. One well-conducted meta-analysis of treatments of specific phobias (Choy et al., 2007) found that active therapies (the majority of which were exposure based) had a large effect when compared to no treatment. The average person who got treatment was better off, after treatment, than 84% of those who had received no treatment. The same study also found that exposure-based therapies were more effective than non-exposure-based therapies. Therapy can also have generalisable effects such as improvements in relationships and increased self confidence, and it has been noted that exposure has cognitive as well as behavioural effects (Butler, 1989).

Section summary

This section has looked at how specific phobias are treated. We have seen that if phobias can be learnt then it must be possible to un-learn them. We have also learnt, however, that this is usually achieved by exposing someone to the object of their fear, rather than by purely attempting to 'unpick' their cognitive biases using cognitive therapy.

Essential questions

Some possible exam questions that stem from this chapter are:

- What is a specific phobia and how can it be treated?
- How has learning theory informed the treatment of phobias?
- Are phobias the result of maladaptive cognitions?
- Are learning theories and preparedness incompatible explanations of specific phobias?
- Does the success of exposure therapy mean that cognitions are not important in specific phobias?

Further reading

www.anxietyuk.org.uk/ (Anxiety UK is a UK-based charity for sufferers of all kinds of anxiety disorder. This great, reliable website is written largely by sufferers of anxiety disorders, and is checked by leading psychologists. It contains lots of information on what it is like to have an anxiety disorder, and about treatment.)

http://phobialist.com/ (This website is produced by a non-psychologist who has a strong interest in phobias, and focuses more on theories about phobias than on treatment.)

Bennett-Levy, J., Richards, D., Farrand, P., Christensen, H., Griffiths, K., Kavanagh, D., et al. (2010). *Oxford Guide to Low Intensity CBT Interventions*. Oxford: Oxford University Press. (If you want to know more about cognitive-behavioural treatments for phobias, there are lots of 'introduction to CBT'-type books around, and most will have a chapter on phobias. This good, modern one also gives you a feel for the realities of delivering psychological interventions in a hard-pressed public health service.)

Butler, G. (1989). Phobic disorders. In K. Hawton, P.M. Salkovskis, J. Kirk and D.M. Clark (eds), *Cognitive Behaviour Therapy for Psychiatric Problems: A Practical Guide*. Oxford: Oxford University Press. (This is a good, clear account of how therapy for specific phobias is put in place: it may look like quite an old reference, but things really haven't changed that much!)

Fisak, B., & Grills-Taquechel, A. E. (2007). Parental modeling, reinforcement, and information transfer: Risk factors in the development of child anxiety? *Clinical Child and Family Psychology Review*, 10(3): 213–231. (This paper nicely reviews the literature on the vicarious learning and negative information pathways to fear acquisition, with a particular focus on how parents might transmit fears to their children in this way.)

Wermter, A.-K., Laucht, M., Schimmelmann, B., Banaschweski, T., Sonuga-Barke, E., Rietschel, M., & Becker, K. (2010). From nature versus nurture, via nature and nurture, to gene × environment interaction in mental disorders. *European Child & Adolescent Psychiatry*, 19(3): 199–210. (An accessible overview of the gene–environment story.)

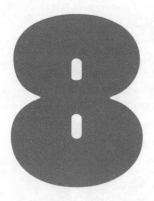

PANIC DISORDER AND SOCIAL ANXIETY DISORDER

General introduction

This chapter progresses our understanding of anxiety disorders by looking at two closely related disorders: panic disorder and social anxiety disorder (known as 'Social Phobia' in *ICD*-10). First, we will look at how clinicians diagnose these disorders before considering explanations of them. We examine the two most influential explanations for panic disorder: biological and cognitive. You will see that biological explanations are based on the idea that the fight-or-flight mechanism is oversensitive in people with panic disorder, and cognitive models describe the cognitive processes involved in a panic attack. Next we will look at explanations for social anxiety disorder, focusing on cognitions and how they lead people with this disorder to interpret social situations in a negative way. Finally, we'll find out how panic disorder and social anxiety disorders are treated, and consider the effectiveness of those treatments.

Assessment targets

At the end of the chapter, you should ask yourself the following questions:

- Can I explain the key diagnostic criteria for social anxiety disorder and panic disorder?
- Can I explain the similarities and differences between models of panic disorder and social anxiety disorder?
- Can I explain biological theories of panic disorder and demonstrate awareness of their limitations?

- Can I explain the cognitive biases that contribute to social anxiety disorder and panic disorder?
- Do I understand how social anxiety disorder and panic disorder are treated and can I relate the therapeutic techniques back to the theories on which they are based?

Section 1: How are panic disorder and social anxiety disorder diagnosed and how do they differ from each other?

This section will look at how clinical psychologists diagnose social anxiety disorder and panic disorder and explore some of the problems with the diagnostic criteria. As we've mentioned in previous chapters, it is important that psychological disorders are accurately diagnosed, but the process of classification can be very difficult. While reading this section, ask yourself whether panic disorder and social anxiety disorder should be thought of as different disorders, and whether they seem distinct from the specific phobias described in Chapter 7.

We will start by looking at the history of panic disorder and social anxiety disorder before describing their respective *ICD*-10 criteria and some of the problems with these.

Historical background

In early versions of the *DSM*, panic disorder and social anxiety disorder were treated as a single disorder, and in fact it was only the discovery that social anxiety disorder with panic attacks responded to different drugs from those for social anxiety disorder without panic attacks (Klein, 1964) that led to them being distinguished. Even though they respond to different drugs, theoretical models and treatments for the two disorders have a substantial overlap, which is why we will consider these syndromes together.

Diagnosis of panic disorder

A panic attack is a discrete period in which there is a sudden onset of intense fearfulness, with symptoms of breathlessness, palpitations, dizziness, trembling, nausea, feelings of choking, derealisation, chest pain, skin prickling, and many others (see Box 8.1). The individual usually fears that they are experiencing a severe physical or mental breakdown. This sort of experience is common in the majority of anxiety disorders. In fact a large percentage of us will experience a panic attack like this at some point in our lives. However, for most people these attacks remain merely an uncomfortable inconvenience, do not threaten normal activities, and remain isolated within the stressful period. So what distinguishes these people from those with panic disorder? The ICD-10 criteria for panic disorder are listed in Box 8.1.

Box 8.1   Essential diagnosis

Panic disorder

The *ICD*-10 (World Health Organisation, 1992) diagnostic criteria for panic disorder (episodic paroxysmal anxiety) are as follows:

A. Recurrent panic attacks, that are not consistently associated with a specific situation or object, and often occurring spontaneously (i.e. the episodes are unpredictable). The panic attacks are not associated with marked exertion or with exposure to dangerous or life-threatening situations.

B. A panic attack is characterized by all of the following:

   (a) it is a discrete episode of intense fear or discomfort;
   (b) it starts abruptly;
   (c) it reaches a crescendo within a few minutes and lasts at least some minutes;
   (d) at least four symptoms must be present from the list below, one of which must be from items (1) to (4):

Autonomic arousal symptoms

   (1) Palpitations or pounding heart, or accelerated heart rate.
   (2) Sweating.
   (3) Trembling or shaking.
   (4) Dry mouth (not due to medication or dehydration).

Symptoms concerning chest and abdomen

   (5) Difficulty breathing.
   (6) Feeling of choking.
   (7) Chest pain or discomfort.
   (8) Nausea or abdominal distress (e.g. churning in stomach).

Symptoms concerning brain and mind

   (9) Feeling dizzy, unsteady, faint or light-headed.
   (10) Feelings that objects are unreal (derealization), or that one's self is distant or "not really here" (depersonalization).
   (11) Fear of losing control, going crazy, or passing out.
   (12) Fear of dying.

General symptoms

   (13) Hot flushes or cold chills.
   (14) Numbness or tingling sensations.

C. Most commonly used exclusion criteria: not due to a physical disorder, organic mental disorder, or other mental disorders such as schizophrenia and related disorders, affective disorders, or somatoform disorders.

The severity of panic disorder can also be specified based on the frequency of panic attacks.

It is important to note that the panic attacks should be spontaneous/unpredictable, in other words the person cannot identify a particular stimulus or situation that causes them to panic. If a particular stimulus could be identified, then the clinician should consider a diagnosis of a specific phobia instead. The panic attacks must also be recurrent: a one-off panic attack, or even occasional panic attacks, will not attract a diagnosis because so many people will experience this.

Another similarity with other diagnostic criteria is that the symptoms must not be better explained by an alternative diagnosis. This comes back to the point that the diagnostic criteria should result in mutually exclusive groups of people (see Chapter 1). For example, if the panic attack is triggered by a specific stimulus (such as seeing a spider), then it may be better explained as a specific phobia in which panic is triggered by the feared stimulus. Alternatively, there could be a medical condition that better accounts for the panic attacks, although a diagnosis of panic disorder should not be immediately excluded, even if the person has a condition that is probably contributing to their panic disorder. For example, having an overactive thyroid (hyperthyroidism) is known to increase the risk of having panic attacks. However, someone *may* still qualify for a diagnosis of panic disorder, even though their panic attacks were initially caused by hyperthyroidism. Moreover, some people find that they still have significant panic attacks even after their illness is successfully treated. (When you have finished reading this chapter, try to work out why this might be.)

There are some problems with the *ICD*-10 criteria, however. Unlike the *DSM*-5 criteria, the *ICD*-10 does not require distress between panic attacks (e.g. concern or worry about having another panic attack). Therefore this would cover someone who had lots of panic-type symptoms, but was not worried about them (perhaps they ascribed them to too much caffeine or 'excitement'). Do you think that this is how it should be?

Box 8.2   Essential experience

Rob, 30, vividly remembered having his first panic attack when he was in his early teens. He was in assembly at school, it was a hot day, and he was feeling stressed about exams. He started to feel a bit funny and needed some air, but couldn't get out because he was stuck in the middle of the room. Since then he has frequently felt something happen to

(Continued)

(Continued)

his body 'out of the blue': in particular, he notes his heart beating fast, his palms and brow sweating, feeling short of breath and feeling dizzy. These attacks start abruptly, last around 15 minutes, and occur two or three times a week. At the time Rob feels like something terrible is happening inside his body and is terrified that he will lose control at best, or die at worst. On one occasion he experienced a panic attack when on a busy train, and he now no longer uses the London Underground because he fears the same pattern of events happening again.

Diagnosis of social anxiety disorder

Social anxiety disorder often includes panic attacks, but differs from panic disorder in that it is specifically social situations that trigger the anxiety. Most sufferers of social anxiety disorder can interact comfortably with certain people (such as close friends and family members), but will experience extreme anxiety in a variety of other situations. You will sometimes see social anxiety disorder referred to as 'generalised', meaning that it is triggered by a wide range of situations, or 'non-generalised', meaning that a more limited set of situations will act as triggers.

Most of us can relate to feeling anxious in certain social contexts, such as giving a presentation to a psychology seminar group. Even if we are very socially confident people, it is likely that we will have experienced some social anxiety on occasion.

Try this now: think of the most embarrassing thing that has ever happened to you. What did your body feel like? What thoughts were going through your head? What did you do in response?

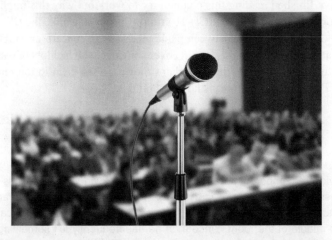

Figure 8.1 Most of us get a few butterflies when we have to give a presentation, but for people with social anxiety disorder, the anxiety can be overwhelming

Keep those thoughts, feelings and behaviour in your mind as you read the rest of this chapter. People with full-blown social anxiety don't just feel like this on rare occasions, but frequently, as part of their daily life. However, given that we almost all experience social anxiety on occasion, how does having social anxiety disorder differ? Box 8.3 outlines the *ICD*-10 diagnostic criteria for social anxiety disorder, or as it is known in the *ICD*, 'Social Phobia'.

Box 8.3   Essential diagnosis

Social phobia

The *ICD*-10 (World Health Organisation, 1992) diagnostic criteria for social phobia are as follows:

A. Either (1) or (2):

>   (1) marked fear of being the focus of attention, or fear of behaving in a way that will be embarrassing or humiliating;
>   (2) marked avoidance of being the focus of attention or situations in which there is fear of behaving in an embarrassing or humiliating way.

These fears are manifested in social situations, such as eating or speaking in public; encountering known individuals in public; or entering or enduring small group situations, such as parties, meetings and classrooms.

B. At least two symptoms of anxiety in the feared situation at some time since the onset of the disorder:

Autonomic arousal symptoms

>   (1) Palpitations or pounding heart, or accelerated heart rate.
>   (2) Sweating.
>   (3) Trembling or shaking.
>   (4) Dry mouth (not due to medication or dehydration).

Symptoms concerning chest and abdomen

>   (5) Difficulty breathing.
>   (6) Feeling of choking.
>   (7) Chest pain or discomfort.
>   (8) Nausea or abdominal distress (e.g. churning in stomach).

(Continued)

(Continued)

Symptoms concerning brain and mind

(9) Feeling dizzy, unsteady, faint or light-headed.
(10) Feelings that objects are unreal (derealization), or that one's self is distant or "not really here" (depersonalization).
(11) Fear of losing control, going crazy, or passing out.
(12) Fear of dying.

General symptoms

(13) Hot flushes or cold chills.
(14) Numbness or tingling sensations.

And, in addition, one of the following symptoms:

(1) Blushing.
(2) Fear of vomiting.
(3) Urgency or fear of micturition or defecation.

C. Significant emotional distress due to the symptoms or to the avoidance.
D. Recognition that the symptoms or the avoidance are excessive or unreasonable.
E. Symptoms are restricted to or predominate in the feared situation or when thinking about it.
F. Most commonly used exclusion criteria: Criteria A and B are not due to delusions, hallucinations, or other symptoms of disorders such as organic mental disorders, schizophrenia and related disorders, affective disorders, or obsessive compulsive disorder, and are not secondary to cultural beliefs.

In fact, if you look at the *ICD*-10 criteria, there isn't a lot to discriminate normal performance anxiety from social anxiety disorder, in terms of the actual anxiety experienced at the time. However, most people do not avoid the situations that make them feel anxious, and do not experience severe emotional distress as a result of the avoidance or their symptoms.

Box 8.4   Essential experience

Erica had always been shy, but in her teens things got really bad. She sometimes got teased at school about her acne and lack of fashionable clothes, and she began to really worry about this. Whenever she had to speak to anyone who wasn't a close friend or relative, she felt really nervous. Her mouth felt dry, and she was sure that she would just talk nonsense. She began avoiding certain situations where she felt self-conscious and might get teased, such as school social events. She put heavy make-up on her skin, and soon got that she couldn't leave the house without it. She let her hair grow long, and hid behind it whenever she had to speak to someone.

Prevalence, comorbidity and course of the disorders

Isolated panic attacks are very common: up to a quarter of the population will have the odd panic attack now and then. However, full panic disorder would only be diagnosed in around 2% or 3% of the population in a 12-month period (Kessler et al., 2006). Panic disorder, like all anxiety disorders, often has its onset in childhood or more commonly adolescence, and it is highly comorbid with other anxiety disorders: most people with panic disorder have (or will at some point have) another anxiety disorder too (e.g. Skapinakis et al., 2011).

Social anxiety disorder is more common than panic disorder, and, indeed, has been reported to be the third most common psychological disorder, after major depression (Chapter 5) and substance use disorder (Chapter 9). It is thought to affect around 6% to 7% of the population in any 12-month period (Kessler et al., 2005) and typically begins during adolescence (Grant et al., 2005), although children can present with it too. As well as being very common, social anxiety disorder is also a very persistent disorder. In one study that followed sufferers over a 12-year period only 37% lost their diagnosis, which was a much lower rate than other disorders (Bruce et al., 2005).

Section summary

In this section, you have learnt the key diagnostic features of social anxiety and panic disorder, and seen how they overlap with each other. We have recognised that occasional panic attacks and anxiety about social situations are fairly common in healthy people, but these symptoms cause severe distress and impairment of normal functioning in people who have the disorders.

Section 2: Can we explain panic disorder?

This section looks at various theories of panic disorder, first by looking at biological explanations, and then by focusing on cognitive behavioural theories. Note that these theories are not necessarily mutually exclusive. Sometimes the same phenomena can be explained on a number of levels and this is true of panic disorder.

Born to panic? Biological theories of panic

One of the most basic survival responses in humans (and indeed many other animals) is the 'fight-flight' response. We covered the fight-flight response in detail in Chapter 7, but to recap, the basic idea is that when faced with danger (e.g. a large tiger dressed in a dinner jacket waving a knife and fork at us) our body does various things to help us out: it increases the blood flow to our muscles (by increasing heart rate) and releases glucose and hormones so that fats are more quickly broken down into protein and sugars (the body's source of energy). It slows non-urgent activities such as digestion, and reduces the production of saliva and mucus to increase the size of the air passages to our lungs. The net effect is that our body becomes prepared to expend energy either in defence or by running away. If our body didn't do this, then when the aforementioned tiger came after us, we'd be slower to run away because we'd still be digesting our last meal, we couldn't get energy quick enough and so we'd soon become tired, and the mucus in our airways would prevent us getting sufficient air to keep on running! In short, the tiger would be very happy and we'd end our days passing through its digestive system! These sensations should be familiar to you – they are what we experience when we are anxious or feel threatened.

Box 8.5   The physiology of fear

The autonomic nervous system (ANS)

The ANS is the system in the body that controls visceral functions, such as heart rate, breathing, sexual arousal and digestion. Importantly, it controls the adrenal glands, heart, intestines and stomach. This system is kept in balance by two (usually) opposing subsystems.

The *sympathetic nervous system* creates physiological arousal when required. For example, it increases heart rate and activates glands to secrete hormones (such as the adrenal gland to produce adrenalin).

The *parasympathetic nervous system* inhibits physiological arousal. The parasympathetic nervous system tends to be dominant most of the time, and regulates basic functions such as digestion. However, in times of stress the parasympathetic nervous system takes a back seat, and the sympathetic nervous system tends to become dominant.

The fight-flight response is controlled by the autonomic nervous system (see Box 8.5 above). Ordinarily, fight-flight responses are inhibited by the parasympathetic nervous system until some external threat comes along, at which point the sympathetic nervous system leaps into action. The biological theories of panic are all based, to some extent, on people's failure to regulate their fight-flight response. For example, Rapee et al. (1992) found that if panic disorder patients purposely hyperventilate, or inhale carbon dioxide (CO_2), they are much more likely to have a panic attack (around 45% to 65% of them will do so) than healthy participants, *and* more than patients who have other anxiety disorders but not panic disorder. Therefore, some have suggested that panic disorder is the result of an overactive fight-flight response (McNally, 1990).

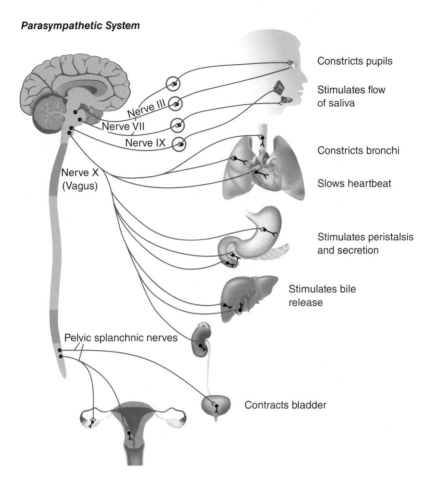

Parasympathetic System

Constricts pupils

Stimulates flow
of saliva

Nerve III

Nerve VII

Nerve IX

Constricts bronchi

Nerve X
(Vagus)

Slows heartbeat

Stimulates peristalsis
and secretion

Stimulates bile
release

Pelvic splanchnic nerves

Contracts bladder

Figure 8.2   The parasympathetic nervous system

Klein (1993) noted that processes that can induce panic (e.g. hyperventilation and inhaling CO_2) involve an increase in levels of carbon dioxide to the brain. He therefore proposed the 'suffocation false alarm theory', which suggests that panic disorder sufferers' brains are particularly sensitive to increases in CO_2. Humans need oxygen to survive, which fortunately for us is in abundant quantities in the air that we breathe on Earth. There is a little carbon dioxide in our normal atmosphere, but not much, and our bodies have evolved to cope with it. However, Klein suggests that panic disorder sufferers' brains interpret an increase in CO_2 as meaning that oxygen levels may soon become too low, and they will then suffocate, which triggers a full-blown fight-flight response.

There is also evidence for differences in physiology in panic patients' brains. The limbic system is the information pathway between the brain stem (which receives signals about

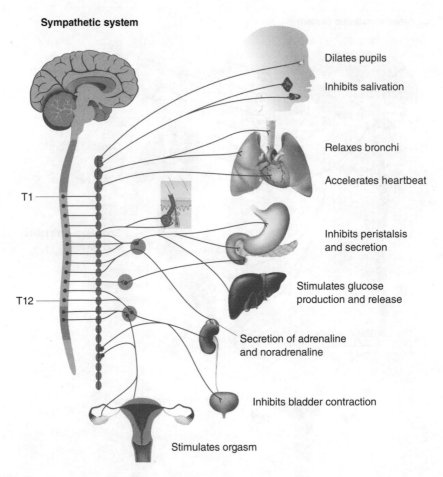

Sympathetic system

Dilates pupils

Inhibits salivation

Relaxes bronchi

Accelerates heartbeat

T1

Inhibits peristalsis
and secretion

Stimulates glucose
production and release

T12

Secretion of adrenaline
and noradrenaline

Inhibits bladder contraction

Stimulates orgasm

Figure 8.3 The sympathetic nervous system

bodily functions) and the cortex (where these signals are interpreted). This information pathway relies on noradrenergic neurotransmitters for communication, and Reiman et al. (1986) have found increased activity levels of these neurotransmitters (e.g. norepinephrine) in the limbic system of panic disorder patients who were having panic attacks. However, it's difficult to know whether this increased activation caused the panic or was merely a by-product of it. Likewise, panic disorder sufferers may have a deficiency in some neurotransmitters (e.g. serotonin) in the limbic system, which makes the fight-flight response hyperactive (so the threshold for a panic attack is permanently reduced). As for the other anxiety disorders, there appears to be a particular issue with the amygdala in those who have panic disorder, with studies showing reduced volume and reduced glucose metabolism in their amygdalae, compared to those without panic disorder (Roy-Byrne et al., 2006).

So are we born to panic? Well, it certainly seems that there is a physiological component to the disorder, but does that mean that it is inevitable in some people? The genetic research would suggest that this is not the case, with estimates of heritability from twin studies coming in at around 30% to 40% (Hettema, 2001), thus leaving a substantial role for environmental influences.

Thinking ourselves into a panic: Clark's cognitive model of panic disorder

Probably the most influential explanation of panic disorder is Clark's (1986) cognitive model. Clark believed that even though panic attacks appear, to the sufferer, to come out of the blue, there is usually a *trigger stimulus* or stimuli. These stimuli can be either external (e.g. a crowded supermarket) or internal (i.e. thoughts, body sensations, or images). The notable thing about these trigger stimuli is that they are perceived as threatening, and are seen as predictors of impending danger. This is the starting point for Clark's model, as shown in Figure 8.1. This perceived threat creates apprehension, which is associated with a variety of bodily sensations, such as an increase in heart rate and sweating. The key to the *panic cycle* is that these bodily sensations are then interpreted in a catastrophic way; for example, the increase in heart rate could be seen as indicative of an oncoming heart attack, or the fuzzy feelings in the head might be seen as impending loss of control or insanity. This process of *catastrophic misinterpretation* increases the perceived threat, and therefore the apprehension experienced. Now that the apprehension is even greater, the bodily sensations increase again and are again interpreted catastrophically, leading to an even greater perceived threat. It's easy to see how this process quickly becomes a vicious circle that culminates in a panic attack.

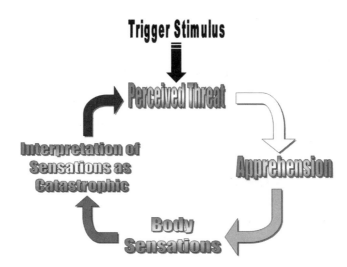

Figure 8.4   Clark's panic cycle (1986)

Box 8.6   Safety behaviours (Salkovskis et al., 1996)

These are behaviours that anxiety disorder sufferers sometimes engage in, because they believe that they will prevent some negative outcome. Typically these behaviours are counter-productive, because they prevent the person from gathering accurate information about the true state of affairs, and instead reinforce their biased view of reality.

An example in someone with social anxiety disorder might be avoiding eye contact to prevent them from seeing a negative expression that they fear might be on the face of the person in front of them. In doing this the sufferer never finds out whether people they are talking to really are looking angry, bored or disgusted (as they assume they are).

Another example that is sometimes seen in people with panic disorder is breathing into a paper bag. Breathing in and out from a paper bag helps to stabilise levels of CO_2 in the bloodstream and can therefore cut short a panic attack. While this is a good short-term fix, it can have negative long-term consequences. In not seeing a panic attack through to the bitter end, the sufferer never finds out that although it is highly unpleasant, they won't come to any harm in a panic attack. They won't die, go mad, or lose control. And because these negative beliefs are not properly challenged, future panic attacks are more likely (take a look at Figure 8.1: can you see why?). Also, this means that the individual must always have access to a paper bag, which although only a minor inconvenience, does mean that the person is never really 'free' from their difficulties.

Clark identified two other important mechanisms that are not in Figure 8.1. First, Clark suggested that once someone has developed the tendency to interpret bodily sensations catastrophically ('Oh no, my heart is beating fast again, maybe I'm going to have a heart attack') they will begin to repeatedly scan their bodies for sensations that might prove their worst fears. This is called *hypervigilance*. This internal focus allows these people to notice sensations that others would not, and interpret them as further evidence of some physical or mental disorder. So, for instance, it has been shown that people with panic disorder are often very tuned into their heart rate, and are much better at estimating their heart rate than controls (Ehlers, 1993). Second, Clark noticed that as with many anxious people, panic disorder sufferers engage in *safety behaviours* (see Box 8.6). For example, someone preoccupied with having a heart attack might avoid exercise, believing that this will help prevent a heart attack. Of course, this behaviour merely prevents the person from discovering that an occasional increased heart rate and skipped beats are perfectly normal sensations.

Box 8.7   Essential debate

How useful is Clark's cognitive model of panic disorder?

It is very difficult to prove models like this, but there is some evidence that this one has some explanatory power. So do people with panic disorder misinterpret their bodily sensations as signs of impending physical disaster more than other people? Clark et al. (1994) showed that successful treatment of panic disorder reduces the level of misinterpretation of bodily sensations, suggesting that this might be the case. However, technically this doesn't tell us whether panic causes misinterpretation or vice versa.

One very useful aspect of this model is that it accounts for both panic triggered by a state of heightened anxiety (i.e. some event unrelated to the panic attack heightens anxiety, or the anticipation of a panic attack) and panic that appears to occur randomly.[1] On the other hand, although it may be an excellent description of how individual panic attacks escalate, it does not explain why some people who have a panic attack go on to develop panic disorder, whereas others do not. Also, although most of the supporting research shows that panic disorder sufferers do indeed show all of the cognitive biases suggested in Clark's model, it isn't entirely clear whether these biases cause panic disorder, or whether having panic disorder creates these biases and they maintain the disorder. We also know next to nothing about how these biases develop (Field & Lester, 2010). There is very little research that has looked at whether these cognitive biases are driven by biological mechanisms or are learnt through experience or some combination of these. However, there is some evidence for both genetic and environmental influences on their development. For instance, Eley et al. (2008) showed that 30% of the variance in the way that 8 year old twins interpreted ambiguous, potentially threatening information was explained by genetic factors.

Box 8.8   Essential research

Do catastrophic misinterpretations of physical sensations cause panic attacks? Clinical psychologist Ron Rapee and colleagues set out to answer this question using a nifty little experiment (Rapee et al., 1986). They got 16 people with panic disorder and 16 people with social anxiety disorder (who were clearly anxious, but who did *not* have

(Continued)

---

[1]In reality panic attacks are rarely random: according to Clark's (1986) model they are usually triggered by some event such as standing up quickly, or palpitations caused by drinking too much caffeine, or by some threat that has been perceived outside of someone's conscious awareness.

(Continued)

panic attacks) into the lab. They asked them all to breathe in gas through a mask. The gas was a mixture of 50% oxygen and 50% carbon dioxide, which is harmless in small doses, but produces physical sensations that are similar to those experienced in panic attacks. Before breathing the gas they told half of the participants (half the people with social anxiety disorder and half with panic disorder) what they were breathing, and they described, in detail, the physical symptoms that it could be expected to produce: they were also told that these sensations were just caused by the gas, and would be short-lived and harmless. The remaining participants were told that the gas may briefly change their heart rate, but were told nothing else. After breathing the gas, some interesting differences between the groups emerged. Of those with panic disorder, most who were in the minimal explanation condition reported having catastrophic cognitions about the symptoms they were feeling: they reported that the symptoms felt very panic-like, and indeed many had actual panic attacks. However, of those with panic disorder who had the effects of the gas explained to them in detail, very few reported catastrophic misinterpretations of their symptoms, and very few had actual panic attacks. The authors took this as evidence that making misinterpretations about physical sensations can trigger panic. So what do you think happened to the people with social anxiety disorder? Well, very little actually. These were people who, although anxious, were not prone to interpreting physical sensations catastrophically, and when they got the symptoms caused by the gas, they didn't think these were anything to worry about and were therefore unlikely to experience panic, regardless of whether they had received information about the effects of the gas or not. Note, however, that the study was rather small, using only 16 people with panic disorder.

Section summary

In this section you have learned about about the biological and psychological processes that are involved in panic disorder, and have seen how these processes interact. Overall, it seems likely that both biological and cognitive factors are important determinants of panic disorder, and theoretical models based on these factors are useful. In the next section, we will look at models of social anxiety disorder.

Section 3: Can we explain social anxiety disorder?

Most of us will experience some degree of anxiety in certain social situations (e.g. when we're about to have a job interview), yet for some this anxiety will extend to situations that most of us will not find threatening (e.g. going to a party). As for all disorders, explanatory models of social anxiety disorder exist on a number of overlapping levels, including the molecular, genetic, structural and cognitive. As you might expect, there is research exploring genetic contributors to social anxiety disorder, and a meta-analysis of twin studies produced a mean heritability estimate of .65 (Beatty et al., 2002). Likewise, there is research exploring the neurocircuitry of the disorder. This tends to show that the usual suspects, the limbic and paralimbic areas, show increased activity, as they do in other anxiety disorders. In social anxiety disorder specifically, the amygdala, which is responsible for detecting and acting on danger, seems to be hyperactive when patients see threatening (or potentially threatening) stimuli, in particular faces, or when a patient is expecting to do something threatening, such as give a presentation (Freitas-Ferrari et al., 2010). Interestingly, when social anxiety disorder is treated, imaging studies show a reduction in this amygdala hyperactivity, and this is not just the case for drug treatment, but also for cognitive behaviour therapy (Furmark et al., 2002)!

The remainder of this section will focus on the cognitive approach to understanding social anxiety disorder, and will cover Clark (yes, him again) and Wells's (1995) influential cognitive model of social anxiety disorder. This is probably the dominant cognitive model, although other models, including Rapee and Heimberg's (1997), make very similar predictions. By the end of this section you should have some idea of the psychological processes that underlie this disorder.

The cognitive model of social anxiety disorder

The cognitive theory of social anxiety disorder proposed by Clark and Wells (1995) has three stages.

Before a social interaction: on the basis of early experiences, people with social anxiety disorder develop a set of assumptions about themselves, and about social situations that affect the way in which they interpret situations. For example, Hackmann and colleagues (2000) found that clients with social anxiety disorder frequently report experiencing negative, distorted images when in anxiety-evoking situations, and that these images are commonly linked to memories of adverse social events at the time of onset. An example of this is a teenage boy who remembered being mocked by 'friends' for being sweaty, and began to experience severe social anxiety afterwards. These assumptions lead some people to interpret normal social interactions in a very negative way. So, for example, in one of our lectures the authors might interpret the fact that some students are yawning and staring into space as meaning that they are being very boring (as apposed to a more positive interpretation such as 'All of my students have hangovers this morning'). These assumptions, and the perceived social threat resulting from them, trigger an anxiety response, which is characterised by three interlinking components: somatic and cognitive symptoms, safety behaviours, and how the person processes themselves as a social object (see Figure 8.5).

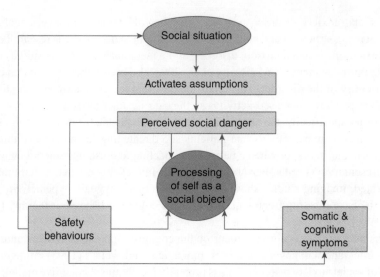

Figure 8.5   Clark and Wells's (1995) model of social anxiety disorder

People with social anxiety disorder also tend to engage in detailed thinking about the possible negative outcomes of social interactions prior to entering them (this has been called a *pre-mortem*). Recollections of past failures, negative images of themselves, and predictions of poor performance and rejection dominate these thoughts. This pre-mortem can lead to complete avoidance of the situation, or simply put the person in a 'negative processing' state, in which failure is expected and signs of social success are dismissed or simply not seen.

During a social interaction: Figure 8.5 shows Clark and Wells's (1995) model of social anxiety disorder, which involves similar core processes to Clark's model of panic disorder:

- *Somatic and cognitive symptoms*: these are reflexive responses triggered by the perception of threat (e.g. blushing, trembling, increased heart rate, mental blanks, lack of concentration, palpitations). Any one of these behaviours can be taken as further evidence of a threat. This, in turn, can lead to further anxiety in much the same way that the vicious circle in panic disorder is established (e.g. trembling, which is interpreted as obvious and embarrassing, leads to further anxiety, which leads to more trembling).
- *Safety behaviours*: as with panic disorder sufferers, socially anxious individuals engage in safety behaviours to reduce the social threat and prevent feared outcomes. These behaviours are often directly related to the outcomes that people fear (e.g. avoiding eye contact, grasping a cup or glass tightly to avoid their hand shaking, or avoiding speaking for fear of being evaluated negatively because of saying something stupid). These behaviours often have detrimental effects: for example, reducing eye contact and avoiding talking can be perceived as being bored by the

conversation, and clutching a glass tightly can actually increase trembling and might increase the risk of spillage. As such, safety behaviours can prevent disconfirmation of false beliefs and can even increase the likelihood of the negative outcome (see Box 8.10).

- *Processing of the self as a social object*: the crucial component of this model is that individuals with social anxiety disorder show a shift in attention. When they believe that they are under social scrutiny, they focus inwardly and monitor their behaviours. The interoceptive information that this yields is used to construct an impression of what they believe others think of them. They form mental images of themselves as if from an external perspective (called the observer perspective), that is, as if they were someone else looking at them. For example, a socially anxious person might assume that others notice that they are trembling and consequently think badly of them, and they will then form a mental image of themself trembling, which is viewed from an external perspective. As such, they end up in a closed-feedback loop in which internally generated information heightens their belief in the danger of a negative evaluation, and disconfirming information is ignored or avoided.

After a social interaction (post-event processing): after a social interaction, the anxiety does not necessarily subside. Social phobics tend to conduct a post-mortem of the social event, which typically involves thinking about the negative or ambiguous signs of social acceptance. The preoccupation will be with anxious feelings and negative self-perceptions and the ambiguous information will be reinterpreted as negative.

Box 8.9   Essential debate

Is the Clark and Wells's (1995) model of social anxiety disorder useful?

This model has quite a lot of empirical support. For example, when entering a social situation, socially anxious individuals seem to shift their attentional focus towards detailed monitoring and observation of themselves as a social object, to the neglect of external information (see Holmes & Mathews, 2010 for a review of the fascinating topic of imagery in psychological disorders). This tends to make them aware of the somatic and cognitive symptoms triggered by the perception of threat (e.g. blushing, trembling, increased heart rate, mental blanks, lack of concentration, palpitations). These reflexive behaviours are usually taken as further evidence of threat and create further anxiety (see Roth et al., 2001; Wells & Papageorgiou, 2001). Furthermore, people with social anxiety disorder use in-situation safety behaviours as coping strategies to reduce the risk of negative evaluations

(Continued)

(Continued)

by others (see Essential research Box 8.10 below and Wells et al., 1995). The role of post-event processing has also been supported by a neat experimental study by Cody and Teachman (2010) and by Rachman et al. (2000). Cody and Teachman (2010) studied students who scored high or low on measures of social anxiety and then video-recorded them whilst they gave an unprepared presentation. They were then given false feedback on their presentation (with mixed positive and negative comments). They also watched a presentation given by another student, and saw their (false) feedback, which was of similar quality, and also quite mixed. They were then given a memory test for the feedback shortly afterwards, and two days afterwards. The more socially anxious students showed a tendency to remember their own feedback as less good than that of the other students, even though it was in fact very similar. And over the course of the next two days, their memories of the negative feedback on their own presentations became even more negative, which was not the case for the less socially anxious students. Rachman et al. (2000) handed out a post-event processing questionnaire and found a significant association between engaging in post-event processing and experiencing social anxiety. In individuals with social anxiety disorder, recollections of the social event tended to be recurrent, and individuals with elevated levels of social anxiety spent long periods of time thinking about unsatisfactory social events in the past.

Additionally, post-mortem thoughts have an intrusive quality that interferes with an individual's ability to concentrate. Despite efforts to resist thinking about past events, socially anxious people have reported difficulty in forgetting or suppressing this information (Fehm & Margraf, 2002).

Box 8.10   Essential research

Safety behaviours

We have talked a lot about safety behaviours, but do they really stop anxious people from getting over their fears? Psychologist Adrian Wells and his colleagues decided to find out (Wells et al., 1995). They recruited eight participants with social anxiety disorder, and quizzed them about their fears and the safety behaviours that might be supporting them. So, for example, one participant reported having fears about drinking in public, in case she shook (and presumably spilt the drink) or 'went to pieces'. In order to prevent this happening, she used a number of safety behaviours: she held the cup with both hands, she gripped tightly, she moved slowly, she avoided using a saucer, she distracted herself, sat down when possible, used a mug (instead of a cup) when possible, and tried to relax. Can you see how these things may have actually made her feel worse? And can you also see how doing all of these things might have stopped her from finding out whether she would really shake and spill her drink and lose control?

Having identified the various fears and safety behaviours, the psychologists asked the participants to do two things: they entered their feared situation (e.g. drinking in public) once whilst using their safety behaviours, and once whilst dropping all of their safety behaviours. The results were interesting. In the situations where participants dispensed with their safety behaviours, they reported feeling much less anxious than they did in the situations where they used them. And in the situation where they dropped their safety behaviours, their belief that their feared catastrophe would come true also reduced, much more than it did in the situation where they faced their fear but kept their safety behaviours. The authors took these findings as evidence that safety behaviours can maintain anxiety, even when the person is engaging in exposure to their feared situation.

It's easy to see many similarities between the cognitive models of panic disorder and social anxiety disorder: both involve safety behaviours and bodily sensations as well as a cognitive bias in how threat is perceived. This is interesting, given that panic disorder and social anxiety disorder are treated as different disorders. Perhaps these similarities tell us that some common processes underlie the disorders. If this is the case, is there a value in distinguishing the disorders? Also, like the cognitive model of panic disorder, the cognitive model of social anxiety disorder does a good job of describing what happens to a social phobic when they are placed in a social situation, but it does little to tell us why social anxiety happens in the first place. How do social anxiety disorder and panic disorder develop? Why do some of us get it and some not? These are the questions that researchers are trying to address and which we touched on in Chapter 3.

Section summary

In this section we have explored the main psychological model of social anxiety disorder and have seen that this arises as a result of the same sort of processes as the other anxiety disorders, namely avoidance and biases in the interpretation of information, memory and attention. In the next section we will look at the treatments for social anxiety disorder and panic disorder.

Section 4: How are panic disorder and social anxiety disorder treated?

We've had a look at some of the main theories of how panic disorder and social anxiety disorder are maintained. The final part of this chapter examines how aspects of these models can be applied in therapeutic settings to help sufferers overcome their problem. We'll also look at the extent to which these therapies are effective.

Box 8.11   Essential experience

Behavioural experiments

As we have seen in this chapter, and in previous chapters, avoidance (see Box 7.5 in Chapter 7) is absolutely key to understanding anxiety disorders. People with anxiety disorders usually avoid stimuli (objects, places, situations) because they fear that if they encounter a certain stimulus something bad will happen. Overcoming this avoidance is fundamental to treating anxiety disorders, and so any cognitive behavioural intervention will include a substantial element of *exposure* to the feared stimulus. Exposure can be done in a very behavioural way, that is, the client will just be encouraged to approach the feared stimulus and stay there until they feel comfortable with it. This works fairly well. However, in recent years psychologists have increased the level of use of cognitive therapy during exposure, and now use the opportunity to conduct a 'behavioural experiment'. In a behavioural experiment, the client and the psychologist use the exposure to test out whether anything bad is going to happen to the client. So, for example, one of Sam's clients, a 16 year old called Tom, had social anxiety disorder, and was very worried about eating in public. In particular, he was worried that he would spill food on the floor and that this would be terrible. To start the behavioural experiment, Sam worked with Tom to work out exactly what he thought was going to happen if he spilt food. It turned out that he thought everyone in the café would turn and glare or laugh at him. He also thought that the staff would storm over and tell him off loudly. As the next stage of the behavioural experiment, Sam and Tom set out to find out whether this predicted catastrophe would come true. They went to a café, and bought Tom a large fizzy drink. After sitting for a minute or two, and going over what Tom expected to happen (and a few nudges from Sam), he deliberately spilt the drink all over the table and all over the floor. Sam and Tom looked around, ready to count up how many people were glaring and how many were laughing. Can you guess how many? Of course, not one person glared, and not one person laughed. A couple of people glanced over, but were clearly not that interested and soon went back to their own far more fascinating lives. Sam and Tom then waited for the staff's response. Would they come over and yell at Tom? After about five minutes someone wandered over with a mop, and after a cursory nod in Sam and Tom's direction, cleared up the mess. Tom's predictions had clearly not come true, and as a final stage of the behavioural experiment, Sam and Tom discussed what he had learnt, namely that our worst fears may not be totally accurate representations of reality, and that although testing them out feels scary beforehand, it feels great after.

Treatment of panic disorder

The National Institute for Clinical Excellence (NICE) has published guidance on how panic disorder should be treated in the UK's National Health Service (NICE, 2011). They suggest that, as a first line, all clients with panic disorder should be offered Cognitive Behaviour Therapy (CBT). If clients cannot be persuaded to have CBT, or if it does not work (or, as is sadly often the case, it is not available locally), then SSRI medication is recommended.

Drug therapy

SSRIs (or tricyclic antidepressants)   NICE suggests that CBT should always be tried as the first line of treatment for people with panic disorder, and that medication should only be used if CBT is not effective.

If the recourse to medication is taken, then NICE recommends that an SSRI drug should be used. If someone can't take SSRIs for some reason, or if the SSRIs do not work, then NICE recommends a trial of imipramine or clomipramine, which are an older class of drugs known as tricyclic antidepressants. These work fairly well (NICE, 2011) but have a number of unpleasant side effects, and potentially fatal interactions with some common foodstuffs, so tend to be used as a last resort these days.

Benzodiazepines and beta blockers   Before SSRIs were widely available, two other classes of drugs, benzodiazepines and beta blockers, were commonly prescribed for panic disorder. However, these drugs are addictive, and people can build a tolerance so they will then need increasing doses to have an effect. These drugs have some nasty withdrawal symptoms including irritability, anxiety, insomnia, seizures and paranoia, which means that some people never manage to come off them. They also show a 90% relapse rate when people do stop taking them, and interfere with cognitive functioning (hindering driving, work etc.), so it seems that they just suppress the symptoms without really solving the problem. It is therefore no wonder that NICE (who are normally very cautious about these things) say that benzodiazepines should not be prescribed for panic disorder.

Beta blockers (e.g. Propanolol) target beta receptors, which can be found throughout the body, particularly those areas that are under the control of the sympathetic nervous system. As a result, taking beta blockers can dampen down some of the symptoms of anxiety, and thus reduce panic attacks. However, they have a number of side effects, and a lot of people (e.g. those with asthma, which is frequently comorbid with panic disorder) shouldn't take them, so they are not so widely used nowadays.

Cognitive Behaviour Therapy for panic disorder

CBT works by addressing the cognitive components of Clark's panic disorder model. First of all, the triggers for panic attacks are identified. Despite what clients often think, panic attacks don't come out of the blue, but are usually triggered by something: sometimes this can be obvious, such as criticism from a boss. Sometimes, however, it can be subtle, such as an internal event that the client is barely aware of, for example a slight increase in heart rate. Diaries and structured interviews can help a therapist identify these events and build up a personalised idea of what is triggering the vicious circle.

Next, the therapist will begin some cognitive restructuring to try to loosen some of the problematic beliefs that the client is carrying. They will try to use evidence from the client's own life to challenge their troublesome beliefs. So, for example, if I were starting to have a panic attack in a lecture, some external event (such as a student asking a question) might distract me enough to stop the panic cycle. The therapist could then question my assumption that I was going to have a heart attack by asking me 'Is someone asking you a question a good cure for heart disease?'. The therapist will also use 'psychoeducation' to challenge some of their client's beliefs. So, for example, Clark (in Clark & Fairburn, 2007) points out that panic disorder patients who experience purely left-side pain can benefit from being given medical evidence that this type of pain is more likely to come from a panic attack than it is from a genuine heart condition. Psychologists should also educate their clients about the fight-flight response, thus helping them to understand the true reasons for the nasty symptoms that they get when they are having a panic attack. The intention is for clients to realise that these symptoms are not a sign of serious harm, and therefore to cut into the vicious cycle outlined in Figure 8.1.

Once a client is ready (i.e. when some of their most harmful beliefs have been softened up, and they have a good, trusting relationship with the psychologist), the psychologist will begin to introduce behavioural experiments (see Box 8.11) to test out some of the client's key beliefs. In the case of panic disorder, the therapist will aim to use behavioural experiments to test out their catastrophic misinterpretations of the bodily sensations of anxiety. So, for example, the therapist will often attempt to induce a panic attack in their client, to test out their belief that their racing heart means that they are about to have a heart attack, or that a spinning head means that they are about to go mad. When clients normally have panic attacks, they will usually do something to 'stop' their worst fears coming true, such as lying down, or breathing slowly and carefully. These safety behaviours mean that they never find out that their worst fears are untrue. So in this behavioural experiment, the therapist makes sure that the client does not engage in their safety behaviours, and *really* tests out whether their worst fears will come true.

Treatment of social anxiety disorder

NICE (2013a) has also published a document detailing how social anxiety disorder should be treated. As a first line approach, it is stated that clients should be offered CBT. If this is not wanted or available, then a client should be offered a self-help guide, and be given some support in working through it. Only if this fails should medication be considered, and this should be an SSRI.

Drug therapy

The NICE guideline for social anxiety disorder recommends that drug therapy should only be offered if CBT doesn't work, or if the client cannot be persuaded to try it. The evidence suggests that SSRIs are the most effective drug (NICE, 2013a), but that they are not as effective as good CBT (Clark et al., 2003).

Cognitive Behaviour Therapy for social anxiety disorder

Therapy using CBT focuses on core areas of the cognitive model of social anxiety disorder. The psychologist begins by discussing recent situations where the client has felt socially anxious, drawing out their specific fears and specific safety behaviours, and their use of the observer perspective. Once this is done, the psychologist will draw a simplified version of Figure 8.2. for the client, inserting that client's own idiosyncratic details. This process is done collaboratively, with the psychologist explaining each step, and the aim is to have the client agree that it is a good representation of what happens when they are feeling socially anxious.

The psychologist may then do a little cognitive work, in an attempt to loosen some of the client's core beliefs. For example, a socially anxious client might believe that everyone must find them interesting, otherwise they are a failure. The psychologist would ask the client to think about whether this is realistic, and whether they can think of people who not everyone finds interesting, but who are, nevertheless, successful people.

Pretty soon the psychologist will want to get to work on exposing the client to their worst fears. As we have seen already, avoidance is at the core of anxiety disorders and exposure is the key to overcoming them. So, the psychologist will set up situations where the client can test out their worst fears. For instance, if someone is very afraid of giving presentations, the psychologist might find a group of people (e.g. other people who work in the clinic) to form an audience, and the client will be asked to give a presentation to them. This will be set up as a behavioural experiment, and the client will be asked, before entering the situation, to predict the outcome in some detail. For instance, they may predict that they will vomit, and that they will be so boring that people will leave. The client will then give the presentation, and afterwards, together with the psychologist, will review whether these feared catastrophes came true. However, as we have seen above, sometimes exposure efforts such as this are scuppered by the client's use of safety behaviours. So, for instance, this client might 'avoid' vomiting by not eating for six hours before the presentation (and in doing so, make themself dizzy with hunger). If they survived the presentation without throwing up, they might well ascribe this success to their empty stomach, which is not what the psychologist wants. So the psychologist will ask the client to make sure that they engage in the exposure without using any of their usual safety behaviours. In this instance, the psychologist might actually provide some food for the client to eat immediately before they give their presentation.

Often, in treating people with social anxiety disorder, it is helpful to get them into the habit of trying to obtain objective feedback on their social performance, rather than simply relying on the way that they feel (terrible) to infer how they are actually appearing to others. So in the example we have been discussing here, the 'audience' watching the presentation may be asked to give their ratings of the client's performance. Alternatively, video feedback can be very helpful. Here, the client is video recorded doing the thing that scares them. They are then asked to describe, in detail, how they think that they appear on the video. Therefore a client who feels that they blush easily and that this is very obvious would be asked to show (using paint charts, easily available from DIY shops) what colour red they will appear on the video. They may also be asked to show how much they shake, or predict how many times they will stumble over their words, or to give detailed predictions of whatever other calamities they might fear. They will then watch the video and check carefully, guided by the psychologist, to see whether their predictions were correct. Unless the client really does have some social skill deficits (in which case the psychologist should have taken a different approach entirely), their fears will prove unfounded. The results of these exposure or feedback exercises will then be used to discuss whether the client really looks as bad as they think they do, and to open a discussion about how they might be overusing their physical feelings to infer how they appear to other people.

As is always the case for CBT, the client will be asked to carry out homework. They will be asked to continue to test out their fears, whilst being careful not to engage in safety behaviours. For example, someone who is afraid of falling over in public will be asked to go and deliberately trip, to see whether their worst fears come true (will people really point and laugh?). Alternatively, they may carry out a mini-survey amongst friends to test out whether their assumptions about other people's views and behaviours are correct. So, for example, someone who was worried about looking shaky, in case people thought he was 'falling apart', might survey friends to see what they would think if they saw someone who was a bit shaky. In most cases people will give fairly benign answers to this sort of question, such as 'I would think they were cold', and this can go some way to dispelling a client's fears.

How successful is therapy?

Panic disorder

There are now many studies that have investigated the effectiveness of CBT for panic disorder, and these show that CBT is very effective for this condition (e.g. Bergström et al., 2010; Clark et al., 1999; Gloster et al., 2011). For example, Bergström et al. (2010) compared group CBT with an internet-based self-help version, and found that around 63% of participants who had received the group CBT had recovered by the end of treatment, and surprisingly, so were 60% of those who received the internet treatment. At a six-month follow-up the results were maintained, and indeed those receiving the internet-based treatment were doing better than those who had group CBT. However, in researching this book we could find no systematic review or meta-analysis that had pulled all of these trials together.

A systematic review of the evidence for SSRIs found that they were better than a placebo, but flagged up the fact that the placebo effect was very large in this group of patients (Mochcovitch & Nardi, 2010). Finally, one systematic review (Furukawa et al., 2006) compared outcomes for people receiving medication and CBT with people who only received CBT. They found that while in the short term taking medication and CBT together produced better outcomes than CBT by itself, in the long term the outcomes for these two groups were very similar.

Social anxiety disorder

Powers and colleagues (2008) gathered together 32 treatment trials, and conducted a meta-analysis of psychological treatments for social anxiety disorder (most of which were cognitive behavioural in orientation). They concluded that when compared to a placebo treatment psychological treatments were better, and when compared to getting nothing at all they were much better. The average person who received a psychological treatment was better than 80% of those who received nothing, and better than 66% of those who received a placebo treatment. When they looked at the follow-up data (although typically only following up to a year at most) they found that these good results were maintained.

Fedoroff and Taylor (2001) also conducted a meta-analysis of studies that carried out trials of treatments for social anxiety disorder. However, they also included pharmacological treatments, and concluded that medication was the 'most consistently effective' intervention, just having the edge over psychological therapies. Yet they were unable to find sufficient data to draw conclusions about the long-term usefulness of medications, and as discussed in Chapter 2, there is concern that many clients relapse soon after they stop taking their medication.

Section summary

In this section we have looked at the main treatment approaches for panic disorder and social anxiety disorder, and have seen that there are useful psychological and pharmacological approaches to both. For both disorders, psychological (CBT) approaches focus on reducing avoidance to the feared stimulus, whilst being careful that the client does not engage in safety behaviours. However, we have also seen that no treatments are perfect, and far more research is needed.

Essential questions

- What is panic disorder and how can it be treated?
- What is social anxiety disorder and how is it treated?
- Should panic disorder and social anxiety disorder be thought of as different disorders?
- Is panic disorder caused by an overactive fight-flight mechanism?
- Compare the cognitive models for panic disorder and social anxiety disorder.
- What are the similarities (and differences) in the treatment of panic disorder and social anxiety disorder?

Further reading

www.nopanic.org.uk (Organisation for sufferers of panic and other anxiety disorders.)

www.social-anxiety.org.uk/ (Organisation for sufferers of social anxiety disorder.)

Clark, D. M. (1997). Panic disorder and social phobia. In D. M. Clark and C. G. Fairburn (eds), *Science and Practice of Cognitive Behaviour Therapy*. Oxford: Oxford University Press, pp. 121–153. (An old book, but still gives one of the clearest summaries of how CBT for social phobia and panic disorder should proceed.)

Wells, A. (1997). *Cognitive Therapy of Anxiety Disorders: A Practice Manual and Conceptual Guide*. Chichester, UK: Wiley. (This has chapters on panic disorder and social anxiety disorder, and gives a bit more detail on what CBT for panic and social phobia look like.)

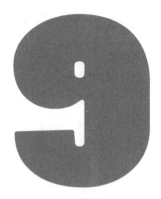

SUBSTANCE USE DISORDERS

General introduction

This chapter begins with an introduction to the clinical description and diagnosis of substance use disorders (SUDs), and we consider the distinction between what is colloquially referred to as 'addiction' versus less severe forms of SUDs. In the subsequent sections we discuss how SUDs develop. Importantly, not everyone who uses substances will develop an SUD, so we also consider individual differences and risk factors that increase the vulnerability to SUDs. Each time a person uses a substance it is ultimately a voluntary behaviour, so we consider the roles of choice and basic learning processes before discussing the psychological and biological theories that explain how addiction distorts these processes. In the final section we evaluate treatments for SUDs, and show how the effectiveness of various treatments can be understood in the context of psychological and biological theories.

Assessment targets

At the end of the chapter, you should ask yourself the following questions:

- Can I explain the diagnostic criteria for substance use disorders?
- Could I explain why any account of substance use disorder has to strike a delicate balance between 'choice' and a loss of control/compulsion?
- Can I critically evaluate the importance of brain adaptations and cognitive processes in substance use disorders?
- Can I explain why some people are at greater risk of developing substance use disorders than others?
- Do I understand how substance use disorders are treated, and can I relate these treatments back to their theoretical models?

Section 1: What is substance use disorder?

Diagnosis of substance use disorder

First, some history: earlier versions of the *DSM* and the *ICD* favoured the diagnostic label 'addiction', but this fell out of favour because it was perceived to imply character weaknesses or moral failure. We could write an entire book on how medical and societal views of 'addiction' have evolved over time (but don't worry, we won't!). Currently, the terms 'dependence' (*ICD*-10) and 'substance use disorder' (*DSM*-5) are used. The *ICD*-10 diagnostic criteria for 'dependence syndrome' are described in Box 9.1.

Box 9.1   Essential diagnosis

Substance dependence

ICD-10 (World Health Organisation, 1992) describes dependence syndrome as a 'cluster of physiological, cognitive and behavioural phenomena in which the use of a substance … takes on a much higher priority … than other behaviours that once had greater value'. In particular, a diagnosis of dependence can be made if at least three of the following have been present together at some time during the previous year:

(a)   A strong desire or sense of compulsion to take the substance.
(b)   Difficulties in controlling substance-taking behaviour in terms of onset, termination, or levels of use.
(c)   Physiological withdrawal when substance use is ceased or reduced.
(d)   Tolerance, such that higher doses are needed to produce the same effect.
(e)   Preoccupation with substance use, as manifested by the neglect of alternative pleasures or interests because of substance use, and the increased amount of time devoted to obtaining or taking the substance, or recovering from its effects.
(f)   Persisting with substance use despite clear evidence of overtly harmful consequences, such as physical harm as a result of substance use. For this criterion to be met, the user should be aware of the harm and that it was probably caused by substance use.

The *ICD*-10 also recognises the 'harmful use' of substances as a distinct diagnostic category characterised by substance use that is harmful to health but which does not meet the criteria for dependence syndrome. The previous version of the *DSM* (*DSM-IV*) also recognised the distinction between dependence and harmful use (abuse), but this distinction was abolished in *DSM*-5, which has combined abuse and dependence into a single diagnosis of 'substance use disorder'. The *DSM*-5 (American Psychiatric Association, 2013) criteria for substance use disorders are similar to those shown in Box 9.1. However, because it is a broader and more inclusive diagnosis, patients need to meet fewer criteria (2 out of 11) compared to the *ICD*-10 diagnosis of dependence. Finally, both the *ICD*-10 and *DSM*-5 diagnostic criteria have the usual requirement that substance use leads to distress and/or the impairment of social or occupational functioning.

Looking at the diagnostic criteria in Box 9.1, we can see that only two of the criteria relate to the physical changes that occur as a result of long-term substance use (tolerance and withdrawal). The others can be summarised as health-related or occupational harms arising from drug use, as well as a 'loss of control'. Someone would warrant this diagnosis if they continued to use drugs when these were causing them obvious harm in one way or another, and if they wanted to stop or at least 'cut down' but found it difficult to do so.

When the next version of the *ICD* (*ICD*-11) is published in 2017, the World Health Organisation may go the same way as the American Psychiatric Association (APA) and abolish the distinction between dependence and harmful substance use (abuse). Although still hotly debated (Hasin, 2012), the available evidence suggests that the distinction is neither meaningful nor helpful in practice. This is because substance use disorders exist on a continuum: the stereotypical 'addict', a person who has lost everything because of alcohol but keeps drinking anyway, would lie at the extreme end of this diagnostic continuum, whereas someone who has one glass of wine on a Friday night and abstains the rest of the time would not meet the criteria at all, and the (more common) person who drinks a little more than they should but generally functions normally might meet the *DSM* criteria for alcohol use disorder, albeit at the bottom of the continuum (see Box 9.2). For this reason, we are going to stick with the *DSM* terminology of 'substance use disorder' in this chapter.

Box 9.2   Essential experience

The UK government recommends that women should drink no more than two to three units of alcohol per day, because regular consumption above these levels is likely to be harmful to health. 'Sam' (which may or may not be her real name) abstains from alcohol on most days of the week, but every Friday night she goes out with friends in Brighton and they each drink a bottle of wine (10 units). What additional information would you need in order to decide whether Sam meets the criteria for alcohol use disorder?

Prevalence and harms associated with substance use disorder

It is difficult to estimate how common SUD is. Approximately 22% of adults in the UK smoke tobacco and most of them will meet the criteria for dependence (i.e. they are 'addicted') (Giovino et al., 2012). British government statistics from 2013 indicate that 39% of men and

27% of women in the UK drink alcohol at unsafe levels, and they would probably meet the criteria for alcohol use disorder at the lower end of the spectrum. However, only about 5% of the population would be diagnosed with alcohol dependence ('alcoholism', in old money) (The NHS Information Centre, 2013). Rates of dependence on illegal drugs (most commonly heroin, cocaine and cannabis) are relatively rare, affecting less than 5% of the population (Degenhardt & Hall, 2012).

All of these figures vary between countries. In predominantly Muslim countries the rates of alcohol use disorder tend to be much lower, whereas in developing countries the incidence of tobacco smoking is much higher (Degenhardt & Hall, 2012; Giovino et al., 2012). This illustrates a broader point: these estimates fluctuate over time in response to changes in government policies (e.g. bans on smoking in public places in many countries have reduced the number of people who smoke), social norms around substance use, pricing and taxation, changes in the legal status of drugs, and the discovery of new drugs. Given their negative impact on physical and mental health, SUDs of one form or another pose a major public health problem in most nations, as well as having devastating consequences for those afflicted by them.

Section summary

We have shown how SUD is diagnosed and we have distilled its core features: the negative consequences of substance use, physical adaptations (tolerance and withdrawal) and, most importantly, the loss of control over drug use. We have demonstrated that SUD in one form or another is common, but severe SUD ('addiction') is fortunately quite rare.

Section 2: How does substance use disorder develop?

There is a baffling range of theories surrounding SUD, and at first glance you might wonder how you could possibly make sense of them all. However, as with other disorders, it is important to realise that many of the theories represent different levels of analysis, from the basic cellular level, moving up to brain dysfunction and associated psychological changes, right up to very broad economic or sociological models. This means that a lot of these theories are actually completely compatible with each other, even though they might initially appear to be completely unrelated (for a general picture of this issue, see Chapter 1). We start with a discussion of learning processes and show how this links with the notion of substance use as 'choice', because this is a good framework on which to build everything else.

Basic learning processes: Classical and operant conditioning

Reinforcement and punishment are central concepts in operant (instrumental) conditioning. If an organism performs a behaviour that leads to a positive outcome, that behaviour is more likely to be repeated in the future (*reinforcement*). If a given behaviour leads to a negative outcome, that behaviour is less likely to be repeated in the future (*punishment*). So, if you give me a Snickers bar each time I perform a star jump, I will perform lots of star jumps for you. If I lick an electric fence once, I probably won't do it again. We also make the distinction between positive and negative reinforcement. A behaviour is positively reinforced if it produces a positive outcome, such as the delivery of peanut-based chocolate bars. But if I have a headache, aspirin functions as a negative reinforcer: it *takes away* my unpleasant headache, but it wouldn't be reinforcing if I didn't have a headache. The link with substance use should be fairly clear: if we were to perform the behaviour of injecting heroin, or drinking alcohol, a positive outcome (euphoria or feeling 'high') would follow pretty much immediately, and we would be more likely to repeat that behaviour in the future (*positive reinforcement*). Whereas if someone is 'addicted', they may experience an unpleasant withdrawal syndrome whenever they stop taking the drug. If they take the drug, the withdrawal syndrome goes away and they feel 'normal' again (*negative reinforcement*).

Classical (Pavlovian) conditioning is also important. Drugs such as alcohol and heroin function as unconditioned stimuli (US), and whenever people take them they will always do so in the presence of drug-related 'cues'. For example, cues such as the sight, smell and taste of beer (and simply being in a pub) are reliably paired with the effects of alcohol (US), and therefore those cues should function as conditioned stimuli (CS). In classical conditioning, when a CS and US are consistently paired with each other, the CS becomes able to elicit a conditioned response (CR). In Pavlov's classic experiment, a bell (CS) was consistently paired with the delivery of food (US) to dogs. After multiple pairings, the dogs started to salivate (CR) whenever they heard the bell. In a similar way, perhaps you can think of certain people who begin drooling whenever they pass a pub!

Classical and operant conditioning also interact in important ways, such as Pavlovian to Instrumental Transfer (PIT), whereby a classically conditioned stimulus (CS) that has been paired with a drug can initiate instrumental responding for that same drug. This process might explain how classically conditioned cues can influence voluntary (operant) behaviour. For example, if someone with alcohol dependence walks past a crowded bar, the bar functions as a CS which elicits a representation of the outcome (the pleasurable effects of alcohol), and this causes the person to perform the operant response that yields the outcome (walking into a bar, ordering a drink and drinking it) (Hogarth et al., 2013).

It is also important to understand how 'habits' develop from an instrumental learning perspective. As described above, voluntary behaviour is controlled by stimulus-outcome-response (S-O-R) relationships. We perceive a stimulus (e.g. a pint of beer) which makes us think of the outcome (in this case, feeling the effects of alcohol), and if we are motivated by that outcome, we perform the necessary response (drinking the beer). But with repeated performance of this behaviour, direct associative links are formed between the stimulus and the response. When a stimulus can elicit a response without retrieving the outcome (S–R learning) we call this habitual behaviour (Hogarth et al., 2013).

Addiction theorists have argued that the positive reinforcing (Stewart et al., 1984) or the negative reinforcing (Wikler, 1948) properties of drugs can explain why SUD develops. These two explanations are not necessarily in competition with each other, because we can acknowledge that both types of reinforcement are important. It is likely that positive reinforcement is more significant for drugs that produce marked euphoria and a fairly mild withdrawal syndrome (e.g. cocaine, cannabis), whereas negative reinforcement might be more important for other drugs such as nicotine (smokers report that once they start, they continue to smoke in order to counteract withdrawal). It is also plausible that positive reinforcement is particularly vital in the early stages of SUD, but as it progresses in severity and withdrawal starts to kick in, then negative reinforcement might be more important. With regard to classical conditioning, it has been well established that the presentation of substance-related cues (such as the sight of syringes, or vodka bottles) to substance users leads to a variety of reactions, including increased physiological arousal and a subjective craving to use the drug (Carter & Tiffany, 1999). Once we add in the concepts of habit formation and Pavlovian-to-Instrumental Transfer, we can see how these basic learning processes are likely to play a key role in the development of SUDs.

Despite this, these processes are not sufficient to explain the development of SUD. If they were, anyone who ever tried a drug would become 'addicted'. This is clearly not the case, because most people who experiment with drugs do not go on to become addicted. There are also other criticisms, which apply equally to 'choice' models of SUD, and we turn to those next.

Choice

'Efforts to understand addiction have crystallized into a cold war between the disease model and an alternative model based on the exercise of choice.' (Lewis, 2011)

Historically, SUD was viewed as a kind of moral failure and some people still hold this view (see www.guardian.co.uk/books/2012/oct/21/peter-hitchens-addiction-drugs-war). In essence, the argument goes like this: 'Drugs make people feel good. If they don't stop using drugs when their life starts to fall apart, this is because they are selfish and weak. They could stop if they really wanted to.' Indeed, if you think about your own substance use (see Box 9.3) you might agree that choice is involved each time a person takes a drug, and therefore people should be able to stop using drugs if they choose to.

Box 9.3   Essential debate

Do people choose to become addicted?

Think of the last time you took a drug. This might be the last time you drank alcohol or coffee, or smoked a cigarette, or did something else that you wouldn't tell the vicar about. Did it feel like a choice? Perhaps you engaged in some kind of private, internal negotiation ('My friends are going to the pub for a beer, and a beer would taste nice', 'But I have

---

to go home and finish writing my book!', 'But a beer would taste nice!', 'But the book won't write itself!', and so on), and eventually you made your decision to have a beer. Now think of a stereotypical alcoholic: someone who is severely dependent on alcohol, who has lost their family, job and home because of it. Yet here they are, still drinking alcohol. Do they drink because they choose to do so? Are they different from you, and if so how? This issue is depicted really well in the 2012 movie *Flight*.

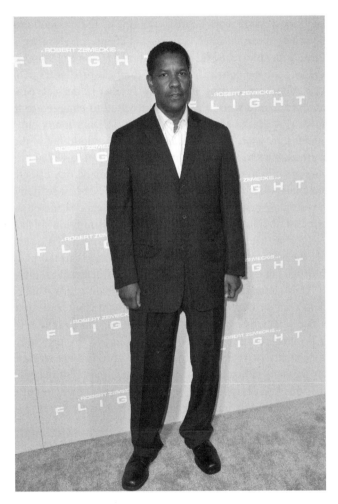

Figure 9.1   The 2012 movie *Flight* stars Denzel Washington as an airline pilot who struggles to overcome alcohol dependence

After having read the material in Box 9.3, you might form an opinion along these lines: 'People choose to start using drugs, but if they use them repeatedly then a disease called "addiction" develops, and this means that when they decide they want to stop using drugs, they cannot do this and therefore their behaviour is out of control.' In other words, drug use becomes *compulsive* because addicted people cannot stop themselves from doing it even though they want to stop, in the same way that someone with obsessive-compulsive disorder might feel *compelled* to repeatedly wash their hands.

The concept of addiction as a 'disease', in which repeated substance use somehow changes the brain causing people to lose control of their behaviour, is the dominant paradigm among those who research addiction, and in the majority of psychologists, doctors, nurses and counsellors who treat it. There is no single disease model of addiction, but we will cover the most important ones later in this chapter. Before we go there, can we defend the notion that people 'choose' to be addicted? There is some evidence that we can. In SUD there is good evidence that one of the best predictors of prognosis (abstinence or at least a reduction in drug use in the future) is the degree of motivation to change the behaviour: people who are really motivated to change are the ones who are most likely to do so (Prochaska et al., 1992). When SUD sufferers enter treatment they are often ambivalent: they want help to change their behaviour, but at the same time they have a lingering attachment to their current lifestyle that involves getting high, or using drugs to take away emotional distress (Miller, 1996). Indeed one effective treatment for SUD, motivational interviewing (discussed later), works because it increases people's motivation to change their behaviour. There is also evidence at the population level that increasing the price of alcohol and tobacco reduces consumption of those substances in that population (Skog & Melberg, 2006), but more intriguing is evidence that people with SUDs adjust their consumption in response to changes in the price of drugs: they consume more if drugs get cheaper, and consume less if drugs get more expensive (Petry & Bickel, 1998). This shows us that drug users are treating drugs much like any other commodity, such as cream cakes or televisions. Finally, it is interesting to note that token economies are a fairly effective treatment for addiction. For example, if cocaine addicts receive cash for proving that they have not used cocaine (by providing a cocaine-free urine sample), then many of them are able to give up (Higgins et al., 1994). We don't know of any trials in which schizophrenic patients were paid if they could prove that their auditory hallucinations had disappeared, but we can't see it being an effective treatment. If SUD can be 'cured' simply by increasing people's motivation to stop using drugs, does that mean that it isn't a disease?

Some people think so. For example, in *The Myth of Addiction*, Davies (1992) argues that drug users try to mislead clinicians about their drug use being 'out of control' for a variety of reasons, including to minimise personal blame or avoid going to prison. Other people such as doctors and politicians are happy to go along with this because it medicalises a problem that would otherwise be a moral problem indicative of a rotten society, etc. This is a very cynical view of addiction that minimises the suffering and despair associated with it. Despite these observations and arguments, 'loss of control' is a central feature of most theories of addiction, even though most theorists would accept that people can exert some control over their substance use if the incentives for doing so are powerful enough.

Finally, we should make some general observations on choice. People (including those who are 'addicted') are surprisingly unaware of the factors that influence their behaviour, but they are very good at thinking back and coming up with a convincing explanation for why they behaved in the way that they did (Nisbett & Wilson, 1977). What did you have for breakfast this morning? Did you weigh up all of the alternatives and make an informed choice, or did you just find yourself eating it? If we accept the view that people are not as in control of their behaviour as they might like to think, or even aware of the things that influence their behaviour, then there is no reason to believe that drug use is amenable to rational choice. Returning to Box 9.3, maybe the last time you (who are not 'addicted') took a drug, you were not as in control of your behaviour as you would like to believe.

Risk factors for addiction

Most people who use a drug once will not become addicted to it. This is evidently true when we think of alcohol, a drug which many people will consume all their lives without becoming alcoholics. Before we move on to discuss biological and psychological theories of addiction, we need to ask why some people develop SUDs and others do not.

Genetic influences: Are we born addicted?

According to Agrawal and Lynskey (2008), SUDs run in families: a person who has a close relative (parent or sibling) with SUD is at a greatly increased risk of being diagnosed with it themselves. However, family studies don't tell us whether this increased risk for SUD is transmitted through genetic factors, or if shared environmental factors are to blame. Other types of evidence have confirmed that genetic factors play a key role. Adoption studies reveal that an adoptee who had an alcohol-dependent biological parent is at a greatly increased risk of developing an alcohol use disorder compared to an adoptee who did not have an alcohol-dependent biological parent. Numerous twin studies (see Chapter 3) have demonstrated that heritability estimates for various types of SUDs, including alcohol use disorder, nicotine dependence and illicit drug use (most commonly heroin or cocaine) disorder, range between 30% and 70%.

There are some other things to note about the heritability of SUD. First is that we might ask if the heritable risk for one type of SUD (e.g. alcohol use disorder) puts someone at increased risk for alcohol use disorder in particular, or for all types of SUD. The answer is a bit of both: someone with an alcohol-dependent parent, for example, is at a greatly increased risk of developing alcohol use disorder, and also at elevated risk for developing any kind of SUD, although the increased risk for alcohol use disorder is more marked. The second important issue is that there are heritable influences on both initial experimentation with drugs (usually during adolescence) and on the development of substance use disorders (which usually only

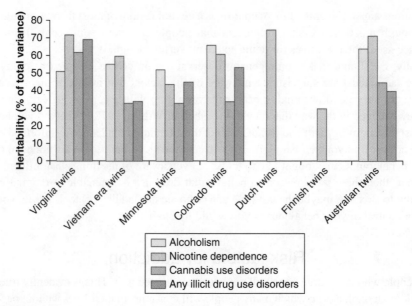

Figure 9.2 Heritability estimates for different substance use disorders (Agrawal & Lynskey, 2008)

become apparent during adulthood). However, these heritable influences tend to overlap with each other, such that an increased familial risk for SUD tends to manifest itself as earlier and more frequent experimentation with drugs, as well as an increased risk of developing SUD in later life (Agrawal & Lynskey, 2008).

Given that we have been successful at establishing that there is some kind of heritable influence on the risk of developing SUD, you might be wondering if we have discovered an 'addiction gene' yet. The answer is we have not, and the likelihood is we never will discover a single gene that increases the risk of one type of SUD (e.g. alcoholism), and it seems even more unlikely that there exists a single gene for addiction in general. As with the other disorders covered in the book, this whole area of research is full of examples of seemingly revolutionary discoveries of genes that appear to confer an increased risk for the development of alcohol use disorder (for example), followed by a long period of failures to replicate the effects and a lot of frantic backpedalling (Ho et al., 2010). Having said this, several candidate gene polymorphisms (mutations) have been identified for different *characteristics* of people with SUDs (endophenotypes), and it seems that each individual gene variant may explain a tiny (typically less than 1%) proportion of the familial risk for that SUD. To give some examples, different genes seem to influence the subjective response to alcohol, the rate at which alcohol is metabolised, and 'disinhibited' personality traits. Each of these factors, in isolation, is related to the risk for developing an alcohol use disorder (Edenberg, 2011).

Traumatic life events

If you were to ask any addiction counsellor what they think are the determinants of SUD, one thing would come up every time: childhood sexual abuse. The evidence supports this view: people who suffered abuse as children are at a greatly increased risk of developing SUDs as adults, and the degree of increased risk is directly proportional to the severity of the abuse during childhood: sexual abuse confers a greater risk than physical abuse, which in turn is associated with a greater risk than neglect (Andersen & Teicher, 2009). There is much speculation about why this might be the case, but one explanation is that severe stressors experienced during childhood, while the brain is still developing, may effectively serve to 're-wire' the brain so that people are less able to cope with negative emotions (and to regulate their mood in general), as well as less able to control and suppress their drives (Andersen & Teicher, 2009). It is not difficult to see how this combination might lead people to start using drugs in order to make themselves feel better, but then be unable to stop once their drug use becomes problematic.

When we combine the strong evidence for effects of childhood abuse on SUDs with the evidence that SUDs are heritable, we can see why being raised by an alcoholic parent leads to a greatly increased risk that a child will develop SUD in later life, because an alcoholic parent is, arguably, more likely to at least neglect their child, and perhaps more likely to physically abuse them as well. It is also very notable that severe life stressors are known to precede the development of SUDs in adults, which might occur because people turn to drugs in order to cope with their negative emotions (Brady et al., 2004).

Section summary

In this section we have introduced the basic learning mechanisms and decision-making processes (choices) that are involved in substance use. In the next section we discuss theoretical models that try to account for how these processes become subverted or 'hijacked' in SUD. We have also discussed risk factors for addiction that might help to explain why not everyone who uses drugs becomes dependent on them. We have shown that SUDs are heritable, although we don't yet have a full picture of how this genetic influence might exert its effect. It is also clear that adverse life events, particularly traumatic events during during childhood, increase the risk.

Section 3: Brain and cognitive mechanisms in SUD

The most frequently identified flaw in 'choice' accounts of SUD (Heyman, 1996) is that this is defined by the presence of a 'loss of control, or compulsive substance use: both the *ICD*-10 and *DSM*-5 criteria are explicit in that they refer to continued substance use even when people say that they would rather abstain. As described above, some people take issue with this because even if sufferers claim that they would rather abstain, they might not be telling the truth! Furthermore, motivational ambivalence is a well-documented feature of SUD sufferers in treatment: they might claim that they want to abstain, and mean it, but they often have a lingering attachment to their lifestyle in which drug use plays a major role. A more fundamental concern is that as SUD progresses, the negative consequences of drug use appear to outweigh the positives. For example, tolerance develops, meaning that the 'high' might not be as good as it used to be, whereas the costs rack up: poor health, loss of job, relationship problems, and so on. At some stage drug users reach a point at which the negatives outweigh the positives, and surely if drug use were simply down to choice, people would choose to stop. This is also the limitation of a simple operant (instrumental) conditioning account: if a voluntary behaviour (taking drugs) produces more negative consequences than positive consequences, that behaviour should extinguish of its own accord.

Theories of compulsive drug use fall into many categories, but here we will focus on the models that have been most influential over the past 20 years or so. These can be broken down into neurobiological and cognitive models.

Biological theories

Drugs of abuse (alcohol, heroin, cocaine, nicotine etc.) have a variety of different actions in the brain, but one thing that they have in common is that they all stimulate dopamine release in the brain's 'reward system', a pathway called the mesolimbic dopamine system that includes the nucleus accumbens, ventral tegmental area, and some regions of the prefrontal cortex. Other things which are rewarding, such as the consumption of sugary foods, also stimulate dopamine release in this system. Therefore this dopamine system was once widely held to be the brain's 'pleasure centre', although this simplistic view has since been challenged.

If both drugs and 'natural' rewards (such as food) stimulate dopamine release in the mesolimbic dopamine system, then why are we more likely to become addicted to drugs than natural rewards? We might speculate that the magnitude of dopamine release produced by drugs is larger than that produced by natural rewards. However, this isn't the case: the surge in dopamine produced by nicotine (for example) is pretty similar to that produced by food. The dopamine activity produced by food and nicotine does differ in one important way though: with repeated administration of food, the 'spike' in dopamine release tends to decline in magnitude, a process known as habituation, whereas the spike in dopamine release produced by nicotine tends to remain fairly consistent, even with repeated administrations. Some evidence suggests that drug-induced dopamine release may even increase with repeated administration, a process known as 'sensitization' (Boileau et al., 2006).

Dopamine plays a key role in classical conditioning. If we expose rats to pairings between a conditioned stimulus (CS) and an unconditioned stimulus (US) – let's say a tone and delivery of food pellets respectively – then we will initially observe that dopamine activity is unaffected by the CS, but we see a big spike in dopamine activity when the rat is eating the food pellets. However, after repeated CS–US pairings, an interesting shift occurs: the spike in dopamine activity now peaks whenever the CS is presented, whereas we may see no change at all in dopamine activity when the rat is consuming the food pellet. So it appears that dopamine release peaks when organisms *expect to receive a reward*, but not when they are actually consuming it (Schultz, 2013)!

One of the most influential models of SUD attempts to make sense of addiction by reframing the role of dopamine. In their incentive-sensitisation theory, Robinson and Berridge (1993) proposed that repeated drug use leads to a sensitised (progressively increasing) spike in activity in the mesolimbic dopamine system. Importantly, this dopamine response is not seen when the person (or lab rat) is experiencing the effect of the drug, but when they are exposed to drug-related cues (such as the sight of syringes, or white powder). According to the theory, this exaggerated dopamine response to drug-related cues manifests itself as increased 'incentive salience': the cues have powerful incentive motivational properties, which increase the motivation to consume the drug (which addicts experience as 'craving') and thereby also increase the instrumental responding to the drug. Robinson and Berridge called this process drug 'wanting', and they distinguished it from drug 'liking', which is the degree of subjective pleasure that addicts experience when they take the drug. Therefore the theory proposes that dopamine dysfunction lies at the root of addiction, but this has nothing to do with the pleasure produced by drug effects, and everything to do with abnormal learning about the motivational properties of drug-related cues. In principle, this model can explain one of the core features of SUD: why addicts are increasingly motivated to take a drug, even when they are enjoying the effects less and less.

A competing model, the 'hedonic homeostatic dysregulation' theory, also proposes that a malfunction of the dopamine system lies at the heart of SUD. Koob and Le Moal (1997) proposed that repeated drug use, which produces repeated spikes of dopamine activity, eventually leads to the long-term suppression of the dopamine function. According to this theory the brain adapts to the repeated increases in dopamine activity, which are followed by decreases in dopamine activity during drug withdrawal by lowering the 'set point' or the 'normal' level of dopamine activity. This theory proposes that dopamine is involved in the regulation of mood, and so the consequence of this lowered set point is that addicts become increasingly miserable and unable to experience pleasure. The only respite comes when they take drugs, which briefly returns the dopamine to an acceptable level, but in the long term only exacerbates the underlying problem.

These two models make quite different predictions yet both can call on evidence in their favour. On the one hand, there is evidence for dopaminergic sensitisation as a result of repeated drug use in laboratory animals (Robinson & Berridge, 1993), and the notion that people can 'want' drugs even when they no longer 'like' their effects has considerable intuitive appeal when we consider the core features of SUD (see Box 9.1). On the other hand, studies of brain function suggest that dopamine activity in the mesolimbic system is suppressed in addicts (which is more consistent with the hedonic homeostatic dysregulation model), and that when addicts are given a drug which increases dopamine function they show a blunted rather than a sensitised dopamine response compared to non-addicts who are given the same drug (Murphy et al., 2012; Volkow et al., 2004). This is clearly not consistent with predictions made by incentive-sensitisation theory. In addition, some studies suggest that rising dopamine levels are associated with euphoria ('liking') rather than craving ('wanting') when cocaine addicts are given cocaine while in an fMRI scanner (Volkow et al., 2004), although this pattern of results has been questioned (Murphy et al., 2012).

There is still considerable debate about which of these two models is 'correct', although they may both explain something about addiction: dopamine sensitisation might occur in the early stages of SUD, whereas hedonic homeostatic dysregulation could be more important in the later stages. Another suggestion is that the dopaminergic response to drug-related *cues* is sensitised (as predicted by incentive-sensitisation theory), whereas the dopaminergic response during the *consumption* of rewards is blunted (as predicted by hedonic homeostatic dysregulation theory). If this is the case, people with SUDs would be powerfully motivated by drug-related cues, but would get reduced enjoyment when they actually consume things that healthy people would find rewarding (Murphy et al., 2012).

Other models of SUD suggest dysfunction in other areas of the brain, in addition to the reward system. For example, Jentsch and Taylor (1999) proposed that repeated drug use led to sensitisation in the mesolimbic dopamine system, resulting in increased 'wanting' and compulsive behaviour produced by drug-associated cues, but this is combined with damage to areas of the prefrontal cortex, which manifests itself as reduced control over motivational states. According to this model, and others like it, the brains of people with SUD become reconfigured such that they have increased the motivation to use drugs, combined with a reduced ability to suppress that motivation and control their drug use. There is compelling evidence that people with SUD have reduced function in the prefrontal cortex, and this is associated with poor performance on behavioural tests of self-control (Murphy et al., 2012). However, it is hard to say whether this is a *result* of drug use over many years, or whether people with SUD had a dysfunctional prefrontal cortex *before* they started using drugs, in which case this pattern of brain activation (which is associated with poor self-control) might be a risk factor for the development of SUD, as suggested by some studies (e.g. Giancola & Tarter, 1999, and see Box 9.4). Importantly, there is evidence from laboratory animals that repeated exposure to some drugs, such as cocaine, can damage the prefrontal cortex and cause corresponding decreases in self-control (Simon et al., 2007).

Box 9.4   Essential research

Using twin studies to untangle the relationships between cocaine dependence, brain abnormalities and poor self-control

People with cocaine dependence perform badly on laboratory tests for self-control and this is associated with impaired functioning of the prefrontal cortex. However, it is unclear whether this arises as a consequence of cocaine use over a long period of time, or whether the heritable risk for addiction (see Section 2) causes abnormalities in brain structure and function that lead to poor self-control and make people more likely to become addicted to cocaine in the first place. Twin studies are one way to investigate this issue. In an ingenious study, Ersche et al. (2012) looked at 50 pairs of identical twins, one of whom was dependent on cocaine and the other not. They also included 50 healthy volunteers for comparison. They found that, compared to the healthy volunteers, both cocaine-dependent individuals and their twins (who did not use cocaine) performed poorly on a test of self-control (the stop-signal task) and they had abnormally structured sub-regions of the prefrontal cortex (the regions that were active when they completed this task).

This study suggests that instead of being a consequence of cocaine use, the 'brain damage' and associated impairments in self-control that are associated with cocaine addiction may actually represent part of the heritable 'endophenotype' for cocaine addiction. However, this study also revealed that the severity of brain damage was associated with the number of years that the cocaine users had been addicted, which alongside animal research demonstrates that cocaine almost certainly does have toxic effects in the brain. Overall, the study shows that previous researchers probably underestimated the degree to which brain and psychological dysfunction is evident *before* people start using cocaine, and this is heritable. However, it doesn't mean that taking lots of cocaine is not harmful to the brain!

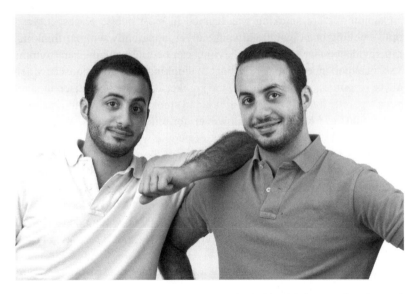

Figure 9.3 An important twin study suggests that heritable risk for cocaine dependence is associated with impaired self-control and subtle abnormalities of brain structure

Finally, there is a general acceptance that some kind of dopamine dysfunction is implicated in SUD, but we also know that this is not the only neurotransmitter to be involved. Other neurotransmitter systems also adapt to repeated drug use, including glutamate, GABA, opioids and acetylcholine (Koob & Volkow, 2010). It seems likely that long-term changes in the function of these neurotransmitters, and their interactions with dopamine, also play a key role in our understanding of SUD.

Cognitive theories

Tiffany (1990) proposed a model of automaticity in SUD that has been very influential. It is essentially a formal model of the development of habits which were introduced earlier in the chapter. The central argument is that drug use starts out as completely voluntary, or *non-automatic*, in the sense that people perform the behaviour (e.g. raising a wine glass to the lips and drinking) because they are motivated to achieve an outcome (in this case, feeling the effects of alcohol). But with repeated performance of these actions, self-administration of drugs becomes *automatic*: people take drugs habitually, without even thinking about the consequences of their actions. The theory states that in the experienced drug user most instances of drug use are automatic, although non-automatic processes play a role some of the time. Another important prediction made by the model is that subjective craving is not a very important determinant of drug use: normally drug use is automatic, but people only experience craving when they have to engage non-automatic processes in order to obtain and then take drugs.

Tiffany's model has considerable intuitive appeal when we think about some addictions. For example, before smoking was banned in most public places, it was common to see people smoking one cigarette after the other, apparently without thinking. Indeed, there is some evidence that smoking behaviour can be understood as an 'automatic' process because, in experienced smokers, the act of smoking does not impose any demands on their cognitive resources, in other words, the smoker is so well-practised at smoking that they can get a cigarette out of the pack, light it and smoke it almost without expending any mental effort at all (Field et al., 2006). However, for other addictions, we have to question how widely the model can be applied. Think of people who are addicted to illegal drugs: a lot of planning is required to obtain the drug from their dealer, and in deciding where to take it, out of sight of the police. This is also true of many alcoholics, who have to go to considerable effort to disguise their drinking from others. Now that smoking has been banned in public places this is now also true for smokers, who might have to walk quite far to find somewhere that they can smoke. So even if we acknowledge that habitual or automatic processes might play a role in addiction, it is likely that they play a less important role than Tiffany originally proposed.

Another limitation of Tiffany's model is that it assumes that most SUD sufferers are automatons, robotically injecting heroin into their groin whenever they see a syringe (to give an extreme example). But there is no role for motivation in all of this: according to the model, people don't compulsively take drugs because of some problem with their motivation to use the drug (or their lack of ability to control themselves), they simply do so because S–R habits have become so entrenched. This absence of a motivational influence on SUD has been criticised by proponents of dual-process models.

According to the dual-process theory of addiction (Stacy & Wiers, 2010), SUDs develop as the result of an imbalance between controlled and automatic processes. Controlled processes are flexible, slow and rule-based and they include rational decision-making processes, including 'choice'. We know that controlled processes are important in SUD; for example, people are more likely to drink alcohol to excess if their outcome expectancies (their beliefs about the effects of alcohol) are primarily positive rather than negative (Jones et al., 2001). Furthermore, these outcome expectancies are formed during youth and they predict drinking behaviour in adolescents (Jester et al., 2014). Beliefs about the effects of alcohol (and other drugs) partially determine people's *intentions* to use drugs, and these in turn predict actual behaviour (Kuther, 2002). However, as discussed previously, the contribution of such controlled processes to drug use in SUD sufferers has been questioned, not least because we diagnose an SUD when people express an intention to stop using drugs, but they continue to use them anyway.

In contrast to controlled processes, automatic processes are inflexible, fast and formed by learned associations. Dual-process theory proposes that automatic processes reflect an incentive learning process (so there is much overlap with many biological theories, such as those of Jentsch & Taylor, 1999; Robinson & Berridge, 1993), and they are able to produce spontaneous behaviour before people have time to consider the consequences of their actions. Some examples of automatic processes include attentional biases for drug-related cues, automatic drug-related memory associations, and automatic approach tendencies evoked by drug-related cues, all of which are present in people with SUDs (Stacy & Wiers, 2010). Importantly, these automatic processing biases may predict future drug use and they can be modified, helping people to recover from SUD (Stacy & Wiers, 2010) (see Box 9.7). However, some researchers, including one of your authors, are sceptical about the clinical relevance of these automatic processes in addiction (Field et al., 2014).

You might be thinking here, is drug use a controlled process or an automatic process? The answer is, it could be both. The essence of dual-process models is that when people start using drugs, they do so as a result of controlled processes: if they think that using drugs would be a good idea, they are likely to do it. However, with repeated experience of drug use, automatic processes start to develop, and these might become more important determinants of drug use as SUD progresses in severity. SUD sufferers should eventually reach a point at which the controlled processes say 'Stop', but by this point their automatic processes, which say 'Go', have become so strengthened that they lead the individual to drug use, even when the controlled processes operating in their 'rational brain' are screaming otherwise.

One final, notable feature of dual-process models is that they may account for individual differences in the determinants of drug use. Executive function refers to a broad set of cognitive functions, which determine how we can flexibly modify our behaviour in response to environmental demands. Arguably the most important aspect of executive function is working memory capacity, which can be defined as the extent of our ability to hold information in our consciousness. Various studies have shown that working memory capacity moderates the relationships between automatic and controlled processes, and drug use. In people with a good working memory, drug use seems to be tightly coupled to controlled processes (such as outcome expectancies) whereas it is unrelated to automatic processes. However, the reverse is true for people with a poor working memory, in whom drug use is more closely related to automatic rather than controlled processes (Wiers et al., 2010). One way to interpret these results is to say that people with a good working memory are better able to evaluate the pros and cons of drug use before they make a decision (to use drugs, or to abstain this time). On the other hand, people with a poor working memory are not able to do this, so their behaviour is determined by automatic processes, and they are more likely to act on the first impulse that pops into their head!

Section summary

In this section we have introduced diverse theories of SUD that come from many different areas of psychology and neuroscience. It is clear that no single theory of SUD can explain all of the evidence, but most of these theories are useful for explaining aspects of SUD, or for explaining the biological or cognitive changes that occur when someone becomes addicted. Crucially, it should be clear that these theories do not necessarily have to compete with each other. For example, basic conditioning processes such as Pavlovian to Instrumental Transfer are a useful starting point, and both the incentive-sensitisation theory and dual-process model can explain how PIT might play an important role in SUD. The difference between the models is that incentive-sensitisation theory explains this in terms of biological adaptations, whereas dual-process models explain this from within a cognitive framework. It is also clear that the key notions of 'choice' versus compulsion can be integrated within each of these models.

Section 4: How are substance use disorders treated?

Assessment of SUD

The type and intensity of treatment that a client receives will depend on their goals (to reduce substance use, or to give up entirely) and an assessment of the severity of their SUD. For illegal substances (such as heroin and cocaine) the client may be required by the courts to aim for complete abstinence. Depending on the case formulation, a clinician might recommend that a client should undergo detoxification (a common first step in the case of alcoholism and heroin addiction), before receiving a psychological intervention such as Cognitive Behavioural Therapy (CBT) and/or motivational interviewing. Patients may also be prescribed a substitute medication, or referred to a 'self-help' group. Unfortunately, there is much inconsistency in the type of treatment that people can expect to receive, if they get any help at all, and there is huge regional variation in this within the UK.

Pharmacological (drug) treatments

Many pharmacological treatments for SUDs work by substituting a safe prescribed medication for the more harmful drug that people are addicted to. For example, nicotine replacement therapy (NRT), in the form of chewing gum, patches, inhalers and so on, provides the nicotine that smokers are addicted to, in a form that is perfectly safe. There is nothing harmful in nicotine as such, but what is harmful to health is obtaining that nicotine by repeatedly inhaling it in the form of hot smoke. Smokers are encouraged to use NRT for a few months after they quit, gradually reducing the dose until they feel confident that they will not return to smoking. Importantly, it is an effective treatment: about 5% of smokers who try to quit without any help will succeed in the long term, but using NRT can double the chance of long-term success (Stead et al., 2012). How should you interpret these figures? On the one hand, you could say that NRT doubles the chances of quitting smoking; on the other hand, you could correctly point out that most people will struggle to give up, whether they use NRT or not (if we take the baseline figure of 5%, doubling it gives us 10%, which means that 90% of smokers who use NRT are still unable to stop smoking). Other drugs, such as varenicline (which seems to reduce the severity of nicotine withdrawal as well as blocking the effects of smoked tobacco) and bupropion (a form of antidepressant), have come onto the market in recent years, and these are at least as effective as NRT, with some studies showing that they are slightly better than NRT, especially when used in combination with it (Henningfield and colleagues, 2005).

Substitution therapies for opioid use disorder (heroin addiction) include methadone and buprenorphine. Both drugs stimulate the same endogenous opioid receptors that are activated by heroin, and therefore when people take these drugs this minimises their withdrawal symptoms and produces a fairly mild euphoria. Buprenorphine is preferable to methadone because of the reduced danger of overdosing on the drug, and also because if people take heroin when they are on buprenorphine, it 'blocks' the high produced by heroin. These drugs are useful in the sense that they reduce the amount of heroin that is used, and they also reduce risky behaviours such as sharing syringes with others, and so we can see a reduction in HIV infections as a result. However, use of these drugs is controversial because they do not 'cure' opioid use disorder: many people end up taking the drugs for years or even decades, and some critics believe that they simply prolong the duration of the disorder (Watson & Lingford-Hughes, 2007).

Although there is no straightforward substitute medication for alcohol use disorder, a variety of medications are prescribed to patients to help them maintain abstinence (or in some cases, reduce their drinking to safe levels) after they have completed alcohol detoxification. For example, naltrexone, which blocks opioid receptors, works by blocking the pleasure that people feel when they drink alcohol, and it seems to improve outcomes in patients in whom alcohol use disorder is not too severe (Jonas et al., 2014). Another drug, acamprosate, has a complicated mechanism of action, but one suggestion is that it partially 'resets' the GABA and glutamate systems that have become dysregulated after long periods of heavy drinking. Acamprosate is most suitable for severely dependent alcoholics who have a goal of stopping drinking entirely, in whom it reduces the risk of relapse compared to a placebo (Jonas et al., 2014). Finally, disulfiram works by disrupting the metabolism of alcohol in the liver, such that if people drink alcohol when they are maintained on disulfiram, this leads to a build-up of acetaldehyde, which causes a very unpleasant reaction including hot flushes, nausea and vomiting. One way of understanding the mechanism of action of this drug is that it gives people a hangover the moment they drink alcohol – in other words, all the pain with none of the pleasure – and you can probably imagine why this would deter people from drinking! Importantly, the drug seems to work because it changes expectancies about what will happen if alcohol is consumed, rather than through any direct re-learning of the consequences of alcohol consumption. If its use is properly monitored by clinicians, disulfiram can reduce the risk of relapse to heavy drinking (Watson & Lingford-Hughes, 2007).

So how do these drug treatments relate to theories of SUD? We can see that many work by relieving withdrawal or by blocking the positive effects of a substance if it is taken. From a simple operant conditioning perspective, we would expect these kinds of drugs to work because they reduce either the negative or positive reinforcing properties of the substance (or in the case of disulfiram, they 'punish' substance use). However, in Section 3 we saw that many theories of SUD propose key roles for dysfunction of dopamine brain circuits. So why don't we prescribe dopaminergic drugs (such as dopamine antagonists, used for the treatment of schizophrenia; see Chapter 4) for the treatment of SUD? The answer is that this approach has been tried, but with very limited success in the clinic. It has proven difficult to find a suitable drug that does not have unpleasant withdrawal symptoms and which SUD sufferers would be willing to take for long periods (Heidbreder & Newman, 2010).

Psychological treatments

Motivational interviewing and the related *motivational enhancement therapy* are commonly offered to SUD patients (particularly alcohol and heroin users). There is some debate over whether it is sufficient as a 'standalone' treatment, or whether it should mainly be used to encourage clients to engage in more intensive treatment. Either way, the goal of motivational interviewing is to encourage clients to recognise that they are ambivalent about their drug use (they want to stop but they also feel that they have good reasons for continuing to use drugs), and to gently encourage people to see the benefits of quitting, or at least cutting down. One notable feature of this treatment is that unlike CBT it does not take the form of an 'expert' clinician giving structured advice to a client. Instead, the client is encouraged to see the negative side of their drug use, and to develop their own motivation to quit (see Box 9.5 for an example). It does, however, require some patience on the part of both therapist and client, because the therapist can become frustrated when they perceive that the client is unaware of the harm that drug use is causing, and the client then becomes annoyed that the therapist cannot see their point of view. Yet there is good evidence that it is an effective treatment for a variety of SUDs, particularly alcohol use disorder (Smedslund et al., 2011), and encouragingly it can be combined with other types of treatment such as cognitive-behaviour therapy (CBT).

Box 9.5   Essential experience

Motivational interviewing (MI) for alcohol dependence (Hall, 2012)

A male patient, 52 years of age, who drinks heavily and has expressed the desire to reduce drinking, continues to drink heavily.

It is easy to conclude that this patient lacks motivation, his judgment is impaired, or he simply does not understand the effects of alcohol on his health. These conclusions may naturally lead the practitioner to adopt a paternalistic therapeutic style and warn the patient of the risks to his health. In subsequent consultations, when these strategies don't work, it is easy to give up hope that he will change his drinking, characterise him as 'unmotivated', and drop the subject altogether. In MI, the opposite approach is taken, where the patient's motivation is targeted by the practitioner. Using the spirit of MI, the practitioner avoids an authoritarian stance, and respects the autonomy of the patient by accepting he has the responsibility to change his drinking – or not. Motivational interviewing emphasises eliciting reasons for change from the patient, rather than advising them of the reasons why they should change their drinking. What concerns does he have about the effects of his drinking? What future goals or personal values are impacted by his drinking? The apparent 'lack of motivation' evident in the patient would be constructed as 'unresolved ambivalence' within an MI framework. The practitioner would therefore work on understanding this ambivalence, by exploring the pros and cons of continuing to drink alcohol. They would then work on resolving this ambivalence, by connecting the things the patient cares about with their motivation for change. For example, drinking may impact on the patient's values about being a loving partner and father or being healthy and strong. A discussion of how continuing to drink (maintaining the status quo) will impact his future goals to travel in retirement or have a good relationship with his children may be the focus. The practitioner would emphasise that the decision to change is 'up to him'; however, they would work with the patient to increase his confidence that he can change (self-efficacy).

The goal of CBT for SUDs is to encourage clients to recognise how their cognitions and behaviours can lead them to drug use, and then to practise ways to modify their beliefs such that drug use becomes less likely. (The general principles of CBT for various different disorders are covered in Chapter 2.) When CBT is applied to the treatment of SUDs, the overall goal is to get sufferers to recognise how their (faulty) cognitions can lead to substance use, and to formulate and then repeatedly practise techniques in order to counteract those cognitions. For example, a client may claim that they drink alcohol when stressed because they think that the alcohol will reduce their stress. A clinician may encourage the client to think of other ways to reduce their stress using alternative behaviours (e.g. going for a walk or reading a novel), and then to practise doing those things each time they are tempted to drink when stressed. There is good evidence that CBT is a reasonably effective treatment for alcohol use disorders, although surprisingly, it seems that the beneficial effects on drinking behaviour may not be mediated by changes in cognition (Morgenstern & Longabaugh, 2000). CBT may also improve outcomes in other SUDs, such as tobacco- and opiate-use disorders, although the evidence here is more mixed.

Many SUD sufferers receive 'treatment' from self-help groups, and in a lot of cases these treatments do not involve any input from clinicians such as clinical psychologists or psychiatrists. For example, you have probably heard of Alcoholics' Anonymous, and the related organisations Narcotics Anonymous, Gamblers Anonymous, etc., which are charitable organisations, usually run by recovering addicts. In the case of Alcoholics Anonymous (AA), clients are paired with a 'sponsor', that is, a recovered alcoholic who provides moral support and encouragement to abstain from drinking with adherence to the '12 steps', a spiritual or quasi-religious doctrine which emphasises a need to recognise the drinking problem over which they have no control. There is some evidence that affiliation with AA can help people to maintain abstinence in the long term (Ferri et al., 2006), although there is also evidence that some people, such as committed atheists, do not respond well to AA involvement, presumably because they are put off by the strong spiritual component!

The final treatment that we discuss is cue exposure therapy, the aim of which is to reduce or eliminate reactivity to drug cues. In Section 2 we showed how classical conditioning could play an important role in the development of SUDs: the rewarding effects of drugs are an unconditioned stimulus (US) which is reliably paired with drug-related 'cues' such as the sight and smell of beer. Therefore, those cues should function as conditioned stimuli (CS) and be capable of eliciting conditioned responses (CR) which could ultimately increase drug-taking behaviour. In cue exposure therapy, the patient is repeatedly exposed to drug-related cues, but they are not able to take the drug. In principle, this 'extinction' training should mask the associative relationship between the CS and US, and lead to extinction of the CR (a reduction in cue reactivity), and ultimately reduce the risk of relapse in patients who are attempting to quit. Based on the success of this kind of treatment in phobias (see Chapter 7), we might hope that it would prove similarly useful for the treatment of SUDs. Unfortunately, it does not: although cue exposure therapy does reduce the degree of cue reactivity when measured in clinical or research settings, there is no convincing evidence that it helps people to abstain from drug use in the long term. This might be because extinction is context-dependent, so any progress (reduced cue reactivity) that is seen in the clinic is immediately eradicated as soon as people return to their old environments in which they used to take drugs (Conklin & Tiffany, 2002). We need to conduct further research to find out whether cue exposure therapy can be an effective treatment for SUDs, but for now we have to think of it as a theoretically well-informed treatment that just does not seem to work in practice.

Box 9.6   Essential treatment

New SUD treatments on the horizon

In Section 3 we discussed dual-process models of SUDs, which suggest that it is important to tackle automatic cognitive processes. One example of an automatic cognitive process is the behavioural approach response that is elicited automatically by drug-related cues. In two recent studies, Wiers and colleagues (2011) and Eberl et al. (2013) looked at alcoholics in treatment and randomly assigned them to one of two groups, both of which repeatedly performed a task in which they had to categorise alcohol-related and neutral images by making an approach or an avoidance movement to the picture with a joystick. The experimental treatment group were always asked to make an avoidance movement when they saw alcohol pictures, whereas the control group approached alcohol pictures half the time, and avoided them half the time. The goal of this treatment was to weaken or reverse automatic alcohol approach responses in the experimental treatment group. In both studies the researchers showed that the treatment improved outcomes, because a higher proportion of patients in the experimental group (compared to the control group) were still abstinent from alcohol one year after receiving the treatment. Furthermore, this outcome was mediated by changes in the automatic approach responses: patients were less likely to relapse if they showed large reductions in automatic approach responses over the course of treatment. It remains to be seen whether this type of treatment could work in other groups of SUD sufferers, or whether it could be combined with other types of treatment, but this promising technique suggests that there is hope for the future.

This is far from a complete list of psychological treatments for SUDs, as we do not have space here to cover some of the other 'talking therapies' that have been shown to be effective, such as marital therapy. Some recent developments include those based on dual process models of addiction, which aim to counteract biases that operate in automatic processes (see Box 9.6). We end this section by attempting to answer a question you might have: Which type of treatment is most effective? To answer this question we need to call on randomised controlled trials (RCTs) in which people are randomly allocated to receive treatment A, or treatment B (and so on), or some kind of control treatment. For example, in Project MATCH alcohol-dependent patients were randomly assigned to receive CBT, motivational interviewing, or '12 step' therapy which is a structured version of the key components of AA. This study revealed no overall 'winner', as all the treatments were more effective than no treatment at all, but there was no consistent difference between treatments (Allen et al., 1997). Many other studies have shown the same kind of effect: any kind of psychosocial treatment for SUD is better than none at all, but there is no treatment which has been consistently shown to be better than the alternatives. This equivalence of psychological treatments for SUDs has been dubbed the

'Dodo bird verdict' after an episode in *Alice in Wonderland* in which the dodo bird's verdict on being asked to judge the winner of a competition was 'Everybody has won, so all shall have prizes'. One explanation for the equivalent effectiveness of treatments which are built on such enormously different assumptions is that unspecified, 'non-specific' aspects of being in treatment (such as the empathy expressed by counsellors) are actually the most important determinants of whether or not SUD sufferers manage to remain abstinent (Morgenstern & Longabaugh, 2000).

Section summary

This section has discussed the treatment of SUDs. We have shown that pharmacotherapies can be used to minimise drug withdrawal or block the pleasurable effects of drugs, and that psychological treatments that aim to tackle the motivation to abstain, or help people identify maladaptive cognitions, can also be useful. However, we don't have a good understanding of *how* psychological treatments help, and there is quite a big gulf between our theories of SUD and the techniques we use to treat them!

Essential questions

Some possible exam questions that stem from this chapter are:

- Do people choose to become addicted?
- Can we effectively treat substance use disorders with pharmacotherapies?
- How can we link biological, learning and cognitive theories of substance use disorders?
- Are substance use disorders a product of genes, the environment, or both?

Further reading

Ryan, F. (2013). *Cognitive Therapy for Addiction: Motivation and Change*. Oxford: Wiley-Blackwell. (Excellent blend of evidence about cognitive processes in addiction, with more practical information on how to apply this knowledge to CBT.)

Watson, B., & Lingford-Hughes, A. (2007). Pharmacological treatment of addiction. *Psychiatry*, 6(7): 309–312. (A brief but comprehensive review of drug treatments.)

West, R., & Brown, J. (2013). *Theory of Addiction* (2nd edition). Oxford: Wiley-Blackwell. (This is a fairly short but comprehensive book on theoretical models of addiction, which contains lots of useful examples.)

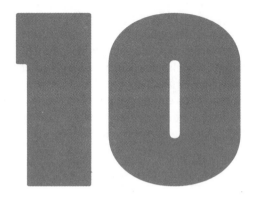

EATING DISORDERS

General introduction

In this chapter we consider three eating disorders: anorexia nervosa, bulimia nervosa and binge eating disorder. Although the disorders are distinct from each other, there are many similarities between them, and some patients meet the criteria for different disorders at different times. We will show that heritable factors, biological changes and socio-cultural pressures to be thin play a significant role, and that these factors contribute to psychological characteristics that initiate and then maintain the symptoms of eating disorders. Finally, we will discuss the diverse ways in which eating disorders are treated, and highlight successes and failures in the search for effective treatments.

Assessment targets

At the end of the chapter, you should ask yourself the following questions:

- Can I explain the diagnostic criteria for eating disorders, discuss the overlap between them and explain how they have changed over time?
- Do I understand how abnormalities of neurotransmitter function and disturbances in different brain circuits lead to the development of eating disorder symptoms?
- Can I explain and evaluate psychological models of eating disorders?
- Can I explain why neither heritable biological influences nor cultural pressures to be thin are adequate explanations for eating disorders by themselves?
- Do I understand how eating disorders are treated, and can I relate treatments back to theoretical models?

Section 1: What are eating disorders?

In this section we will look at how eating disorders are diagnosed, and consider how the categorisation of eating disorders has evolved over time. We will also discuss the relatively recent diagnostic category of binge-eating disorder, which is new for *DSM*-5 (American Psychiatric Association, 2013a), and think about the relationship between eating disorders and obesity.

The *ICD*-10 recognises two 'important and clear cut syndromes': anorexia nervosa and bulimia nervosa (World Health Organisation, 1992). The diagnostic criteria for these disorders are shown in Boxes 10.1 and 10.2.

Box 10.1   Essential diagnosis

Anorexia nervosa

The *ICD*-10 (World Health Organisation, 1992) describes anorexia nervosa as a disorder characterised by deliberate weight loss. To warrant this diagnosis, all of the following criteria must be met:

A. Weight loss (or in children a lack of weight gain), leading to a body weight at least 15% below the normal or expected weight for age and height.
B. The weight loss is self-induced by avoidance of 'fattening foods'.
C. A self-perception of being 'too fat', with an intrusive dread of fatness, which leads to a self-imposed low weight threshold.
D. Widespread endocrine disorder, which manifests in women as amenorrhoea (menstruation stops) and in men as a loss of sexual interest.

The *DSM*-5 criteria for anorexia nervosa are similar, although *DSM*-5 also distinguishes between restricting and binge-eating/purging types of anorexia. These are characterised by different strategies to lose weight. In restricting-type anorexia, the individual severely reduces their food intake. In the binge-eating purging type, the individual engages in excessive food intake ('binge eating'; see Box 10.3), followed by vomiting or the misuse of laxatives.

Box 10.2   Essential diagnosis

Bulimia nervosa

The *ICD*-10 (World Health Organisation, 1992) describes bulimia nervosa as a disorder characterised by repeated bouts of overeating and an excessive preoccupation with the control of body weight, which leads the patient to adopt extreme measures in order to control their weight. To warrant this diagnosis, all of the following criteria must be met:

1. Recurrent episodes of overeating (at least twice per week over a period of three months) in which large amounts of food are consumed over a short period of time.
2. Persistent preoccupation with eating and a strong desire or craving to eat.
3. The patient attempts to counteract the 'fattening' effect of food by one or more of the following:

    o self-induced vomiting
    o self-induced purging
    o alternating periods of starvation
    o use of drugs such as appetite suppressants

4. A self-perception of being 'too fat', with an intrusive dread of fatness.

The *DSM*-5 criteria (American Psychiatric Association, 2013a) are similar, although they explicitly specify that patients should feel a lack of control over eating during binge-eating episodes.

Shortly before *DSM*-5 was published (in 2013), Fairburn and Cooper (2011) argued that the 'clinical reality' of the diagnosis of eating disorders was very different from that set out in *ICD*-10 and *DSM-IV*. This is because at least half of patients who present with symptoms of an eating disorder receive a diagnosis of 'eating disorder not otherwise specified' (EDNOS), a diagnostic category in *DSM-IV* that has been retained in *DSM*-5 (although now relabelled as 'Other Specified Feeding or Eating Disorder', or OSFED). These diagnostic labels were intended for patients with eating disorder symptoms who didn't quite meet the diagnostic criteria for one of the two 'classic' disorders (anorexia or bulimia), and it was anticipated that most patients would receive one of the more specific diagnoses. As Fairburn and Cooper (2011) pointed out, in reality, most patients with eating disorder symptoms receive an EDNOS diagnosis, and relatively few are diagnosed with the 'classic' disorders.

The *DSM*-5 has come some way to addressing these problems, because it recognises binge-eating disorder as a separate disorder (see Box 10.3). According to Fairburn and Cooper (2011), many of the patients who would have received a diagnosis of EDNOS before 2013 can now receive a diagnosis of binge-eating disorder. This is an important step forward because this more specific diagnosis means that patients are more likely to receive appropriate treatment. Some researchers (Fairburn & Cooper, 2011; Keel et al., 2012) have suggested that we could further reduce EDNOS diagnoses by introducing even more distinct types of eating disorder, including 'purging disorder' or 'restrained eating disorder'. However, even these proposed disorders are not clearly distinct from each other: there is a lot of overlap between them, as there is between the two 'classic' disorders of anorexia and bulimia. When you look at it this way, the solution that was adopted for *DSM*-5 (a recognition of binge-eating disorder, in order to reduce the number of EDNOS diagnoses) was perhaps a good compromise!

Box 10.3   Essential diagnosis

Binge-eating disorder

The *DSM*-5 (American Psychiatric Association, 2013a) criteria for binge-eating disorder include those for bulimia (excessive eating and feelings of loss of control) and the duration of symptoms is the same (three months). However, binge-eating disorder has the following characteristic symptoms:

- Binge-eating episodes are associated with three or more of the following: eating much more quickly than normal; eating until feeling uncomfortably full; eating large amounts of food when not feeling hungry; eating alone due to embarrassment about how much one is eating; feeling disgusted, depressed or guilty about eating.
- Marked distress regarding binge eating.
- Importantly, binge eating is *not* associated with the use of compensatory behaviours such as vomiting or excessive exercise that are seen in bulimia.

Treasure and colleagues (2010) argued that the core symptoms of all eating disorders can be characterised as: disturbances in eating behaviour, which can involve abnormalities in what goes in (e.g. restricting food intake, bingeing) and what comes out (purging or misuse of laxatives); an obsession with body image or body weight (e.g. repeated weighing, preoccupation with weight and shape, fear of weight gain); being severely underweight; and physical changes that are associated with starvation such as compromised immune responses, low body temperature and disruptions to the menstrual cycle (in women). These symptoms are present to different degrees in all of the different disorders, and for this reason the 'transdiagnostic' approach is extremely influential among clinicians (Fairburn et al., 2003). According to this approach, common mechanisms underlie all disorders and therefore their assessment and treatment should be informed by the individual patient's specific symptoms rather than the official diagnosis they receive. This is a good example of a 'symptom-based approach' (see Chapter 1) that has been widely adopted, at least in the UK.

Despite the influence of the transdiagnostic model, the majority of the research into eating disorders has focused on specific diagnostic categories, and the structure of this chapter reflects this. To help you tell the disorders apart, remember that anorexic patients are usually underweight, whereas for bulimic patients their body weight is not important for diagnosis. Binge-eating disorder differs from bulimia because there is no inappropriate compensatory behaviour (e.g. vomiting or excessive exercise), whereas compensatory behaviours must be present to warrant a diagnosis of bulimia (Striegel-Moore & Franko, 2008).

Box 10.4 Essential experience (from Field, 2003)

Clare's mum noticed that Clare had stopped having periods and that for nearly a year now her weight had been steadily dropping. What her mother didn't realise was that Clare had started to restrict her eating because she found herself preoccupied with her body weight and calorific intake. In particular, she hated the shape of her bum and thighs, and was intensely fearful of gaining weight. Although, objectively, her body shape was normal, Clare's perception of herself was completely distorted and she began to exercise profusely to try to achieve the body shape she wanted. She remembers beginning to worry about her appearance after being bullied in school. She now has very low self-esteem and often contemplates killing herself. Recently she has begun to induce vomiting after eating.

Box 10.5 Essential debate

Is obesity an eating disorder, or a consequence of one?

In the USA, approximately two-thirds of adults are overweight (defined as a BMI of 25 or above) and about half of these are classified as obese (a BMI of 30 or higher). Some projections indicate that more than half of the population in the UK and other Western countries will be obese by 2050 (www.bbc.co.uk/news/health-25708278). Overweight and obesity lead to other medical conditions including diabetes and high blood pressure. Given their increasing prevalence, it is no surprise that for many Western countries, tackling the obesity epidemic is the top public health priority (Malik et al., 2013).

People usually become overweight as a result of a 'positive energy balance', that is, they consume more calories than they expend. This is the result of a plentiful and cheap supply of food that is high in calories, fat and sugar, combined with decreased physical activity as a result of increasing urbanisation. It is a complex problem that does not have a simple solution, but some have suggested that overeating in particular could be attributed to an eating disorder. In support of this, binge-eating disorder is twice as common in people who are overweight (3%) compared to people who are not (1.5%) (Striegel-Moore & Franko, 2008). Some reports also suggest that the prevalence of binge-eating disorder in people who are overweight is much higher than this (possibly up to 20%). Whatever the exact figure, researchers agree that even though binge-eating disorder is more common among people who are overweight, the vast majority of people who are overweight do not have the disorder (Ziauddeen et al., 2012), and therefore it is obviously not the primary determinant of obesity.

(Continued)

(Continued)

In summary, even though eating disorders (particularly binge-eating disorder) are a plausible cause of excessive eating, broader societal factors such as the overabundance of cheap, high calorie food are the more likely explanation for the high rates of overweight and obesity across the world.

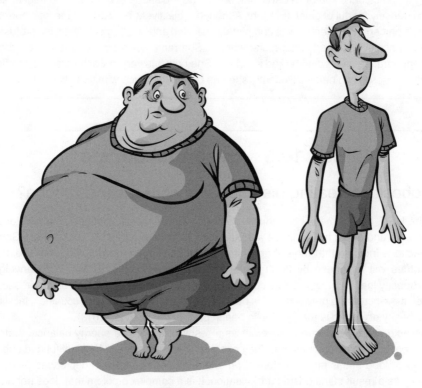

Figure 10.1 Should obesity be added to the list of eating disorders?

Prevalence, consequences, course and outcome of eating disorders

Anorexia nervosa is rare: the 12-month prevalence in females is 0.4% (American Psychiatric Association, 2013), with lifetime prevalence around 0.6% (Treasure et al., 2010). It is even less common in males, to the extent that prevalence in males is difficult to estimate. However, in eating disorder clinics females tend to outnumber males by 10 to 1. Symptoms first appear during adolescence or early adulthood, often after an attempt to control weight by dieting.

Sadly, the risk of premature death is greatly increased in people who suffer from anorexia (Arcelus et al., 2011) and this is mainly attributable to starvation (10% of sufferers) or suicide (0.1% of sufferers). After the initial diagnosis, a recurrence of symptoms in the short term is common, although most sufferers experience a remission of symptoms within five years of initially receiving treatment (Keel & Brown, 2010).

Bulimia nervosa is more common, affecting 1% to 1.5% of females within a 12–month period (12-month prevalence) (American Psychiatric Association, 2013a), and the lifetime prevalence is estimated at 1% (Treasure et al., 2010). The same 10 to 1 female:male ratio is seen as with anorexia. Stressful life events may initially trigger the symptoms, although binge eating and purging behaviour commonly occur during or after the individual tries to lose weight by dieting. Patients who are diagnosed with bulimia exhibit disturbed eating behaviour for several years, although most patients experience at least a partial recovery several years after first presenting with symptoms (Keel & Brown, 2010).

Binge-eating disorder is probably the most common eating disorder, affecting 1.6% of females and 0.8% of males over a 12-month period. Lifetime prevalence is estimated at 3% (Treasure et al., 2010). In contrast to anorexia and bulimia (symptoms of which appear after the individual goes on a diet), binge-eating episodes usually occur *before* the individual attempts to diet. The prognosis for binge-eating disorder is much better than that for either anorexia or bulimia: most sufferers experience a full remission of symptoms within a few years of their initial diagnosis, if not sooner (Keel & Brown, 2010). Treatments for binge-eating disorder also tend to be much more effective than those for anorexia or bulimia (see Section 4).

Importantly, many individuals will initially be diagnosed with bulimia but will subsequently transition into anorexia or binge-eating disorder (Treasure et al., 2010). However, it is rare for someone to be diagnosed with binge-eating disorder and subsequently transition to anorexia (Keel & Brown, 2010). Therefore, even though these appear to be distinct disorders when compared cross-sectionally (Keel et al., 2012), over time it is common for signs and symptoms to change so that the specific diagnosis that patients receive can differ from one point in time to another. The instability of specific diagnoses over time is entirely consistent with the 'transdiagnostic' approach (Fairburn et al., 2003). It is fortunate that this approach is widely used to guide assessment and treatment of eating disorders, at least in the UK.

As with other psychological disorders, psychiatric co-morbidity is common, with much higher rates of mood and anxiety disorders, and autism spectrum disorders, in patients with eating disorders (Jacobi et al., 2004).

Section summary

In this section we have shown how eating disorders are defined and categorised according to *ICD*-10 and *DSM*-5. There appear to be at least three distinct eating disorders, although there is considerable overlap between these, with core symptoms of eating disorders being disturbances in eating behaviour (e.g. restricting food intake, bingeing or purging), an obsession with body image or body weight (e.g. repeated weighing, preoccupation with weight and shape, fear of weight gain), and being severely underweight (in the case of anorexia only). These symptoms are present to different degrees in the different disorders, and some patients seem to transition from one diagnosis to another over time. Having said this, most research into the causes of the disorders assumes that these are distinct from one another.

Section 2: How do eating disorders develop?

Heritability

Eating disorders run in families. For example, family studies show that the first-degree relatives of women with anorexia nervosa are 11 times more likely than the relatives of unaffected controls to have anorexia themselves (Trace et al., 2013). Twin and family studies indicate heritability estimates ranging between 28% and 83% for eating disorders, although estimates for anorexia tend to be considerably higher than those for bulimia and binge-eating disorder (Trace et al., 2013). It is notable that genetic transmission does not seem to be disorder-specific: a family history of any particular eating disorder (e.g. bulimia) is associated with an increased risk of both that disorder and other eating disorders (e.g. anorexia, binge-eating disorder). Furthermore, the genetic risk for eating disorders is shared with the risk for other psychological disorders, including mood disorders, anxiety disorders and substance use disorders, in other words, a person with a first-degree relative who has an eating disorder is at increased risk of developing an eating disorder, as well as a range of other psychological disorders, themselves.

As with other psychological disorders, little progress has been made when it comes to identifying specific genetic variants that are associated with a risk for eating disorders. Trace et al. (2013) reviewed hundreds of studies which investigated the involvement of genes that influence serotonin, dopamine and opioid activity in the brain, as well as other genes that influence hormones involved in appetite, weight regulation and learning. They reached a fairly pessimistic conclusion: most individual studies did not have sufficient statistical power, and because of this the literature is full of findings that other research groups could not replicate, with very little consistency between studies. Huge sample sizes are needed to reliably detect genetic variants that are associated with relatively rare disorders, and eating disorders *are* fairly rare. Trace et al. emphasised the need for researchers to conduct much more ambitious studies that research the whole genome, in tens of thousand of individuals (termed 'Genome Wide Association Studies'; GWAS), and to focus on different subtypes of eating disorders (e.g. the restricting vs binge-eating/purging subtypes of anorexia). A related avenue for future research may be to study the heritability of individual symptoms of eating disorders, for example purging behaviours versus binge-eating behaviours versus concerns about appearance and body weight. Some early research on this topic suggests higher heritability estimates for binge-eating behaviours compared to concerns about appearance and body weight (Trace et al., 2013).

Prenatal stress and birth trauma

Events that occur before and during birth can increase the risk of eating disorders. Maternal stress is associated with increased risk of the subsequent development of eating disorders in offspring, as are premature birth and complications during birth (Treasure et al., 2010). Epigenetic processes (changes in gene expression that occur as a result of environmental influences; see Chapter 1) may explain some of these effects. For example, stress during early development may fundamentally alter the functioning of the hypothalamic-pituitary axis (HPA axis) in offspring, which can plausibly be linked to the patterns of brain activity that are characteristic of eating disorders (see Section 3) (Campbell et al., 2011). However, research on epigenetic mechanisms involved in psychological disorders, including eating disorders, is only just beginning.

Adverse childhood experiences

In common with other psychological disorders, sexual abuse during childhood may be associated with a slightly increased risk of developing an eating disorder during adolescence, although Jacobi et al. (2004) noted the small number of longitudinal studies that had investigated this. Other adverse life events during childhood (e.g. parental divorce) have also been implicated, and parenting style may also contribute. For example, some studies demonstrate increased incidence of eating disorders in children of parents who had unrealistically high expectations of their children (Karwautz et al., 2001).

Social factors: Cultural transmission of the 'thin ideal'

If you ask people why they think some adolescent girls develop eating disorders, many would attribute blame to the enormous social pressures to be thin, at least in developed countries. And they would have a point. There is a widespread cultural acceptance that the ideal body shape is a very thin one, and that deviating from this body shape is socially unacceptable. There is a clear stigma against being overweight and therefore young women might be highly motivated to attempt to control their weight and to lose weight by dieting (Treasure et al., 2010).

Despite the appeal of attributing eating disorders to a social pressure to be thin, this is not a sufficient explanation for eating disorders because *all* females in Western countries are exposed to these social pressures. Even though many adolescent girls (perhaps the majority) will be concerned about their weight and body shape, and many will repeatedly diet in order to lose weight, most (more than 95%) will never be diagnosed with an eating disorder. For this reason, researchers have studied whether eating disorders can be attributed to individual differences in concerns about body weight and the degree to which people 'internalise' the thin ideal. Longitudinal studies are important here because they can identify the psychological characteristics that are involved in the development of eating disorders *before* those characteristics become confounding symptoms of the disorder itself. Dissatisfaction with one's own body shape and aspirations to be thinner ('the drive for thinness') are good examples of variables that are prone to this type of confounding, because they are clearly symptoms of eating disorders (particularly bulimia and anorexia) but also likely to play a causal role in the development of those disorders.

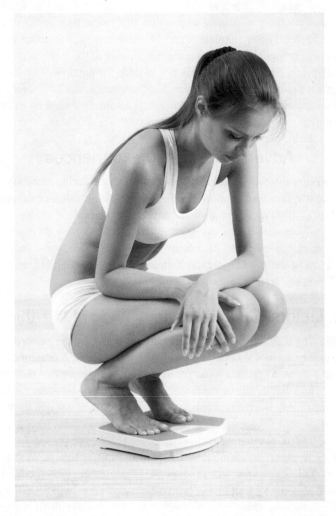

Figure 10.2 Is it simplistic to attribute anorexia to social pressure to be thin?

Wertheim and colleagues (2001) tested adolescent girls in different school years in Australia who were aged 12, 13 or 15 (on average), and followed them up again eight months later. At both time points the participants completed questionnaires that measured the drive for thinness, including restrictive eating behaviours, body dissatisfaction, bulimia symptoms, self-esteem and depression, teasing about weight, and body mass index (BMI). After statistically controlling for all other predictors, their analyses revealed that in the youngest girls body dissatisfaction predicted the drive for thinness (including restrictive eating) at the second assessment eight months later. Conversely, BMI, teasing about weight, and the drive for thinness predicted bulimic symptoms eight months later. Notably, these longitudinal relationships were only seen in the participants in the youngest school year (grade 7). In the slightly older participants (those in grades 8 and 10 at first testing) these longitudinal relationships were not consistently seen, because the psychological constructs tended to be much more stable over time.

The implication of this study, and other similar longitudinal studies (e.g. Neumark-Sztainer et al., 2007), is that in young girls body dissatisfaction, teasing about weight and aspirations to be thin seem to predict other eating disorder symptoms later on. Therefore, some maladaptive ways of thinking about weight may develop in some adolescent girls and then cause an eating disorder to develop. However, in adolescents who are only slightly older, these psychological constructs are fairly stable and they do not change much over time. These findings have clear implications for the timing of prevention interventions for adolescent girls, because these interventions need to be delivered before eating behaviours and dysfunctional beliefs about one's eating behaviour and body shape are firmly established (see Box 10.6).

Box 10.6   Essential research

Can eating disorders be prevented?

Eating disorders, particularly anorexia, are difficult to treat. As we discussed in Chapter 2, prevention is better than cure, so can we do anything to prevent people from developing eating disorders in the first place? A variety of different interventions have been evaluated. A typical one is the *Girl Talk* Peer Support Group, a 10-session school-based programme that has been offered to students aged 12 to 14 in the USA (McVey et al., 2003). This intervention promotes group discussion of the thin ideal promoted by the media, which leads to concerns about body weight and shape. Girls are also encouraged to discuss ways to promote a positive body image and self-esteem, and accept their own body shape and size. Other discussion topics might include the futility and negative consequences of dieting, tips on healthy eating and an active lifestyle, stress management, and forming healthy relationships.

Stice et al. (2007) conducted a meta-analysis of studies which evaluated the effectiveness of prevention interventions such as this one, and they reached some positive conclusions: around half (51%) reduced the risk factors for eating disorders (e.g. internalisation of the thin ideal), and 29% of them led to reductions in the likelihood of developing an eating disorder in the future. These figures compare favourably to comparable figures for interventions designed to reduce problem drinking or sexually transmitted diseases in

(Continued)

(Continued)

young people. Interventions were more likely to be effective if they were targeted at 'at-risk' girls, interactive, targeted at girls aged 15 or above (rather than younger); if they incorporated body acceptance content; and if they were delivered by professionals. Overall, it seems that if the most effective prevention measures were implemented more widely, this could lead to large reductions in the incidence of eating disorders in young women.

However, when we evaluate this research we should bear in mind that these studies identified predictors of low-level eating disorder symptoms in adolescent girls who were generally psychologically healthy: most of them did not actually have an eating disorder. Therefore it is necessary to investigate whether these psychological constructs in healthy individuals can predict who will subsequently be diagnosed with an eating disorder, but this research is difficult to do because eating disorders are so rare (Jacobi et al., 2004). However, we can look at studies of patients who have recovered from eating disorders. For example, Keel et al. (2005) showed that an excessive concern with body weight and shape predicted which anorexic and bulimic patients would subsequently experience a relapse of eating disorder symptoms after initial treatment. This key study suggests that body weight concerns play an important causal role in the persistence of eating disorder symptoms.

This issue has also been investigated using experimental research methods. Groesz and colleagues (2002) conducted a meta-analysis of studies that manipulated exposure to the thin ideal (usually by showing people images of skinny models) on body (dis)satisfaction. Perhaps unsurprisingly, their analysis of 25 studies found a clear effect of exposure to these images on body dissatisfaction: participants reported being much less satisfied with their own body after being exposed to images of skinny models, compared to if they had seen images of average size or overweight models. When we combine these results with those from longitudinal studies, we can speculate on mechanisms through which the social pressure to be thin leads to eating disorder symptoms in adolescent girls: repeated exposure to the 'thin ideal' causes dissatisfaction with one's own body shape, which in turn increases the motivation to be thin, which leads to dieting and/or compensatory behaviours such as purging or excessive exercise. This account has influenced psychological theories of eating disorders (Fairburn et al., 1999), which we discuss in Section 3.

Box 10.7   Essential research

Gene x environment interactions

One environmental risk factor for the development of anorexia nervosa is a parenting style characterised by overly high expectations of their children (Karwautz et al., 2001). A genetic variation that is associated with anorexia relates to the serotonin transporter gene, although the consistency of this evidence has been questioned (Trace et al., 2013). In a recent study, Karwautz et al. (2011) investigated possible interactions between these genetic and environmental risk factors in a group of 128 pairs of sisters, one of whom had anorexia nervosa and one of whom did not.

The results are shown in the graph below, and they show a clear gene x environment (or G×E) interaction: repeated experience of a parenting style characterised by unrealistically high expectations (on the x axis) leads to an increase in the risk of developing anorexia (on the y axis), but these effects are only present in females who possess two short alleles of the serotonin transporter genotype ('SS' genotype) and, to a smaller extent, in those who possess one short and one long allele ('LS' genotype). However, in females who possess two long alleles (LL genotype, green line), the relationship between parenting style and the risk of anorexia is, if anything, reversed.

On the face of it, this represents a very impressive demonstration of an interaction between genetic and environmental risk factors as a cause of anorexia. It is important

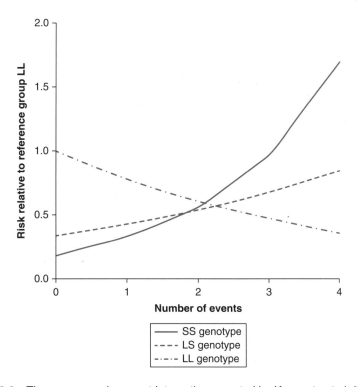

Figure 10.3   The gene x environment interaction reported by Karwautz et al. (2011)

(Continued)

(Continued)

that other researchers attempt to replicate this finding using a much larger sample. While we wait for this replication to appear, it is worth thinking critically about it. If you read the Karwautz et al. (2011) paper, you will see that the researchers measured a large number of environmental risk factors for anorexia, together with a large number of genetic variants that have previously been associated with anorexia. Although they used conservative statistical tests, do you think it is possible that the result shown in the graph could have occurred by chance because the researchers had a very large number of interaction effects that they could study? Research on similar G×E interactions in the depression literature (see Box 5.4 in Chapter 5), which were initially reported very enthusiastically before other researchers struggled to replicate them, may give you pause for thought!

Section summary

In this section we have shown that eating disorders are heritable, but also that twenty-first century Western cultures (in which a thin body shape is highly valued but fattening food is readily available) are conducive to the development of these disorders. As with other psychological disorders we have to be careful about how we interpret heritability estimates, because even a very high heritability estimate leaves a lot of room for environmental influences and gene × environment interactions. As for environmental influences, it is worth remembering that eating disorders are relatively rare, and therefore we need to explain why most people do not develop such disorders despite being exposed to a society in which reminders of the 'thin ideal' are regularly encountered.

Section 3: Brain and cognitive mechanisms in eating disorders

Brain mechanisms involved in appetite and food intake

Treasure et al. (2010) suggest that to understand the biological basis of eating disorders we must consider three biological systems that are involved in appetite and food intake in healthy individuals. First, the homeostatic system, which is centred in the brain stem and lateral hypothalamus, receives signals from the gastrointestinal system and transmits signals of hunger and satiety. It has been well established that electrical stimulation of the lateral hypothalamus leads to hunger and food intake, whereas its removal or deactivation causes feelings of satiety and cessation of food intake.

Second, the hypothalamus is connected to the brain's reward system, a network of subcortical structures, including the nucleus accumbens and ventral tegmental area, that receive input from regions of the prefrontal cortex (see Chapter 9). When food is anticipated and during the early stages of food intake, the reward system is activated and these changes are primarily mediated by increases in *dopamine* activity. Dopamine registers the reward value of food and plays an important role in seeking out food when hungry. But as eating continues, dopamine activity habituates and is replaced by increases in *serotonin* activity in the brain reward system. These increases in serotonin transmission produce feelings of satiety and they normally lead to reductions in food intake (Schwartz et al., 2000).

Finally, signals from the reward system are modulated by the self-regulation system, a network of structures in the prefrontal cortex that are involved in thinking, reasoning and planning for the future (see Chapter 9). These brain structures normally inhibit or 'dampen down' activity in the reward system, which is why healthy people are usually (or at least, sometimes!) able to resist the motivational appeal of tempting food in order to stick to a long-term goal, such as dieting to lose weight.

What's wrong with the brain in eating disorders?

Early research suggested a role for serotonin function in anorexia nervosa because serotonin transmission throughout the brain is dampened in anorexic patients compared to controls (Jacobi et al., 2004). Initially, researchers found it difficult to establish whether this biological deficit was a cause of anorexic symptoms or a consequence of malnutrition and starvation. It is a plausible consequence of starvation because tryptophan, the biological precursor of serotonin (the stuff that the body needs to make serotonin), is obtained from food and therefore severely underweight anorexic patients are unable to produce enough tryptophan. One way to resolve this issue is to look at the brains of recovered anorexic patients. Intriguingly, these studies show *hyper-responsivity* of the serotonin system in formerly anorexic patients, once they regain a healthy weight (Attia, 2010).

Kaye and colleagues (2009) argue that this is crucial to our understanding of anorexia, and that a hyper-responsive serotonin system may be a risk factor for the development of the disorder. Serotonin serves many different functions in the brain, and this picture is complicated because there are many different types of serotonin receptors, each of which will react differently to serotonin and lead to different behavioural outcomes. For example, increased serotonin transmission has been linked to both increased and decreased anxiety, depending on where in the brain the serotonin activity is concentrated and which types of serotonin receptors are being stimulated. On the other hand, increased serotonin activity in the hypothalamus is experienced as satiety. Kaye et al. (2009) propose that individuals who are vulnerable to anorexia (either people who are at risk of developing the disorder in the future, or those who have recovered and regained a healthy weight) have increased extracellular serotonin concentrations, and an imbalance in the number and sensitivity of two types of serotonin receptors (the 5-HT_{1A} and 5-HT_{2A} receptors). This particular pattern of serotonin activity leads to high levels of anxiety, particularly perfectionism and obsessive-compulsive traits, and an exaggerated satiety response. These symptoms are exacerbated whenever food is eaten because eating leads to the production of tryptophan, which leads to the synthesis of more serotonin, which activates the already over-stimulated serotonin receptors. Therefore, the biological consequence of eating (i.e. increased serotonin transmission) is extremely aversive for anorexic patients. This account can explain why symptomatic anorexic patients have reduced serotonin transmission: it is a consequence of self-starvation, something that anorexic patients do deliberately because they have learned that it is an effective way to dampen down activity in their hyperactive serotonin system, and thereby make themselves feel less anxious. The argument is that anorexic patients need to reduce their serotonin activity in order to feel 'normal', and they learn that starvation is a very effective way to do this.

Compelling evidence implicating the serotonin system with anxiety in anorexic patients comes from 'tryptophan depletion' studies. In these studies, participants consume an amino-acid drink that results in reductions in the level of tryptophan and therefore reduces serotonin transmission. In healthy controls tryptophan depletion leads to depressed mood, but in anorexic patients it results in reduced anxiety (Friederich et al., 2013).

While this general account of the role of serotonin in anorexia is widely accepted, the specific details of the underlying changes in serotonin transmission and receptor activity are still being investigated. Researchers hope that a better understanding of these biological changes will lead to new medications for anorexia that might be able to normalise serotonin transmission in the brain (see Section 4).

A deficit in dopamine function has also been implicated in anorexia. Anorexic patients show blunted dopamine transmission, including in the brain's reward system and some regions of the prefrontal cortex. A similar (albeit less severe) deficit is also seen in patients who have recovered from anorexia and have regained a healthy weight, which suggests that this is not merely a short-term consequence of starvation (Kaye et al., 2009). According to Kaye et al. (2009), reduced dopamine transmission may account for some other symptoms of anorexia including anhedonia (the inability to experience pleasure) and compulsive exercising.

Abnormalities of neurotransmitter function are also seen in bulimic patients. Regarding serotonin function, this appears to be hypo-responsive in bulimic patients who are currently symptomatic, but the deficit returns to normal in patients who have recovered (Jacobi et al., 2004). Given that bulimic patients do not tend to be underweight, this deficit in serotonin function is unlikely to be a consequence of nutritional deficits. In patients who are symptomatic, the severity of bulimic symptoms is negatively correlated with serotonin function: the more severe the symptoms, the more hypo-responsive is the serotonin system (Jacobi et al., 2004).

Beyond neurotransmitters: Brain network dysfunction in eating disorders

Kaye et al.'s (2009) account of anorexia starts with the role of anxiety in the disorder, and notes that self-starvation may reduce anxiety because it reduces serotonin transmission. Food-related cues evoke anxiety in anorexic patients, and brain imaging studies reveal that food cues activate an extended 'fear network' that includes the amygdala, anterior cingulate cortex, bilateral medial prefrontal cortex and hippocampus (Kaye et al., 2009). This may occur as a consequence of rapid fear learning for food stimuli, which we would expect if consumption of food leads to an aversive state as a result of increased serotonin activity. In addition to this 'fear of food', Friederich et al. (2013) reviewed evidence showing that anorexic patients exhibit cognitive deficits such as impaired cognitive flexibility, and this has been linked to an imbalance between prefrontal 'control' systems (which function normally) and subcortical motivational systems (which are underactive, perhaps due to reduced dopamine transmission, as discussed previously). The behavioural consequence of this is that anorexic patients should exhibit rigid, over-controlled behaviour and they should be very good at controlling their appetitive motivation (e.g. the motivation to consume food). This is, intriguingly, almost the exact opposite of the pattern of brain activity that characterises substance use disorders (see Chapter 9), and possibly bulimia and binge-eating disorder, as we discuss next.

According to Friederich et al. (2013), the disturbances in brain activity that characterise bulimia nervosa and binge eating disorder are quite different from those seen in anorexia. In healthy controls the reward system is usually activated during anticipation and initial consumption of food, an effect that is driven by increased dopamine transmission in the reward system (see the preceding section). Compared to healthy controls, bulimic patients show a blunted dopaminergic response to food while eating. Some studies have shown that bulimic patients show blunted activation in the reward system to all types of reward (e.g. monetary reward), which is linked to reduced dopamine transmission. Friederich et al. (2013) argue that the evidence suggests hypo-responsive reward circuitry in bulimic patients, which can be compensated for by binge eating. In other words, patients with bulimia have to eat a larger amount of food in order to stimulate their reward system, compared to healthy controls. By contrast, patients with binge-eating disorder show increased dopamine release in the reward system when they are exposed to food cues (e.g. the sight and smell of pizza) and when they are *anticipating* consuming food, a pattern that is not seen in bulimic patients.

Combined with these abnormalities of reward system function, bulimic patients show decreased activation of the prefrontal 'control' network, which includes the lateral prefrontal cortex and anterior cingulate cortex, when they perform tasks that require inhibitory control. Patients who are overweight also show reduced activation of this control network when they are exposed to food-related cues, which suggests a 'disinhibiting' effect of being exposed to food cues, at least in overweight participants.

Taking all of these findings together, Friederich et al. (2013) suggest that bulimic patients need to overeat in order to stimulate their relatively insensitive reward system, whereas patients with binge-eating disorder engage in binge eating because the motivational 'pull' of appetising food is too strong to resist. In addition, the prefrontal control system is relatively weak in these disorders, particularly when exposed to food-related cues, and this means that people find it difficult to resist whatever their reward system is motivating them to do (e.g. overeat). In this regard, the brain mechanisms that underlie bulimia and binge-eating disorder are very similar to those that are thought to underlie substance use disorders (see Chapter 9), which are an exaggerated reward response to the anticipation of drug reward, a blunted reward response during the consumption of drugs, combined with poor inhibitory control. However, we would urge you to be cautious and critical of this research on the brain mechanisms that are implicated in bulimia and binge-eating disorder. Most of the studies are very recent and many findings require replication, particularly those results that seem to be inconsistent across studies. There are also some examples of slightly dodgy intuitive leaps, for example using observations of how obese patients differ from normal weight controls to make assumptions about the psychological processes that underlie binge-eating disorder, even though binge-eating disorder and obesity are actually quite distinct from one another (see Box 10.5).

Box 10.8   Essential debate

Is anorexia a brain disease or an extreme response to the social pressure to be thin?

Widespread cultural acceptance of the 'thin ideal' is regularly blamed for the incidence of anorexia in females. As we showed in the previous section, there is plentiful evidence from longitudinal and experimental studies showing that exposure to the thin ideal leads to dissatisfaction with one's own body shape, and this in turn leads to symptoms of eating disorders such as restrictive eating and compensatory behaviours such as purging and excessive exercise.

However, it is often overlooked that *all* females in Western countries are bombarded with information about the thin ideal, yet anorexia is very rare: fortunately, most adolescent girls will not develop anorexia. Anorexia also has a very stereotyped and predictable clinical presentation, and this means that the symptoms are fairly uniform across individuals and tend to appear within a very specific age range. It is also highly heritable. Furthermore, cases of anorexia have been reported by doctors for (at least) the past few centuries, covering periods in which the 'ideal' female body shape was much larger than it is today. Historical records indicate cases of anorexia in previous centuries that did not have the shape and weight concerns that are typical of cases today (e.g. Parry-Jones & Parry-Jones, 1994). Also, clinicians working in developing countries report the absence of concerns about shape and weight in otherwise 'typical' cases of anorexia (Khandelwal et al., 1995), and weight concerns are not always seen in cases of anorexia even in Western countries (Palmer, 1993).

On this basis, Kaye et al. (2000) argue that anorexia should be seen as a heritable brain disorder, and cultural influences have been exaggerated. We might argue against this reductionist view by pointing out that medications such as antidepressants (e.g. selective serotonin reuptake inhibitors) and antipsychotics (dopamine antagonists) are not effective in the treatment of anorexia (see Section 4). Biological theorists would counter that this is because we do not yet fully understand the neurobiology of anorexia, and that until we do, we cannot create medications that target the complicated biological deficit that underlies anorexia.

Whatever your view on this, the correct explanation, as always, probably lies somewhere between these two extremes, with cultural pressures possibly exaggerating a heritable biological abnormality that predisposes to the disorder.

Psychological theories of eating disorders

Consistent with the biological theories described in the previous section, many psychological theories claim that anorexia is a form of anxiety disorder. More specifically, the symptoms of anorexia arise as a result of dysfunctional attempts to regulate emotion. Recall that biological theories (e.g. Kaye et al., 2009) suggested that a hyperactive serotonin system leads to feelings of anxiety that can only be alleviated by severely restricting food intake. This argument is extended in other theories. For example, Hatch et al. (2010) suggested that patients who are at risk of developing anorexia are hypersensitive to negative stimuli in general. During adolescence, they notice that eating food makes anxiety symptoms worse but restricting food intake leads to an alleviation of anxiety. This then gives rise to to the formation of negative associations with food, such that after a while food-related stimuli are processed as if they were threatening stimuli (e.g. in the same way that a spider phobic would process an image of a spider). Therefore, anorexia might be maintained because food evokes a form of fear response. Evidence in support of the theory comes from cross-sectional studies which show that food cues evoke a response in anorexic patients that is indistinguishable from the response of anxious patients to anxiety-provoking stimuli, in terms of their cognitive processing of those cues (see Treasure et al., 2010) and associated patterns of brain activation (Hatch et al., 2010). However, it is difficult to prove that pathological fear learning is actually the cause of food restriction, or whether it develops as a consequence of the other symptoms of anorexia.

Haynos and Fruzzetti (2011) proposed a similar emotion dysregulation model of anorexia. They argued that anorexic patients are prone to anxiety, particularly when faced with food. Importantly, these fear reactions are exacerbated by the effects of starvation, fatigue (induced by excessive exercise), and the sleep disruption that is an inevitable consequence of starvation. Furthermore, the frustrated reactions of family members to anorexic behaviour ('Why don't you just eat something?') only serve to increase the anxiety even more. It is important to distinguish the immediate from the longer-term effects of starvation on anxiety. In the short term, starvation leads to a temporary reduction in anxiety because it reduces serotonin activity. But in the longer term, starvation makes it more difficult to regulate mood and anxiety, which creates a vicious circle in which self-starvation is the only thing that can alleviate anxiety, all the while increasing the focus on food and the underlying level of anxiety.

As reviewed by Haynos and Fruzzetti (2011), several lines of evidence converge to suggest a deficit in emotion regulation in anorexic patients. Anorexic patients are more likely to use ineffective emotion regulation strategies such as suppression and avoidance. They are also likely to show abnormalities of emotional expression in the form of *alexithymia*. This refers to a style of not paying attention to one's one thoughts and feelings, such that they find it difficult to recognise and describe to others how they are feeling. There is also evidence that anorexic patients are more likely to restrict their food intake when they experience high levels of anxiety. For example, Engel et al. (2005) asked anorexic patients to carry mobile devices so that they could record life events, mood and restrictive eating practices. They found that the affective lability (big fluctuations in negative mood) that occurred in response to life stressors was predictive of restrictive eating practices in the hours after the stressful life event.

This suggests that anorexic patients use restrictive eating as a way to control their negative emotions following aversive experiences. However, this study doesn't confirm that patients engage in self-starvation in a deliberate attempt to control their anxiety levels, because these results could be explained in other ways. For example, high levels of anxiety might suppress appetite to such an extent that people feel too sick to eat. However, the balance of evidence does suggest that anorexic patients restrict their food intake in order to produce at least a short-term reduction in their anxious mood.

One issue with all emotion regulation theories of anorexia, including biological theories (Kaye et al., 2009), is that we cannot be sure that poor emotion regulation is a cause of restrictive eating rather than a consequence of months or years of starvation. However, evidence that close family members of anorexic patients show poor emotion regulation is consistent with the notion that this is a heritable vulnerability marker for anorexia (Kaye et al., 2000). According to Haynos and Fruzzetti (2011), if poor emotion regulation is a central feature of anorexia then it should be directly targeted during treatment. Unfortunately, although emotion regulation is a core component of CBT for bulimia (see Section 4), it is not usually included as a component in psychological therapies for anorexia, apart from in patients with the bingeing/purging subtype of anorexia (e.g. Fairburn et al., 2009). The emotion dysregulation theories discussed in this section suggest that treatments for all types of anorexia (including the restricting type) may benefit from including components that are designed to improve emotion regulation.

Perfectionism and the need for control

Fairburn et al. (1999) proposed a theoretical model for the *maintenance* of anorexia nervosa. According to this, people who are vulnerable to developing anorexia feel the need to control all aspects of their lives, a need that is related to perfectionism and inflexibility, two characteristic traits of anorexia. At some point they realise that dietary restriction is an extremely effective way of controlling body weight. For an individual who feels the need to control their life, restrictive eating behaviours are powerfully reinforced – not only by their highly visible and rapid weight loss, but also by the immediate emotional effect on family members, who are unable to influence the behaviour (i.e. they cannot force the anorexic patient to eat). Furthermore, the 'cultural wisdom' in Western countries is that people who are overweight have poor self-control, and the best way to lose weight is to exercise some self-control and restrict food intake. This strengthens the belief that being able to control food intake is indicative of good self-control in general.

According to the theory, anorexic patients perceive the high level of control that they have over their eating behaviour, and from this they infer that they have a high level of control over their life in general, something that is highly desired and equated with self-worth. Importantly, as body weight falls, it becomes harder to lose more weight and this threatens the sense of self-control, which means that the patient has to try even harder to 'take control' and restrict their food intake even further. Also, anorexics will constantly check their appearance for signs of 'progress' in weight loss ('body checking'), and subtle cognitive biases mean that anorexics perceive themselves as 'fat', and therefore as lacking in self-control, even when they are starving to death. Frequent body checking leads to even more dissatisfaction with one's physical appearance, which strengthens the belief that their body shape is out of control. Finally, starvation leads to a loss of concentration and reduced behavioural flexibility, which exacerbates the feelings of loss of control. The end result of all of these factors is a vicious circle of self-starvation in the pursuit of feelings of self-control.

When evaluating Fairburn's model, it is necessary to remember that it is explicitly framed as a model of the *maintenance* of anorexic symptoms once they develop. Therefore it is completely compatible with theories which suggest that symptoms can develop in response to biological abnormalities (e.g. a hyper-sensitive serotonin system) and associated problems with emotion regulation, which may also maintain the symptoms of the disorder. Fairburn's (1999) model makes a number of specific predictions that can and have been subject to empirical testing. For example, in a recent cross-sectional study Donovan and Penny (2014) showed that healthy adolescents who tried to exert control over their lives in general were more likely to diet. Furthermore, people who strongly equated self-control with their own self-esteem were much more likely to diet. This is consistent with Fairburn's prediction that self-esteem, self-control and dietary restriction are closely linked. However, this cross-sectional study with healthy volunteers (none of whom had an eating disorder) tells us nothing about the causal relationships between dietary restriction and perceived self-control that are central to Fairburn's theory.

Shafran et al. (2007) conducted an elegant experimental study to investigate whether repeated 'body checking' (scrutinising one's own appearance, usually in the mirror) was associated with body dissatisfaction and self-criticism. Sixty women were assigned to either a high body-checking group, who were instructed to critically scrutinise their bodies in a mirror, or a low body-checking group, who were instructed to scrutinise their bodies in a neutral way. In the high body-checking group body dissatisfaction and self-criticism increased, but these did not change in the low body-checking group. This study shows that critical body checking is likely to increase dissatisfaction with one's own appearance, as the theory predicts.

Finally, a strength of the theory is that is strikes a reasonable 'middle ground' between reductionist biological theories which argue that anorexia is the inevitable result of a biological and emotional deficit, and the popular and common-sense view that anorexia results from a societal pressure to be thin. We discussed this debate in Box 10.8. Fairburn's model allows the compromise between these two opposing views because it proposes that the disorder is maintained by the need to exert self-control, something that *can* be independent of the need to conform to a social pressure to be thin. However, in Western societies cultural acceptance of the thin ideal and stigmatisation of overweight can, and usually do, lead to concerns about body shape and the need to be thin.

Section summary

In this section we reviewed biological and psychological mechanisms in eating disorders. Disturbances of brain function are clearly established in anorexia, specifically hypersensitivity of the serotonin system that is linked to high levels of anxiety, which can be alleviated by self-starvation. Bulimia and binge-eating disorder have been linked with abnormalities of serotonin and dopamine function, which are possibly associated with altered responses to the rewarding properties of food. However, this research is in its early stages and it is becoming apparent that large networks of different structures in the brain are likely to be involved in eating disorders. Finally, one influential psychological theory of anorexia is related to the perfectionist traits that are characteristic of the disorder. This theory, which assigns a key role for self-control with regard to restricted food intake, is compatible with both the biological and broader cultural influences on symptoms of the disorder.

Section 4: How are eating disorders treated?

Initial interventions for anorexia

When anorexic patients present for treatment, they are often dangerously underweight. Therefore the first priority for treatment is to prevent patients from starving themselves to death. Seriously underweight patients are usually admitted to hospital where they will receive a structured behavioural intervention, the goal of which is simply to persuade them to eat enough food so they will gain weight. Clinicians are not really attempting to treat the underlying anorexia at this point, for fear of alienating the patient (Kaye et al., 2000). Attia (2010) points out that it is very difficult to conduct research into these kinds of interventions because most anorexic patients are not willing to take part in trials of therapy if the aim of that therapy is to gain weight.

Most patients who receive such behavioural interventions will eventually gain enough weight that they can be discharged from hospital and referred for different types of treatment to tackle the underlying causes of anorexia. Attia (2010) reported a weight gain of 1–2lbs per week in outpatient programmes and 3–4lbs per week in inpatient programmes. Unfortunately, some patients will refuse to gain weight, either by refusing to eat or by eating the food that is provided but then either vomiting it back up or burning off the calories by exercising. In these cases, doctors need to make the decision about whether the patient should be forced to gain weight against their will (e.g. by drip feeding), or whether their wishes should be respected. This is an issue that divides opinion among health professionals, and it boils down to whether you believe that a person who wants to starve themselves to death has the 'mental capacity' to take this decision (Bennett, 2005). As this is not clear cut, some anorexic patients do die of starvation because they cannot be forced to eat against their will.

Pharmacotherapy for eating disorders

In the previous section we showed that abnormalities of serotonin and dopamine function might contribute to the symptoms of eating disorders. Specifically, anorexia may be a consequence of hypersensitive serotonin function, and this is associated with feelings of anxiety, particularly around food, whereas abnormal (underactive) dopamine function in anorexia might underlie other symptoms such as anhedonia and compulsive exercising. In bulimia, dopamine and serotonin function seem to be relatively insensitive, which may explain why bulimic patients need to binge on food in order to gain enjoyment from eating and experience satiety. In binge-eating disorder the dopamine-based reward system may be oversensitive, which means that patients cannot resist the motivational 'pull' of food.

Clinicians can choose from lots of different drugs to increase, decrease or 'normalise' dopamine and serotonin transmission. For example, a crude way to block activity of the dopamine system is to prescribe dopamine antagonist drugs such as haloperidol: these are termed 'antipsychotic' drugs because their primary use is as a treatment for schizophrenia and other psychotic disorders (see Chapter 4). Other potentially useful drugs include different types of antidepressants, particularly selective serotonin reuptake inhibitors (SSRIs) which increase the amount of serotonin in the synapse and effectively increase serotonin activity. SSRIs are commonly used for the treatment of depression (Chapter 5) and generalised anxiety disorder (Chapter 6).

Therefore, there are sound biological reasons for believing that antipsychotics and antidepressants might be useful in the treatment of eating disorders. Furthermore, given that the disorders are characterised by anxious and depressed mood, and some anorexic patients appear delusional (e.g. about their own appearance), it makes sense that drugs which treat these symptoms in other disorders might be useful for the treatment of eating disorders. Randomised controlled trials show that SSRIs have a small beneficial effect on the symptoms of bulimia and some studies suggest that they may also be effective for binge-eating disorder (Kaye et al., 2000). However, although the drugs are effective for the short-term alleviation of symptoms, these symptoms tend to recur once patients stop taking the drugs, and therefore they should be combined with psychological therapy (Kaye et al., 2000).

Unfortunately, despite some initial promising trials, the available evidence suggests that neither antidepressants nor antipsychotics are effective for the treatment of anorexia (Treasure et al., 2010). Most researchers agree that abnormal serotonin function plays a key role in anorexia, so the lack of effectiveness of SSRIs was initially difficult to explain. Researchers now agree that SSRIs are ineffective because serotonin function in emaciated anorexic patients is so depleted that SSRIs (selective serotonin *reuptake inhibitors*) cannot work because there is not enough serotonin in the synapse to prevent the reuptake, and therefore the drugs do not lead to a substantial increase in serotonin function. A further complexity is that the nature of the disturbance in neurotransmitter activity in anorexia is not straightforward, because *some* subtypes of serotonin receptors in *some* brain regions may be hypersensitive, whereas other subtypes, in other brain regions, may be hyposensitive (Kaye et al., 2009). Therefore drugs such as SSRIs, which are not sufficiently specific to different receptor subtypes, may have no net benefit, and we need to design more specific drugs to target the particular neurochemical imbalance that characterises anorexia.

Cognitive behaviour therapy for bulimia

Fairburn et al. (1993) describe a therapy for bulimia based on cognitive behavioural techniques. This therapy can be broken down into three distinct stages:

- In *Stage 1*, the therapist and patient work together to identify the cognitive and emotional causes of binge episodes. This requires the patient to monitor their own eating behaviour and to identify any emotional triggers or maladaptive thoughts that trigger episodes of bingeing. The patient also receives information about the harmful effects of cycles of vomiting, use of laxatives, excessive exercise, and any other 'purging' behaviours. The therapist also 'prescribes' regular eating patterns (e.g. three meals and two snacks per day), and encourages the patient to stick to this in order to eliminate the desire to binge, identifying behaviours that should be applied whenever the patient is tempted to binge (e.g. phoning a friend). Close friends and family members may also be involved at this point, to ensure that the problem is 'out in the open' and to encourage the patient to comply with the advice of the therapist.

- *Stage 2* continues the emphasis on regular meals, identification of triggers of binge episodes, use of alternative behaviours to displace binges, and breaking the cycle of bingeing, purging and dieting. Patients are also encouraged to broaden the types of foods that form their typical diet. Other skills are introduced too: cognitive restructuring and behavioural techniques are used to tackle concerns about body shape and weight, and behavioural experiments are conducted to tackle dysfunctional beliefs. For example, bulimic patients often wear baggy clothes to avoid showing their bodies in public. In such cases, they would be encouraged to wear tighter clothes in order to disprove their 'hypothesis' that other people will remark that they look fat.

- *Stage 3* begins once patients are taking regular meals, and the frequency of bingeing and purging have been drastically reduced. Patients are encouraged to continue to apply the skills they have learned in order to prevent a relapse to bulimic behaviours. The most vital part of this stage is to reassure patients that it is unrealistic for them to expect never to binge again. They should be told that a relapse is likely, but also reminded of the skills they have learned to help them get over these setbacks.

Family therapy for anorexia

'Family Based Treatment', also known as 'Maudsley Family Therapy', is recommended for the treatment of anorexia by the American Psychiatric Association (Couturier et al., 2013). It is recommended for adolescents, but not adults, in the UK (Treasure et al., 2010). During this therapy, the immediate family members of the anorexic patient take responsibility for 'renourishing' the anorexic patient and helping them gain weight. Treatment usually lasts 9–12 months and most of it takes place in the patient's home. Receiving treatment at home may be preferable to conventional therapy in which anorexic patients must be admitted to hospital (so that they can gain weight), because although inpatient hospital treatment does lead to weight gain, extended hospital stays are very disruptive for family and social life and for progress in education. Treatment is usually provided by the family, with input from a therapist, and can be broken down into three stages:

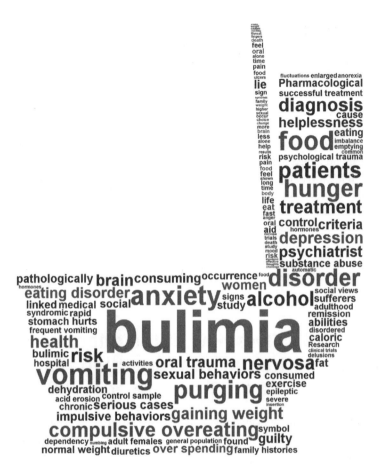

Figure 10.4   CBT aims to help bulimic patients to eat regular meals and reduce purging behaviours

- In the *weight restoration* stage, the therapist works with the family members to ensure that the patient gains weight. This is accomplished by being sympathetic to the patient's ambivalence about food and their concerns about weight gain, while also being firm about the need to eat. The patient is also encouraged to form stronger relationships with their siblings or friends so that they can see what 'normal' eating habits are in people of their own age. The therapist ensures that parents are not critical of their anorexic child, and that they are compassionate but firm. It is notable here that everything that goes on at this stage is pretty much the same as that which would occur if the patient were treated as a hospital inpatient: the main difference is that the treatment is provided in a family setting, by family members.

- The second stage can start once the patient is eating in the way that their parents are encouraging them to, and has started to gain weight. Now the focus shifts to *returning control over eating to the anorexic patient*. This involves a gradual loosening of parental control over eating behaviour whilst making sure that the patient is aware of the importance of gaining weight (slowly) and eating regular meals. Over time the patient exercises more control over what they eat and when they eat, and parental monitoring of this decreases.

- The final stage begins when the patient has almost returned to a healthy weight and they are no longer starving themselves. The focus now is *establishing a healthy adolescent identity*. Parents are involved in helping the anorexic patient to see how their eating disorder has disrupted their normal adolescent development, and they are encouraged to try to think of themselves as a healthy adolescent. As in stage 2, the patient is encouraged to take control over their own eating habits, but they should be guided by ideas about what kinds of behaviours are 'normal' for a person of their age.

How successful is therapy?

Box 10.9   Overview of the effectiveness of different treatments for eating disorders (adapted from Treasure et al., 2010)

(Asterisks indicate quality of evidence: * = poor, ** = moderate, *** = high.)

	Anorexia	Bulimia	BED
Drug treatments			
SSRIs (acute)	No effect*	Small effect***	Small effect**
Antipsychotics	Unclear*	Not studied	Not studied
Topiramate	Not studied	Small effect*	Moderate effect**
Psychological treatments			
CBT	Small effect*	Moderate effect***	Large effect**
Interpersonal psychotherapy	Small effect*	Small effect**	Moderate effect*
Psychodynamic psychotherapy	Small effect*	Unclear*	Not studied

---

Behavioural therapies	Unclear*	Small effect*	Not studied
Family therapy	Moderate effect**	Small effect*	Not studied
Behavioural weight loss therapy	Not studied	Not studied	Moderate effect*

Treasure et al. (2010) summarised the evidence for the effectiveness of drug and psychological therapies for different eating disorders, as well as considering the quality of the evidence. Quality of evidence is important, because if we want to recommend a treatment, we need to know that we are making our recommendation on the basis of good evidence! An overview of their conclusions is shown in Box 10.9, and these conclusions were supported in a more recent review by Hay (2013). We can see that different things seem to be effective for different eating disorders, and that there is no one treatment that is effective across the board. For anorexia, the only thing that is even moderately effective is family therapy, and the quality of evidence for this is reasonably good. Fisher et al. (2010) conducted a meta-analysis of studies that compared family therapy to individual psychotherapy (a similar type of psychological interventions therapy that is delivered by therapists rather than family members) for the treatment of anorexia in both adults and adolescents. They found that both family therapy and individual therapy were better than 'treatment as usual', but there was no difference in the rates of remission from anorexia at the end of treatment between those who received family versus individual therapy.

Couturier et al. (2013) were critical of the review by Fisher et al. (2010) because it combined studies from both adults and adolescents, and therefore neglected the possibility that adolescents might be more receptive to family interventions than adults. Couturier et al. conducted their own meta-analysis that only included studies with adolescent patients. They concluded that the effectiveness of family therapy and comparable individual therapy did not significantly differ at the end of treatment, consistent with the earlier findings from Fisher et al. (2010). However, when they looked at the follow-up data from 6 to 12 months after treatment had ended, family therapy looked significantly better than individual therapy. For example, Lock et al. (2010) reported that 22 of the 61 anorexic patients who had received family-based therapy were in complete remission from anorexia when tested one year after the end of treatment, versus only 11 of the 60 patients who had received comparable psychotherapy delivered on an individual basis.

Why does family therapy seem to be more effective at follow-up, but not immediately after treatment has ended? One plausible explanation is that when family members serve as 'therapists', they continue in this role long after the treatment has officially ended, whether they mean to or not. In contrast, when anorexic patients receive individual treatment from a psychotherapist, that source of support is withdrawn as soon as therapy finishes, and therefore a relapse to previous patterns of disordered eating may be more likely (Couturier et al., 2013)

More recent trials demonstrate that other types of psychological treatments can have small beneficial effects in anorexia, such as CBT (Touyz et al., 2013) and psychodynamic therapy (Zipfel et al., 2014). There is no convincing evidence for the use of medications (particularly antidepressants such as SSRIs, or antipsychotic drugs) for the treatment of anorexia (Mitchell et al., 2013). Treasure et al. (2010) state that there are very few good clinical trials of treatments for anorexia for two main reasons. First, the participants are often withdrawn from the trials because clinicians are unable to stabilise them (i.e. get them up to a healthy weight), which is necessary before any treatment can be started. Second, patients often withdraw from these trials because they find the treatments unacceptable. Therefore it is very difficult to say with confidence what works (and what doesn't work) for anorexia, because it is so difficult to conduct research in this area.

For bulimia there is good quality evidence for the effectiveness of CBT, which has an overall moderate effect. Beneficial effects of treatment are maintained at follow-up, with Fairburn et al. (1995) reporting that 63% of patients had no eating disorder diagnosis an average of six months after therapy. In addition to CBT, Treasure et al. (2010) found evidence that other forms of psychological therapy (interpersonal psychotherapy, psychodynamic therapy, behavioural therapy and family therapy) have a small beneficial effect for patients with bulimia, but the quality of the evidence for these treatments is variable. There are many good quality studies of SSRIs for bulimia, and overall these drugs seem to have a small but robust effect on symptom reduction. However, SSRIs are usually only given for a short period of time (i.e. around eight weeks) and up to 40% of people drop out of treatment if they receive SSRIs with no psychosocial support. Even after treatment has finished, fewer than 20% of patients who had received SSRIs show a complete remission of bulimia symptoms, a similar remission rate to that seen in patients who are given a placebo (Mitchell et al., 2013).

Even though binge-eating disorder was only officially recognised as a psychological disorder in 2013 (when *DSM*-5 was published), treatments for the disorder have been investigated for several years. As a result, several promising treatments have been identified including CBT, psychotherapy and behavioural weight loss therapy, all of which are at least moderately effective and the evidence is reasonably good. Pharmacotherapies including SSRIs and topiramate (an anticonvulsant drug) also seem to be effective. This general pattern was confirmed in a meta-analysis of treatment studies reported by Vocks et al. (2010), who noted that both CBT and antidepressants led to a reduction in binge-eating behaviour but did not result in a reduction in body weight. However, given that excess body weight is not one of the diagnostic criteria for binge-eating disorder, the lack of effect on weight loss is only of concern to those with binge-eating disorder who are also overweight.

It is interesting to note that some treatments seem to be effective for both bulimia and binge-eating disorder, but also that drugs (topiramate and sibutramine) and psychological interventions (behavioural weight loss therapy such as 'Weight Watchers') that are used to help obese people control their appetite are also effective treatments for binge-eating disorder. This takes us back to the issue of overlap between these diagnostic categories, and also the issue of whether overeating that leads to obesity should be considered as an eating disorder, as we discussed in Box 10.5.

Box 10.10 Essential research

Exposure therapy (Koskina et al., 2013)

In bulimia nervosa and binge-eating disorder, overeating may occur because of *cue reactivity*. People may overeat if they are exposed to tempting food cues such as the sight and smell of hot pizza, because that cue has been paired with the rewarding effects of food consumption in the past, which causes that cue to evoke a classically conditioned response including salivation and a desire to eat that food. It may be possible to reduce cue reactivity (and therefore prevent people from binge eating) by exposing them to tempting food cues but not allowing them to eat, an intervention known as *cue exposure with response prevention*, or more simply *exposure therapy*. For details of how this type of treatment has been applied successfully in the treatment of phobias see Chapter 7, although you should also see Chapter 9 for a discussion of why this approach does not seem to be effective for the treatment of substance use disorders.

Koskina et al. (2013) conducted a systematic review of the literature and identified 31 studies that investigated cue exposure therapy for eating disorders. Studies that involved exposure to tempting food cues while preventing binge eating produced some encouraging findings, for example cravings for the food decreased over time. One large trial showed that exposure therapy combined with CBT led to greater reductions in bulimic symptoms at a five-year follow-up, compared to a group that received CBT but no exposure therapy (McIntosh et al., 2011). Koskina et al. (2013) argue that researchers may have lost interest in exposure therapy as a treatment for bulimia because of the clear effectiveness of CBT for the disorder, and because there is no evidence that exposure therapy is superior to CBT. However, they point out that exposure therapy may be worth exploring in combination with CBT, or as an alternative treatment for patients who do not respond to CBT.

Other variations of cue exposure therapy may also be useful for the treatment of eating disorders. For example, if bulimic patients are allowed to binge eat but are prevented from vomiting afterwards, this could break the associative link between binge eating and vomiting. Patients with anorexia experience anxiety when they are exposed to fattening foods or to the sight of their own bodies, and controlled exposure to these stimuli may

(Continued)

(Continued)

lead to reductions in anxiety in the same way that exposure to spiders can help spider phobics overcome their fear (see Chapter 7). However, these applications of cue exposure therapy have not yet been studied in proper randomised controlled trials. Koskina et al. (2013) suggest that these applications of exposure therapy are worth studying more carefully, perhaps in combination with drug treatments or biological interventions such as Transcranial Magnetic Stimulation (TMS; see Box 4.6, Chapter 4) to facilitate learning. This is particularly true for anorexia nervosa, for which very few effective treatments are available.

Essential questions

Some possible exam questions that stem from this chapter are:

- Is anorexia a heritable biological disorder, an inevitable response to a societal pressure to be thin, or a combination of these?
- Critically evaluate biological and psychological theories of eating disorders. To what extent can these theories explain the same phenomena?
- Are treatments for eating disorders effective and what are the prospects for the development of better treatments in the future?

Further reading

Fairburn, C. G., Cooper, Z., & Shafran, R. (2003). Cognitive behaviour therapy for eating disorders: A 'transdiagnostic' theory and treatment. *Behaviour Research and Therapy*, 41(5): 509–528 (A good introduction to the transdiagnostic model, with implications for treatment.)

Kaye, W. H., Fudge, J. L., & Paulus, M. (2009). New insights into symptoms and neuro-circuit function of anorexia nervosa. *Nature Reviews Neuroscience*, 10(8): 573–584. (A well-written overview of the complex issue of biological basis of anorexia: bear in mind that the authors are proposing their own theory in this paper so you should also look at other sources to get a balanced view.)

Treasure, J., Claudino, A. M., & Zucker, N. (2010). Eating disorders. *The Lancet*, 375(9714): 583–593. (Excellent overview of everything, and interesting detail on the medical consequences of anorexia, but a bit light on details of the psychological theories of eating disorders.)

PERSONALITY DISORDERS

General introduction

We begin this chapter by introducing broad issues with the categorisation of personality disorders, and then focus on antisocial and borderline personality disorders in detail. We demonstrate that these disorders are heritable and can be influenced by traumatic events and abnormal attachments during childhood, but we need to be aware of methodological issues that make it difficult to reach straightforward conclusions about their causes. We then discuss psychological and biological models of personality disorders, and show how these have informed the development of psychological therapies. These therapies might be effective for borderline personality disorder, but they don't seem to be very effective for antisocial personality disorder.

Assessment targets

At the end of the chapter, you should ask yourself the following questions:

- Do I understand the diagnostic criteria for personality disorders, and can I explain the controversies that surround their categorisation?
- Can I critically evaluate the roles of childhood trauma, attachment, and genetic influences in the development of personality disorders?
- Can I explain and evaluate biological and psychological models of personality disorders, and relate them back to the ultimate causes of those disorders?
- Can I describe treatments for personality disorders, explain how different treatments overlap, and evaluate their effectiveness?

Section 1: What are personality disorders?

Personality disorders (PDs) are characterised by long-lasting patterns of behaviour and subjective experience that deviate from the norms of the culture in which the person lives. These patterns tend to first appear in adolescence (but there is controversy about whether they should be diagnosed in adolescents), they are stable over time, and they are inflexible. In common with all other psychological disorders, they must cause either distress to the sufferer or impairment of 'normal' functioning. As we will see, the types of behaviours, distress and experience that indicate the presence of PD are very diverse and wide-ranging. You could say that, after excluding other psychological disorders, a person whose personality makes them 'a bit different' from what is considered normal could be considered to have PD.

It is helpful to first consider the general criteria for personality disorders, which are shown in Box 11.1. Bear in mind that these criteria do not describe any particular PD, but they do outline the features that all PDs have in common.

Box 11.1   Essential diagnosis

Personality disorders

According to *ICD*-10 (World Health Organisation, 1992), the general criteria for personality disorder are as follows:

A. Evidence that the individual's characteristic and enduring patterns of inner experience and behaviour deviate markedly as a whole from the culturally expected and accepted range (or 'norm'). Such deviation must be manifest in more than one of the following areas:

   (1) cognition (i.e. ways of perceiving and interpreting things, people and events; forming attitudes and images of self and others);
   (2) affectivity (range, intensity and appropriateness of emotional arousal and response);
   (3) control over impulses and need for gratification;
   (4) relating to others and manner of handling interpersonal situations.

B. The deviation must manifest itself pervasively as behaviour that is inflexible, maladaptive, or otherwise dysfunctional across a broad range of personal and social situations (i.e. not being limited to one specific 'triggering' stimulus or situation).
C. There is personal distress, or adverse impact on the social environment, or both, clearly attributable to the behaviour referred to under (B).

> D. There must be evidence that the deviation is stable and of long duration, having its onset in late childhood or adolescence.
>
> Very similar criteria are described in *DSM*-5 (American Psychiatric Association, 2013a), and both *ICD*-10 and *DSM*-5 specify the importance of excluding brain damage or other psychological disorders as causes of these symptoms.

The German psychiatrist Kurt Schneider (1923) is credited with proposing 10 'psychopathic personality types', and most of these have appeared in successive versions of the *ICD* and *DSM*, albeit with different names (Tyrer, 2013). *ICD*-10 describes seven specific PDs, whereas *DSM*-5 recognizes 10. In *DSM*-5 they are split into three clusters: odd-eccentric, dramatic-emotional and anxious-fearful. The specific PDs in *DSM*-5 are as follows:

Cluster A (the odd-eccentric cluster):

- Paranoid PD (characterised by distrust and suspiciousness of others; also in *ICD*-10).
- Schizoid PD (social detachment and restricted emotional expression; also in *ICD*-10).
- Schizotypal PD (social discomfort, cognitive distortions and eccentric behaviour).

Cluster B (the dramatic-emotional cluster):

- Antisocial PD (see Box 11.2; disregard for the rights and feelings of others; labelled 'Dissocial PD' in *ICD*-10).
- Borderline PD (Box 11.3; unstable relationships, self-image and mood, and marked impulsivity; labelled 'Emotionally Unstable PD, borderline type' in *ICD*-10).
- Histrionic PD (excessive emotionality and attention-seeking; also in *ICD*-10).
- Narcissistic PD (grandiosity, a need for admiration, and lack of empathy).

Cluster C (the anxious-fearful cluster):

- Avoidant PD (social inhibition, feelings of inadequacy, and hypersensitivity to criticism; also in *ICD*-10).
- Dependent PD (submissive and 'clingy' behaviour related to a need to be taken care of; also in *ICD*-10).
- Obsessive-compulsive PD (preoccupation with orderliness, perfectionism, and control over one's environment; also in *ICD*-10 but referred to as 'Anankastic' PD).

In addition to this lengthy list, both *ICD*-10 and *DSM*-5 include formal diagnoses of 'other specified personality disorder' and 'other unspecified personality disorder' which are used when somebody meets the general criteria for PD (see Box 11.1), but doesn't quite meet the criteria for one of the specific disorders listed above. The distinction between these two is that for the 'other specified' diagnosis, the clinician might note, for example, that the person has features of both borderline and schizoid PDs, but they don't quite meet the full criteria for either. The 'other unspecified' diagnosis would be used if the clinician felt that the person met the general criteria for PD, but they could not be any more specific than that (this is a formal way of saying 'This person is a bit odd', and it seems like a pretty unhelpful diagnosis to us). Finally, *DSM*-5 has a further diagnostic category of 'personality change due to another medical condition', which captures the marked personality change that can occur as a result of head injury, infection or substance use for example.

In this book, we will cover antisocial (APD) and borderline (BPD) personality disorders in detail, but we will not discuss the others beyond this section. This is not because we are lazy, but because APD and BPD have been the focus of the majority of PD research, which means that there is lots of evidence related to the psychological processes that underlie the disorders, their causes, and the best ways to treat and manage them (i.e. the things that we are covering in this book). Most of the other PDs have not been studied in as much detail.

Box 11.2   Essential diagnosis

Antisocial personality disorder

The *DSM*-5 (American Psychiatric Association, 2013) criteria for antisocial personality disorder are as follows:

A Pervasive pattern of disregard for and violation of the rights of others, occurring since age 15 years, as indicated by three (or more) of the following:

1. Failure to conform to social norms with respect to lawful behaviours, as indicated by repeatedly performing acts that are grounds for arrest.
2. Deceitfulness, as indicated by repeated lying, use of aliases, or conning others for personal profit or pleasure.
3. Impulsivity or failure to plan ahead.
4. Irritability and aggressiveness, as indicated by repeated physical fights or assaults.
5. Reckless disregard for safety of self or others.
6. Consistent irresponsibility, as indicated by repeated failure to sustain consistent work behaviour or honour financial obligations.
7. Lack of remorse, as indicated by being indifferent to or rationalizing having hurt, mistreated, or stolen from someone.

B. The individual is at least age 18 years.
C. There is evidence of conduct disorder with onset before age 15 years.
D. The occurrence of antisocial behaviour is not exclusively during the course of schizophrenia or bipolar disorder.

The *ICD*-10 criteria for this disorder are similar, although the official label in *ICD*-10 is 'Dissocial' PD (World Health Organisation, 1992).

Box 11.3   Essential diagnosis

Borderline personality disorder

The *DSM*-5 (American Psychiatric Association, 2013a) criteria for borderline personality disorder are as follows:

A. A pervasive pattern of instability and interpersonal relationships, self-image, and affect, and marked impulsivity, beginning by early adulthood and present in a variety of contexts, as indicated by five (or more) of the following:

1. Frantic efforts to avoid real or imagined abandonment.
2. A pattern of unstable and intense interpersonal relationships characterized by alternating between extremes of idealization and devaluation.
3. Identity disturbance: markedly and persistently unstable self-image or sense of self.
4. Impulsivity in at least two areas that are potentially self-damaging, e.g. spending, sex, substance abuse, reckless driving, binge eating.
5. Recurrent suicidal behaviour, gestures, or threats, or self-mutilating behaviour.
6. Affective instability due to a marked reactivity of mood (e.g. intense episodic dysphoria, irritability, or anxiety usually lasting a few hours and only rarely more than a few days).
7. Chronic feelings of emptiness.
8. Inappropriate, intense anger or difficulty controlling anger (e.g. frequent displays of temper, constant anger, recurrent physical fights).
9. Transient, stress-related paranoid ideation or severe dissociative symptoms.

The *ICD*-10 criteria for this disorder are similar, although the official *ICD*-10 label is 'Emotionally unstable PD, Impulsive type' (World Health Organisation, 1992).

Before we move on to a detailed discussion of these two disorders, we must first consider issues of categorisation and diagnosis of PDs, and their overlap with other psychological disorders. This discussion has implications for our understanding of *all* PDs.

Changes and controversies in *DSM*-5

Compared to its previous versions, the publication of *DSM*-5 saw a major change in the way that PDs were categorised. Earlier versions of the *DSM* (3 and 4) were split into five different 'axes' (dimensions). Axis 1 specified the primary diagnosis and this axis incorporated most of the 'clinical disorders' that are covered in this book. All other axes described 'modifiers' which should be considered in order to understand the causes, course and prospects for recovery from the primary diagnosis. Axis 2 incorporated enduring and persistent maladaptive traits, and this included PDs. This distinction is really significant because it has influenced the way in which PDs are perceived in comparison to other psychological disorders. Unlike other 'clinical disorders', these were viewed as permanent features of an individual's psychological makeup that could (and usually did) co-exist with more conventional clinical disorders. A damaging and stigmatising implication of the distinction between axis 1 and 2 disorders was that axis 2 disorders reflected permanent traits that could not be treated, only 'managed' (Limandri, 2012; Trull & Durrett, 2005).

This all changed in *DSM*-5: all mental disorders are now viewed along the same axis. Most researchers have welcomed this change, because there is no convincing evidence for a meaningful distinction between PDs and other mental disorders. However, there is an arguably even bigger issue with the categorisation of PDs, and this was not really addressed in *DSM*-5. Throughout this book we have been critical of the *categorical* (or *diagnostic*) view of psychological disorders espoused in *ICD*-10 and *DSM*-5, which treats each disorder as if it were distinct from other disorders and from 'normal' human experience. According to the *DSM*, you either have a particular disorder or you do not.

This standpoint is particularly problematic when it comes to PDs. The structure of 'normal' personality is captured by the 'Big Five' personality dimensions, which are neuroticism, openness to experience, extraversion, agreeableness and conscientiousness (Costa & McCrae, 1992). Everyone has a personality, and all personalities can be 'boiled down' to a combination of these traits. This raises a critical question: Do PDs reflect some combination of these Big Five traits, possibly with extreme scores on some traits? If so, this would suggest that PDs are at the extremes of 'normal' personality, but there is no qualitative difference.

Saulsman and Page (2004) conducted a meta-analysis of existing studies and showed how the Big Five could be meaningfully applied to PD diagnoses: most personality disorders were characterised by high neuroticism and/or low agreeableness, with other traits discriminating between different disorders. For example, BPD is characterised by high neuroticism, low agreeableness and low conscientiousness, whereas APD is characterised by low agreeableness and low conscientiousness. A large body of subsequent research has confirmed that there is no meaningful qualitative difference between pathological and 'normal' personalities (see also Trull & Durrett, 2005; Tyrer, 2013). As a consequence of these and other findings, researchers have called for categorical approaches to PDs to be replaced by dimensional approaches (Trull & Durrett, 2005). With a dimensional approach, all personality traits operate on a continuum, and people with PDs are at the extreme ends of one or more of those continua.

As *DSM*-5 was being developed, the American Psychiatric Association was wrestling with the categorical versus dimensional distinction for many disorders, and particularly PDs, and this is evident in the addition of section 3 for *DSM*-5. In section 3, a hybrid dimensional-categorical model of PDs is outlined in order 'to encourage further study on how this new methodology could be used to assess personality and diagnose personality disorders in clinical practice' (American Psychiatric Association, 2013b). The proposal, which was very close to being adopted and replacing the categorical approach (Skodol, 2012), was that clinicians would evaluate impairments in personality functioning (how the individual experiences themself as well as others), but they would also assess five pathological personality traits (which overlap with the Big Five, but are not quite the same) that have been implicated in PDs (Skodol, 2012). Distinct constellations of traits should map onto distinct categorical diagnoses. Using this hybrid approach, six different PDs could be distinguished:

- borderline;
- obsessive-compulsive;
- avoidant;
- schizoptypal;
- antisocial;
- narcissistic.

This hybrid dimensional-categorical model was carefully considered by the APA as a radical replacement to the existing categorical model of PDs, and it came very close to replacing the old model in *DSM*-5. However, this (and any dimensional model) has its own problems, some conceptual and some practical (see Millon, 2012). For example, concerns were raised that most clinicians are trained in the medical model of diagnosis (their patients either have a disease, or they do not), and they may be uncomfortable if asked to assess patients using a dimensional approach. Furthermore, with any dimensional approach some kind of cut-off score would need to be applied. For example, a decision may need to be made about what level of neuroticism would indicate that a patient needs treatment. This leads us back to the same problems that plague the categorical, diagnostic approach (Skodol, 2012). After much internal wrangling within the APA, they eventually decided to stick with the existing categorical approach, and relegate the dimensional-categorical model to section 3 of the manual as something in need of more research. Some researchers were very critical of the APA's decision to stick with the status quo. For example, Tyrer (2013) wrote in a scathing commentary, published just before *DSM*-5 was published:

> … (the APA) cannot tolerate it and will return to the old DSM-IV classification when the DSM 5 is published, with the DSM 5 proposal (for a dimensional diagnosis) placed in a parking lot to be revisited by weary travellers at some time in the very distant future.

Tyrer was more positive about the prospects for the *International Classification of Diseases*, the 11th edition of which will be published in 2017. *ICD*-11 is likely to incorporate a dimensional approach to PDs, which will be diagnosed based on the severity of impairment in four different domains of personality. This would mark a break from the way in which PDs are viewed in *DSM*-5. For many clinicians (but not all) this new approach to diagnosis would be very welcome and long overdue.

Other 'personality disorders'

You may be wondering when we will cover the *really interesting* PDs, such as multiple personality disorder and psychopathy. The disorder depicted in fiction and films as 'multiple personality disorder' is officially known as 'Dissociative Identity Disorder' and it belongs in the 'Dissociative Disorders' category in *DSM*-5 (American Psychiatric Association, 2013a): it is not categorised alongside other personality disorders so we do not cover it here. There is controversy over whether it should be recognised as a disorder at all: some researchers claim that most apparent sufferers should be given a different diagnosis, and that over-zealous clinicians are blamed for diagnosing it inappropriately (Boysen & Vanbergen, 2013).

The terms 'psychopathy' and 'sociopathy' are often used interchangeably with antisocial PD. However this is inappropriate, because psychopathy is not (and never has been) recognised as a PD by the *DSM* or *ICD* classification systems. However, the term 'psychopath' is widely used in forensic settings such as prisons and secure psychiatric hospitals. Hare (2003) is widely credited with characterising the disorder and formulating an instrument for assessing it: the Psychopathy Checklist – Revised (PCL-R). Although there is similarity between APD and psychopathy, such as the shared emphasis on antisocial and criminal behaviour, psychopathy is a much narrower diagnosis. Characteristics of psychopathy that are not features of APD include poverty of positive and negative emotions (emotional detachment) and being motivated by thrill-seeking. Some theorists (e.g. Blair et al., 2006) argue that the emotional aspects of psychopathy are crucial to its development and are what distinguish it from APD. According to Hare (2003), the prevalence of APD in forensic settings ranges between 50% and 80%, but only 15% to 25% of prisoners would be diagnosed with psychopathy based on the PCL-R. The discussion in the previous section about categorical versus dimensional diagnosis of PDs also applies to psychopathy: its status as an extreme dimension of 'normal' personality or a distinct personalty type is debated (Trull & Durrett, 2005).

Regardless of the official status of the 'psychopathy' label, PDs are very important in forensic settings. People with an APD diagnosis are at least 10 times more likely than controls to commit a violent crime. Furthermore, incarcerated offenders with a diagnosis of APD are twice as likely to commit another offence after their release from prison, compared to offenders without such a diagnosis (Yu et al., 2012). In the UK, the term 'Dangerous and Severe Personality Disorder' was introduced to replace the term 'psychopathy'. This label was applied to offenders who had a high score on the PCL-R and were deemed a risk to the public, and it was used to justify their 'preventive detention', that is, they had to remain in prison, even after their initial sentence had finished, for the protection of the public. While this makes sense from one perspective, another way of looking at it is that it justifies keeping people in prison on the basis of bad things that they *might* do in future, and all this on the basis of a dubious 'diagnosis'. Following extensive criticism, the DSPD scheme was eventually terminated (Duggan, 2011).

Prevalence, course and comorbidity of personality disorders

PDs are common: according to the APA, between 9% and 15% of adults in the USA have at least one PD (American Psychiatric Association, 2013a). Most patients who are diagnosed with a specific PD meet the criteria for more than one (Skodol, 2012) – which again raises questions about the extent to which the different PDs reflect distinct diagnoses that can be distinguished from each other. The prevalence rates of APD range between 0.2% and 3.3%, although prevalence estimates as high as 80% are seen in forensic settings (see previous section) and in males with severe alcohol use disorder (American Psychiatric Association, 2013a). The population prevalence of BPD is estimated at 1.6% but could be considerably higher (up to 5.9%), rising to about 20% of psychiatric inpatients (American Psychiatric Association, 2013a). Prevalence estimates for the other PDs are also provided in *DSM-5*, and they range between 0.5% (dependent PD) and 7.9% (obsessive-compulsive PD). However, you should treat these prevalence estimates with some scepticism, given the controversy surrounding the validity of the different diagnoses, the fact that many patients will be diagnosed with more than one PD, and the overlap and co-morbidity with other psychological disorders, which we discuss later in this section.

Box 11.4 Essential debate

Are personality disorders stable over time?

Unlike other psychological disorders, PDs are viewed as stable, enduring features of an individual's character that have a chronic course and cannot be effectively treated. This is the main reason why *DSM-IV* distinguished them from most other psychological disorders by placing them on a totally different axis. Although the multi-axial format of *DSM-IV* was discarded in *DSM-5*, the assumption that PDs are stable is still prominent in the *DSM* criteria, which refer to all indicators of PDs as 'enduring' (see Boxes 11.2 and 11.3). Morey and Hopwood (2013) reviewed the results from several large longitudinal studies that investigated the stability of PDs. They concluded that the overall picture was complex, and the stability of PDs depended on various features of the methods used. One of their conclusions was that PD *diagnoses* tended to be unstable over time, whereas PD *dimensions* (particularly personality traits that were central to the disorder) were much more stable over time.

This has some important implications. First, if PD diagnoses are not stable over time, then this removes any meaningful distinction between PDs and other mental disorders and justifies the decision in *DSM-5* to place all mental disorders in the same category. Second, it suggests that the dimensional approach to PDs, which was *not* adopted for *DSM-5*, implies that dimensions of PDs (i.e. personality traits) may be relatively stable. If dimensions of PDs are stable but dimensions of other mental disorders are not, this supports the idea of a clear distinction between disordered personality traits and mental disorders – and therefore they should perhaps be on a separate axis after all! However, other mental disorders such as anxiety and mood disorders are more stable over time than is generally assumed (Morey & Hopwood, 2013). Overall, we can conclude that there is probably no meaningful difference in stability between PDs and other psychological disorders.

As with every other disorder in this book, co-morbidity between PDs and other disorders is very common. For example, the symptoms of schizophrenia and other psychotic disorders (Chapter 4) bear a striking resemblance to those of paranoid, schizotypal and schizoid PDs, with a clear overlap between the positive symptoms of schizophrenia and paranoid and schizotypal PDs, whereas the negative symptoms of schizophrenia are similar to those seen in schizoid PD. Although patients are rarely diagnosed with *both* schizophrenia and one of these PDs, there is evidence for shared vulnerability factors (e.g. heritable risk) for both schizotypal PD and schizophrenia. Also, patients who are diagnosed with schizotypal PD at one point in time are more likely to be diagnosed with schizophrenia at a later point in time (Links & Eynan, 2013). Some researchers have suggested that the trait of schizotypy, which is present to varying degrees in the general population (see Chapter 4), should be thought of as one domain of a continuum of normality, with schizophrenia at the extreme end and schizotypal PD somewhere in the middle (Links & Eynan, 2013). This would suggest a logical change to future versions of the *DSM*, which could combine the diagnostic categories of schizophrenia and schizotypal PD to form a dimensional category.

To give another example, avoidant PD shares many features with social anxiety disorder (Chapter 8), and arguably the most important difference between them is that social anxiety disorder is seen as treatable whereas avoidant PD is held to be stable and enduring. The evidence discussed in Box 11.4 on the (in)stability of PDs suggests that even this distinction may be an illusion, so the case for recognising them as distinct disorders seems weak (Links & Eynan, 2013).

Unlike most other PDs, APD appears to be distinct from other mental disorders. However, the disorder is highly co-morbid with various disorders, including social anxiety disorder, GAD, attention deficit disorder and substance use disorders (the estimated prevalence of APD in severely dependent alcoholics has been estimated at 80%; see Links & Eynan, 2013). Finally, there is a considerable overlap between BPD and bipolar disorder (see Chapter 5): both are characterised by unstable mood, impulsivity, and behavioural dysregulation (Limandri, 2012). *DSM*-5 (American Psychiatric Association, 2013a) specifies that the disorders can be distinguished on the basis of the duration of episodes of mania or depressed mood. However, manic episodes can last for a very long time in some subtypes of bipolar disorder, and in clinical practice it may not be possible to distinguish between the two (Limandri, 2012). Other research suggests that BPD is co-morbid with *all* mood, anxiety and substance use disorders, and it is common for BPD patients to be diagnosed with three or more co-morbid disorders (e.g. alcohol use disorder, generalised anxiety, and bipolar disorder; Links & Eynan, 2013).

Comorbidity between PD and other mental disorders is important: a PD diagnosis usually means a worse prognosis for any co-morbid mental disorders. For example, major depressive disorder (Chapter 5) tends to have a much more chronic course in people who also have a PD diagnosis (Gask et al., 2013).

Section summary

In this section we have introduced the diagnostic category of PDs and provided a detailed description of two specific disorders: antisocial and borderline personality disorders. We have shown that there is a great deal of controversy about the way that PDs are categorised, and we have argued that a dimensional approach may be more useful, although it is not without its own problems. Finally, we also showed that PDs are fairly common and are frequently co-morbid with other mental disorders.

Section 2: How do personality disorders develop?

Heritability

There are substantial heritable influences on both personality traits and PDs. Heritability estimates for personality traits in the general population range between 40% and 60%, whereas heritability estimates for the symptoms of personality disorders range between 30% and 80% (Fontaine & Viding, 2008). Twin studies have yielded heritability estimates ranging between 43% and 69% for APD, although one study that relied on a self-report measure reported a heritability estimate of zero. Heritability estimates for BPD derived from twin studies range between 69% and 77% (Fontaine & Viding, 2008), although a more recent review estimated the heritability of BPD at 40% (Amad et al., 2014). Adoption studies also suggest that PDs are heritable; for example, adopted children of biological parents that had been diagnosed with APD had higher levels of antisocial traits themselves (Fontaine & Viding, 2008). However, the role played by a stressful prenatal environment should not be discounted here (see Chapters 1 and 3).

Although this all seems fairly straightforward, the reality is complex. Conduct disorder in children (see Chapter 3 and Box 3.2) is a precursor of APD in adults, and adult APD is highly co-morbid with substance use disorder (particularly alcohol use disorder). Heritable influences on all of these disorders are shared, and it is not possible to distinguish between these influences (Hicks et al., 2004). This means that an individual who is at increased heritable risk of alcohol use disorder is also at increased risk of conduct disorder and APD, and the converse is also true: heritable risk for APD translates to increased risk for alcohol use disorder. Similarly, there is considerable shared heritability between APD and antisocial and criminal behaviour more generally (Blair et al., 2006). A more promising focus has been the study of heritability of the callous and unemotional traits that underlie *psychopathy*. Several twin studies suggest high heritability estimates for these traits (e.g. fearless dominance and impulsive antisociality) in the general population (see Blair et al., 2006). A similar picture emerges for BPD: there is substantial overlap between genetic vulnerability for BPD and major depressive disorder (see Chapter 5), and heritability estimates for BPD *traits* tend to be higher than those for BPD diagnoses (Amad et al., 2014). A recent study also showed that the severity of the nine different *criteria* for BPD (see Box 11.3) was highly heritable in the general population (Reichborn-Kjennerud et al., 2013). This has implications for the debate about dimensional versus categorical classifications of personality disorders, as this recent heritability research shows us that a more precise understanding of genetic influences can be gained by studying traits rather than categorical diagnoses.

Finally, for all personality disorders, including APD and BPD, the search for specific genetic variants that underlie these disorders has been the familiar story of an apparent breakthrough discovery ('We found the gene for psychopathy!'), followed by several failures to replicate those findings (see Chapter 1). This is unsurprising for numerous reasons; for example, it is implausible that a single genetic variant could account for a personality disorder diagnosis. Multiple different genes, and G × G and G × E interactions (see Chapters 1 and 3) are likely to contribute to the specific traits and behaviours that make up different dimensions of personality disorders (Amad et al., 2014; Calati et al., 2013; Fontaine & Viding, 2008).

Environmental factors

Although high, heritability estimates for PDs are some way off 100%, which suggests a substantial role for environmental influences. The main purpose of twin studies may be to quantify the heritability of psychological characteristics, but these studies can also be used to identify environmental influences that cause one twin to develop a PD but leave the other unaffected (Fontaine & Viding, 2008). For example, Caspi et al. (2004) showed that within MZ twin pairs, if one twin received less warmth and more negative emotional expression from their mother compared to their sibling, they were more likely to exhibit antisocial behaviour later in life.

Psychopathy, APD and antisocial behaviour in general are often attributed to childhood abuse, and particularly sexual abuse (Blair et al., 2006). Consistent with this view, both physical and sexual abuse during childhood and being raised in a violent home or neighbourhood are associated with increased aggressive behaviour later in life, which may result in a diagnosis of conduct disorder (in children) or APD (in adults) (Blair et al., 2006). However, Blair et al. have argued that childhood abuse is unlikely to lead to the affective flattening and emotional detachment that is characteristic of psychopathy, and this view forms part of their neurobiological model of psychopathy, which we discuss in the next section.

The development of BPD has also been attributed to traumatic life events, particularly physical, sexual and emotional abuse during childhood (Sempértegui et al., 2013). Cross-sectional studies in which BPD patients recall their childhood show that up to 90% recall some kind of abuse (Ball & Links, 2009; O'Neill & Frodl, 2012). Yet despite its plausibility, the causal role of childhood abuse in BPD is hotly disputed. For example, approximately 80% of adults who have a history of childhood sexual abuse do not have any form of PD (Amad et al., 2014). On the other hand, Ball and Links (2009) reviewed the evidence and concluded that childhood abuse was likely to play a causal role in BPD. For example, there is a clear 'dose–response' relationship between the severity of recalled childhood abuse and the severity of current symptoms in adults with BPD (Ball & Links, 2009). Their overall conclusion was that childhood abuse is an important contributor to BPD but it is unlikely to be the only cause, it is not specific to BPD (see Chapters 1, 2 and 3), and it is important to consider its interactions with other variables such as temperament before the abuse took place. A notable recent study that used an innovative research design suggests that the apparent causal relationship between childhood abuse and BPD during adulthood does not stand up to scrutiny (Bornovalova et al., 2013; see Box 11.5).

Box 11.5   Essential research

The effect of childhood abuse on BPD (Bornovalova et al., 2013)

The relationship between sexual, physical and emotional abuse during childhood and a diagnosis of BPD during adulthood is well established, but the interpretation of this relationship is a matter of ongoing controversy. For example, children may inherit personality characteristics (such as mood lability) from their parents, and these personality characteristics could predispose to BPD later in life. However, one or both of the child's parents will also have these personality characteristics, and these characteristics in the parents may make them more likely to abuse their own children. If so, this would explain the relationship between childhood abuse and BPD, but it would not mean that childhood abuse was the cause of BPD.

To investigate this issue, Bornovalova et al. (2013) used a longitudinal discordant twin design to follow up more than 1,300 pairs of twins from age 11 to age 24. The crucial comparisons were between MZ and DZ twin pairs that were discordant for childhood abuse (in which one twin was abused, but the other was not). The logic behind this comparison relies on the fact that MZ twins share 100% of genetic material whereas DZ twins share only 50% on average. If common genetic influences account for the association between childhood abuse and BPD (as discussed above), then MZ twins that are discordant for childhood abuse should have similar levels of BPD traits during adulthood. But in discordant DZ twins, the twin that experienced childhood abuse should have higher levels of BPD traits than the unaffected twin, because DZ twin pairs only provide partial control for genetic influences (see Chapter 1 for more discussion of the logic behind this methodology).

The authors found that among MZ pairs, there was no difference in BPD traits during adulthood between the twin that had suffered childhood abuse and the twin that had not. However, among DZ pairs, childhood abuse was associated with increased BPD traits during adulthood. These results are inconsistent with claims that childhood abuse has a direct causal effect on BPD traits during adulthood, because MZ twins that had been abused did not differ from their non-abused siblings in terms of BPD traits during adulthood. Instead, these results (supplemented by other types of analyses reported in the paper) support a 'genetic mediation' model, in which inherited traits increase two things: the likelihood of experiencing abuse during childhood *and* the likelihood of developing BPD traits as an adult. However, if childhood abuse is *not* experienced, this does not seem to make much difference to the appearance of BPD traits as an adult. As the authors explain:

A child who shares a genetic predisposition to impulsivity, aggression, or negative emotionality with his or her parents is also more likely to be reared in a hostile and abusive family environment. (p. 190)

(Continued)

285

> *(Continued)*
>
> This study is significant, but we have to be cautious when interpreting these results. They do *not* mean that childhood abuse is 'harmless'. Indeed, the authors acknowledged that childhood abuse produces many other harmful effects, and they reported additional analyses that show that some types of childhood abuse (emotional and physical) may have a direct, albeit small, causal influence on BPD traits.

Attachment

Although abuse during childhood is rare, other aspects of the parent–child relationship have been the focus of attempts to explain the development of PDs. For example, unpredictable and intrusive parenting has been linked with the development of BPD, whereas ineffective parenting or the loss of a parent have been associated with the development of APD (Laulik and colleagues, 2013).

One of the core features of all PDs is difficulty interacting with other people and in forming close relationships: patients with BPD tend to have relationships that are intense and unstable, whereas patients with APD tend to have a callous disregard for the feelings of other people, and they are more likely to be violent to their partners (Laulik et al., 2013). Early relationships and attachments, particularly the parent–child relationship, have an important impact on relationships with others during adulthood (Bowlby, 1969, 1973). Therefore some researchers (e.g., Fonagy & Bateman, 2008; Levy, 2005) have argued that children who do not form healthy attachments with their parents will find it difficult to form close relationships with other people for the rest of their lives, and this may underlie the development of PDs. These influential theories are well developed for BPD (and they will be discussed in more detail in the next section), but some researchers have argued that unhealthy parent–child attachments could be linked to all personality disorders (Laulik et al., 2013).

Consistent with these theories, 'unhealthy' types of attachment are more prevalent in people with PDs compared to the general population. For example, Levy (2005) estimated that based on interviews, only 6% to 8% of BPD adults have a 'healthy' secure attachment style. This is important because early relationships and attachments, particularly the infant–caregiver relationship, have a significant impact on attachments to others during adulthood, and therefore unhealthy attachments during adulthood may have their roots in the infant–caregiver attachment that was formed during childhood (Bowlby, 1969). Longitudinal studies have generally supported Bowlby's theory by demonstrating that the quality of attachment formed with the primary caregiver is a reliable predictor of attachment style throughout adulthood (Levy, 2005). Most importantly, other longitudinal studies have demonstrated that insecure attachment styles in early adulthood are reliable predictors of BPD symptoms a few years later (Fonagy & Bateman, 2008; Steele & Siever, 2010).

Although there is convincing evidence for a link between early attachment and subsequent PDs, particularly BPD, we should be cautious before inferring that abnormal attachment during childhood is the cause of relationship difficulties and PDs in later life. Recent research using sophisticated longitudinal designs (Bornovalova et al., 2013; see also Box 11.5) suggests an alternative explanation: inherited personality traits such as high neuroticism in childhood may be a precursor of BPD traits later in life, and those same traits held by both the child and its parents may make it difficult for that child to form a healthy attachment with their parents. This could explain the relationship between early attachment and subsequent PDs, but it would not imply any causal relationship between the two. Following a review of the evidence, Steele and Siever (2010) proposed a slightly different mechanism: they argued that genetic transmission of critical personality traits (e.g. high neuroticism) influences the quality of the infant–caregiver attachment, and these traits make it more likely that children of BPD mothers will form disorganised attachments and subsequently develop BPD as a result. However, it isn't inevitable that they will form disorganised attachments, and it is possible that they may form a perfectly healthy attachment with their mother and thus not develop BPD as an adult. Therefore, the gene × environment (G × E) interaction between heritable personality traits (G) and infant–caregiver attachment (E) may be crucial. Overall there are clear links between heritable personality traits in infants, infant–caregiver attachments, and BPD diagnoses in adults. But there are many competing explanations for these associations, and further research, ideally using longitudinal discordant twin designs such as the one described in Box 11.5, is needed in order to resolve these issues.

Section summary

In this section we have shown that heritability estimates for PDs are high, although there is considerable overlap between heritable risk for PDs and that for other psychological disorders. In terms of environmental influences, childhood abuse and insecure attachments formed during childhood are closely linked to PD diagnoses and traits later in life. However, recent research challenges the widely-held view that PDs are the inevitable result of such adverse experiences during childhood. Some researchers believe that the contribution of genetic factors to PDs had been underestimated, and we return to this issue in the next section.

Section 3: Brain and cognitive mechanisms in personality disorders

Antisocial personality disorder and psychopathy

Abnormalities of brain function associated with antisocial behaviour form the basis for theoretical models that will be discussed in this section. It is not easy to integrate and summarise this research because conclusions have been drawn from studies of patients with an APD diagnosis, 'psychopaths' (in forensic settings), children with a diagnosis of conduct disorder (see Chapter 3), and research into aggressive behaviour in healthy individuals. This is reasonable given the overlap between these things, but it means that we must be careful when trying to identify the biological and psychological processes that are *specific* to APD.

James Blair and colleagues (Blair, 2001, 2013; Blair et al., 2006) proposed and subsequently refined a neurobiological model of psychopathy. Their central argument is that psychopathic traits can be broken down into a callous-unemotional component and an impulsive-antisocial component, and these are related to dysfunction in distinct but overlapping networks of brain structures.

Regarding the callous-unemotional component, psychopathy is associated with reduced empathy for emotional distress in others, the biological substrate of which is reduced activity in the amygdala and ventromedial prefrontal cortex (VMPFC). In healthy individuals, their perception of distress in other people leads to activity in the amygdala and VMPFC, which increases arousal and causes the diversion of attention to whatever is the cause of the other person's distress. This has an adaptive function, because it helps us to learn about things in the environment that are unpleasant so that we know to avoid them in the future. For example, if we perceive that another person is fearful, and we see that a spider in the vicinity is the cause of that fear, then we learn that spiders are something to be afraid of and avoided (the contribution of this process to spider phobia was discussed in Chapter 7). In the context of APD, a more important consequence of perceiving distress in other people is that normally this helps people to control their own behaviour towards them. According to the 'violence inhibition mechanism' model (Blair, 2001), as children develop they learn to associate their own aggressive actions with distressed facial expressions in others. Given that perceiving distress in others activates the amygdala and is perceived as aversive, this means that healthy individuals quickly learn to inhibit violence towards others. As argued by Blair (2001: 730):

> The appropriately developing child thus initially finds the pain of others aversive and then, through socialisation, thoughts of acts that cause pain to others aversive also.

According to the theory, these normal reactions to the distress of others and resultant modification of one's own behaviour towards others do not function normally in psychopathy. Many studies have shown that psychopathy is associated with selective impairments in the recognition of and response to facial expressions of distress (fear, sadness and pain), but a normal recognition of and response to facial expressions of anger and disgust. These effects are particularly pronounced for recognition of fearful expressions and are seen in a broad range of antisocial populations (youth with conduct disorder, and adults with APD and/or psychopathy) (Marsh & Blair, 2008). These behavioural impairments are associated with blunted amygdala activity (Blair, 2013). According to the theory, this reduced responsiveness to distress in others (linked to the amygdala) and reduced awareness of the causes of things that cause distress in others (linked to the VMPFC) lead to indifference to others' distress and a lack of awareness of the things that cause them distress (i.e. the psychopath's own violent behaviour). Therefore Blair argues that people with psychopathic traits are more likely to hurt other people because they are insensitive to their distress, but also because they don't understand the things that cause other people to feel distressed.

Regarding the impulsive-antisocial component, psychopathy is associated with deficits in decision making and aspects of reinforcement learning, and these can be attributed to abnormal function in a broader (but overlapping) network of brain structures. This component is associated with psychopathy but is not *specific* to psychopathy, because it is also a feature of APD and other externalising disorders such as ADHD. To give some examples of reinforcement learning deficits, psychopathic traits are associated with deficient 'reversal learning', in which people are initially required to make a response when they see one stimulus and ignore a different stimulus, but are subsequently required to switch and respond to the stimulus that they previously ignored. Another example is aversive conditioning (i.e. learning to associate a stimulus, action or event with negative outcomes), which is also impaired in psychopathy. Deficits in these and other reinforcement learning tasks are associated with reduced function in the VMPFC, dorsomedial prefrontal cortex (DMPFC), amygdala and nucleus accumbens, in psychopathy. Blair (2013) gives an example of how this could lead to aggressive or criminal behaviour: a psychopath might attempt to rob somebody on a street corner even if they had been arrested by the police for robbery on the same street corner the previous day. In these circumstances, it would make sense to find somewhere else to rob innocent members of the public. However, psychopathic individuals are unable to learn from the negative consequences of their behaviour, so they repeat those behaviours.

Research has generally supported Blair's account of the abnormalities of brain function that characterise psychopathy. For example, Yang and Raine (2009) conducted a meta-analysis of brain imaging studies of the prefrontal cortex in APD, and psychopathic and violent individuals. Compared to healthy controls, these individuals had reduced brain volume and functional activity in sub-regions of the prefrontal cortex that were specified by Blair (2013). Kiehl (2006) reviewed the evidence for amygdala dysfunction in psychopathy and concluded that both adult psychopaths and children with psychopathic tendencies had deficits in emotional processing that were closely associated with a hypofunctioning (low functioning) amygdala. For example, Williamson et al. (1991) reported that healthy controls were faster to respond to emotional rather than neutral words, and emotional words evoked distinct patterns of brain activity (event-related potentials; ERPs), as measured by EEG. However, psychopaths failed to show differential reaction times or ERPs to emotional and neutral words. In a recent review of the evidence, Blair (2013) concluded that the evidence for structural and functional abnormalities in the amygdala is compelling, although he acknowledged that the evidence for structural abnormalities of the VMPFC in adult psychopathy is inconsistent across studies.

Finally, Blair (2013) has attempted to explain the development of the neurobiological and psychological characteristics of psychopathy. He argues that reduced volume and function in the amygdala and VMPFC are likely to be heritable rather than the result of environmental influences such as dysfunctional attachment. However, he also suggests that environmental factors (including disorganised attachment) may lead to emotional hyper-responsiveness which could then give rise to different forms of conduct disorder and APD that are *not* associated with psychopathy or callous-unemotional traits (see Blair et al., 2006). Most importantly, Blair argues that environmental factors influence the expression of psychopathic traits: a person with such traits is unlikely to engage in violent criminal behaviour unless they are raised in poverty or exposed to criminal activities that make those behaviours more likely.

Borderline personality disorder

BPD is associated with a number of structural brain changes, particularly a reduction in the size of the hippocampus (O'Neill & Frodl, 2012). Reduced hippocampal volume may underpin some features of BPD such as cognitive deficits, dissociative symptoms and unstable identity (Brambilla et al., 2004). Intriguingly, several studies have shown that hippocampal size is related to (retrospective memories of) childhood trauma: more severe childhood trauma is associated with reduced volume of the hippocampus. Animal studies also show that stress during critical developmental periods leads to shrinkage of the hippocampus, so a causal link between childhood trauma and reduced hippocampal size during adolescence is plausible (O'Neill & Frodl, 2012). However, remember that we need to be careful when interpreting adults' memories of childhood trauma as evidence that childhood trauma is the cause of BPD (see Section 2 of this chapter, and Box 11.5). A further consideration is that other trauma-associated conditions such as post-traumatic stress disorder are also associated with reduced hippocampal volumes, which suggests that this is probably not a specific feature of BPD (O'Neill & Frodl, 2012).

More recent studies suggest that the amygdala and anterior cingulate cortex (ACC) are also smaller than normal in BPD (O'Neill & Frodl, 2012). These brain regions have also been implicated in BPD by scans of brain activity. For example, studies using fMRI revealed that, compared to controls, BPD patients have increased activity in the amygdala combined with reduced activity in the prefrontal cortex, including the ACC, when viewing emotionally unpleasant stimuli. However, in their review of this literature, O'Neill and Frodl (2012) cautioned that very few studies had investigated brain function in BPD and there are many inconsistences in the literature, particularly when different forms of brain imaging (e.g. fMRI vs PET) are used. However, if these findings are confirmed, it may suggest brain mechanisms that underlie symptoms of the disorder: an exaggerated emotional response to threat (which is related to a hypersensitive amygdala) leads to attempts to cope with negative emotions, but these attempts are unlikely to succeed because of hypoactivity in the anterior cingulate and other regions of the prefrontal cortex that are involved in emotion regulation (O'Neill & Frodl, 2012).

Whilst it is important to understand abnormalities of brain function in BPD, this research is in its early stages and has not yet produced a coherent theoretical framework that can explain the development of BPD. Psychological models of BPD attempt to explain how the developmental causes of BPD lead to the core psychological disturbances of the disorder. In an influential model, Peter Fonagy and colleagues (Fonagy & Bateman, 2008; Fonagy & Luyten, 2009) proposed that people who experience disrupted attachment during childhood experience long-lasting problems with *mentalisation*. This can be defined as a form of social cognition that enables us to perceive and interpret the mental states (e.g. emotions, goals and drives) that underlie both our own and others' behaviour. Patients with BPD have inadequate mentalisation and this means that they are unable to make sense of their own feelings, and they misunderstand the feelings and intentions of other people. This gives rise to many of the core symptoms of BPD, including unstable relationships with others, identity disturbance, feelings of emptiness, and paranoia. A further prediction made by the model is that emotionally arousing interactions with close partners lead to further temporary impairments in the ability to mentalise, which creates a vicious cycle of emotional distress.

Evidence in support of the model was reviewed by Fonagy and Luyten (2009). Numerous studies show that, compared to controls, BPD patients have deficits in judging the emotional states or intentions of others. Furthermore, mentalising abilities in adults are related to the quality of the infant–caregiver attachment that they formed as children: children who form secure attachments with their caregiver tend to perform better on 'theory of mind' and other mentalising tasks in later life (Fonagy & Luyten, 2009). However the evidence is not always consistent, and the overall picture is complicated because mentalising is a multifaceted construct, and the aspects of it that are associated with BPD in adults may not be the same as those that develop in children as a result of secure infant–caregiver interactions. Other studies have shown that stressful social interactions lead to different patterns of brain activation in people with secure versus disorganised attachments, and these may reflect a temporary worsening of the ability to mentalise in those with disorganised attachments. Increased activity in the amygdala and reduced activity in the ACC in response to stress in BPD patients, as previously discussed (O'Neill & Frodl, 2012), can be interpreted as evidence for the deactivation of mentalising processes during stressful social interactions (Fonagy & Luyten, 2009).

One of the most significant pieces of evidence in support of the mentalising model of BPD is the apparent success of mentalising-based treatments for BPD, which we discuss in the next section. However, the effectiveness of mentalising-based treatments does not imply that a developmentally-acquired deficit in mentalising is the ultimate cause of BPD, and some critics have argued that there is no compelling evidence that specific mentalising deficits arise as a consequence of disorganised attachment (Steele & Siever, 2010).

Stanley and Siever (2010) proposed a biological model of BPD involving the abnormal functioning of multiple neurotransmitters, hormones and neuropeptides. According to their model, disorganised attachment leads to abnormally low levels of endogenous opioids but over-sensitive opioid receptors, the combination of which results in negative mood and feelings of 'inner emptiness' but a hypersensitive rewarding response to anything that triggers endogenous opioid activity, such as self-harming. There is some evidence in support of this: for example, BPD patients have relatively low levels of endogenous opioids and their metabolites in cerebrospinal fluid, and medications such as naltrexone (which block the effect of endogenous opioids) lead to a reduction in self-harming (Stanley & Siever, 2010). A hormone called oxytocin, which is released in the brain during social interactions and plays an important role in mother–infant bonding, may also function abnormally in BPD, and this could explain other BPD symptoms including alternating between feeling very close to and infatuated with others, but then feeling nothing about them at all. The central features of this model, particularly the roles of endogenous opioids and oxytocin in intimate social interactions and their importance in infant–caregiver attachments, have been well-supported by animal research (Stanley & Siever, 2010). However, there are very few studies of these neurotransmitters and their relationship to symptoms in BPD patients, and this model is unlikely to provide a complete explanation of BPD and its development.

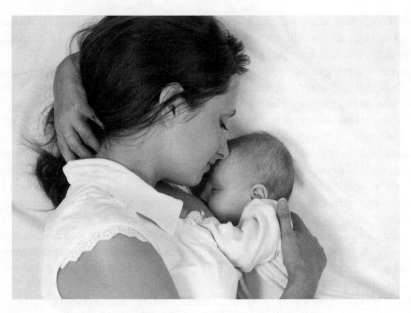

Figure 11.1   One theory of BPD suggests that the hormone oxytocin, that plays an important role in mother–infant bonding, may function abnormally in patients with BPD and this may explain some of the symptoms

Section summary

In this section we have reviewed evidence for abnormalities of brain function in psychopathy, APD and BPD, and evaluated theoretical models that can explain how brain function is related to the psychological characteristics of people with PDs. In turn, core psychological characteristics and their underlying brain substrates can explain the specific symptoms of PDs. We also linked these psychological characteristics to the ultimate causes of personality disorders, particularly heritable influences and childhood experiences. Current models of personality disorders suggest a strong heritable influence on psychopathy and APD, but a more important role for childhood attachment in BPD. However, this is not a clear distinction, and it is likely that both types of PDs are heritable and that early experiences play a role in both.

Section 4: How are personality disorders managed and treated?

The majority of PD patients do not seek treatment, primarily because their 'symptoms' do not cause them distress or because they accept their personality as a defining feature of who they are, rather than a disorder in need of treatment. As we showed in Section 1 of this chapter, in some ways they are right! However, people with some PDs (particularly APD and BPD) tend to cause distress or harm to other people, and many PDs (including BPD) are associated with distress to the person with the PD. Furthermore, as we noted in Section 1, the prognosis for recovery from any mental disorders that are co-morbid with PD is much better if the PD can be managed or treated. Therefore, there is a rationale for identifying effective treatments and offering them to PD patients. APD is usually detected among criminal offenders by forensic psychiatric services (e.g. in prisons), whereas BPD patients often come into contact with treatment services because they seek help for co-morbid conditions such as mood and anxiety disorders.

Clinicians who make a diagnosis of PD often do so with the implicit acknowledgement that there is not much that the clinician can do because the disorder is impossible to treat (Gask et al., 2013). There may be some truth in this in the case of APD, and for this reason people talk about the 'management' of PDs (particularly APD) rather than their treatment. However, there are reasons to be more optimistic about the prospects for improvement in symptoms and quality of life in those with BPD (see Box 11.6).

Box 11.6   Essential experience

The treatment of BPD

Gask et al. (2013) describe the experience of a BPD patient, and how they feel that their life improved as a result of treatment:

> Before therapy I just did not know what was going on in my head. One thing always seemed to affect another: the inability to hold down a job, getting into debt, relationship problems, constantly blaming others, and wondering what the hell was wrong with me.

> My GP was becoming concerned and I willingly accepted a referral to the local psychotherapy department. When I was told that I probably had borderline personality disorder and that a service was available for people with this disorder it was an enormous relief.

> The therapy has been ongoing and has enabled me to feel safe and contained within it. This has helped me to be more open with my therapist and to make sense of my difficult childhood and adolescence and how this has affected my present condition.

> The things that create a better life for people are jobs, relationships, and security. However, for people with personality disorder these are the very situations that can often trigger symptoms. Therapy can show different directions: one you have always known and another way. New ways, however, can also bring new problems.

> It makes me aware that I need to be kind to myself and that healing is an ongoing process.

Treatment of BPD

Gask et al. (2013) identified five treatments for BPD that are effective at reducing symptoms and/or improving quality of life.

Dialectical behaviour therapy (DBT) is a modified form of CBT that incorporates elements of 'mindfulness', a concept drawn from Buddhist philosophy which involves being aware of and accepting one's emotions, thoughts and bodily sensations. The treatment is guided by Linehan's (1993) model of BPD, which asserts that the disorder is the result of poor emotion regulation, a heritable characteristic which is exacerbated by disorganised attachment with the primary caregiver (see Sections 2 and 3). Treatment involves individual sessions with a therapist as well as group therapy, and focuses on skills to improve emotion regulation, tolerance of emotional distress and changing the social environment in order to reduce the occurrence of emotionally distressing interactions. Unlike conventional CBT, it attempts to strike a balance between altering dysfunctional beliefs and emotion regulation strategies, and accepting those beliefs and emotions for what they are (the 'mindfulness' aspect). Several RCTs of DBT for women with BPD who were self-harming showed reductions in anger, depression, self-harm and suicide attempts. Most of these studies compared DBT to treatment as usual, but some studies compared it to other forms of psychotherapy and demonstrated a benefit for DBT (Gask et al., 2013; Lynch et al., 2007; Stoffers et al., 2012).

Mentalisation-based treatment draws heavily on Fonagy's mentalisation theory (Fonagy & Bateman, 2008; Fonagy & Luyten, 2009; see Section 3), which posits that BPD arises because of a disorganised infant–caregiver attachment that results in people being unable to 'mentalise' (understand the emotions, thoughts and intentions of others). Therapy involves individual and group sessions, the goal of which is to improve patients' ability to mentalise. Compared to treatment as usual, it leads to reduced suicidal behaviour and hospitalisations, as well as an improvement in social functioning (Choi-Kain & Gunderson, 2008; Gask et al., 2013), effects that may persist for at least eight years after the end of treatment (Bateman & Fonagy, 2008)

Schema therapy was originally developed for patients with PDs who did not respond to conventional CBT (Young, 2003), and Arntz and van Genderen (2009) have developed a version of the therapy for BPD. It incorporates elements from CBT, attachment theory, humanistic and psychodynamic therapies, and it has several features that distinguish it from other cognitive therapies (see Box 11.8). Therapy involves individual or group sessions with a therapist, the goal of which is firstly to identify dysfunctional 'schema modes' (ways of perceiving and reacting emotionally to the world, themselves and others) and try to find out how those schema modes developed during childhood. Therapy focuses on helping a client to develop awareness of their modes and triggers for the activation of these. They will then work on developing a repertoire of healthy coping strategies. In schema therapy, there is a greater emphasis on experiential change techniques, rather than cognitive behavioural techniques. It also uses a strategy of 'limited reparenting', in which, in a limited, boundaried way, the therapist attempts to meet some of the client's core unmet childhood needs. Meta-analyses of schema therapy show that compared to treatment as usual and other forms of psychotherapy (e.g. transference focused therapy), it improves the core symptoms of BPD, general psychological functioning, and quality of life (Jacob & Arntz, 2013; Sempértegui et al., 2013). Treatment is more beneficial if offered for longer periods of time (ideally over 18 months), and the effects may be maintained for several years after the end of treatment (Jacob & Arntz, 2013).

Box 11.7   Essential treatment

What distinguishes schema therapy from other forms of cognitive therapy? (Jacob & Arntz, 2013)

1. Focus on processing of aversive childhood memories/experiences.
2. Use of 'experiential' techniques such as imagery rescripting, the goal of which is to change the negative emotions that are associated with aversive memories from childhood.
3. The therapeutic relationship as a form of 'limited reparenting', that is, the therapist assumes the role of the patient's parent when recreating aversive childhood experiences.
4. The 'schema mode' model (a schema mode is a distinct way of perceiving the world, for example as 'abandoned child') helps a patient to understand the cause of their current problems.

Transference focused therapy is a form of psychodynamic psychotherapy that involves individual sessions with a therapist. The goal is to identify and resolve internal representations of the self and others that contradict each other (e.g. 'My husband is the best person ever' and 'My husband is a moron', both statements that one of your authors has overheard said about himself in the space of a few minutes). This reduces the core symptoms of BPD, improves psychological functioning and also reduces hospital admissions (Gask et al., 2013; Giesen-Bloo et al., 2006).

Cognitive analytic therapy combines aspects of psychodynamic theory and CBT. This therapy involves brief sessions delivered weekly over (typically) 24 weeks, and it involves the patient and therapist working together (e.g. by making diagrams) to help the patient recognise and then change beliefs and ways of thinking that are contradictory, confusing and distressing. This therapy leads to improved interpersonal functioning and general wellbeing, and also leads to a reduction in dissociative experiences (Gask et al., 2013; Kellett et al., 2013; Mulder & Chanen, 2013).

Which type of therapy is best for BPD?

As discussed above, there is evidence that each of these different forms of psychological therapy can be beneficial, usually when compared to 'treatment as usual' (Budge et al., 2013).

However, in a recent Cochrane review Stoffers et al. (2012) raised concerns about the limited number of high quality clinical trials: this really is an area in which more research is needed! It is difficult to say whether one treatment is better than the others because very few studies have directly compared two types of treatment with each other. Gask et al. (2013) suggested that because many different therapies seem to produce some benefit, it may not be particularly important what type of therapy a person receives. There is some conceptual overlap between mindfulness, mentalisation and affect regulation (Choi-Kain & Gunderson, 2008) and this could explain why treatments that specifically target these 'different' constructs tend to produce similar outcomes (Lynch et al., 2007). Perhaps the most important thing is that the intervention is delivered consistently from week to week, and encourages the development of autonomy (self-reliance) in the patient. Gask et al. (2013) emphasise the importance of any treatment being systematic, and ideally manual-based, so that the patient and therapist have a clear structure to work through. The importance of a good therapeutic alliance between the therapist and patient is recognised as crucial for effective psychological therapies for all psychological disorders (see Chapter 2), but this may be particularly important for BPD (Bateman, 2012).

Management and treatment of APD and psychopathy

APD and psychopathy are often initially detected by forensic specialists, such as forensic psychiatrists and clinical psychologists in prisons and secure hospitals (see the discussion about 'Dangerous and Severe Personality Disorder' in Section 1). In these cases, concerns about minimising risks to the public outweigh concerns about providing 'treatment' for the offender. Psychoanalytic and cognitive therapies have been attempted, but the general consensus is that they do not produce any consistent therapeutic improvement (Reid & Gacono, 2000). Therefore, most clinicians in the UK view APD and psychopathy as 'untreatable', and do not attempt to treat the disorder itself (Duggan, 2011). However, the National Institute for Clinical Excellence (NICE) in the UK recommends group-based cognitive and behavioural interventions such as anger management and violence reduction programmes for the reduction of criminal offending and other antisocial behaviour (Gask et al., 2013).

It is difficult to define a 'typical' *therapeutic community*, but in the context of PD they may involve groups of PD patients and/or criminal offenders who design and then provide intensive interventions for others with PD (Manning, 2010). The community itself decides what constitutes acceptable and unacceptable behaviour, and members who join are required to abide by the rules (Bennett, 2005). There is some suggestion of effectiveness in terms of reduced criminal offending and contact with the police (Gask et al., 2013), although many researchers remain sceptical (Emmelkamp & Vedel, 2010). Gask et al. (2013) pointed out that it is difficult to evaluate the effectiveness of such therapies because of problems with identifying a suitable control treatment. While it is true that randomised controlled trials have not been applied to investigate this issue, other lines of research do give some cause for optimism. For example, a mixed-methods (both quantitative and qualitative) evaluation of once-weekly therapeutic community day services in cities in the North of England showed improvements in mental health and social functioning in people who attended for one year (Barr et al., 2010), and the qualitative part of the study suggested that these improvements were associated with improvements in relationships with other people (Hodge et al., 2010). However, this study was not specifically focused on APD, and indeed other personality disorders were more common than APD in this sample. Furthermore, a famous study of a therapeutic community in a prison setting demonstrated that among psychopaths it increased, rather than decreased, rates of criminal offending after release, compared to a control intervention (Seto & Barbaree, 1999), in other words, it was totally counterproductive.

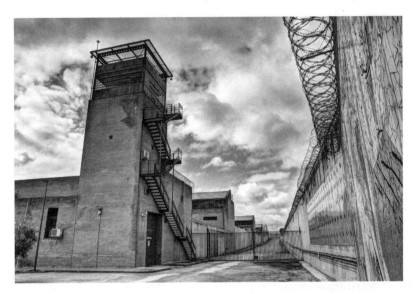

Figure 11.2 Therapeutic communities in prison settings may not reduce the rates of subsequent criminal offending, as intended – they may even have the opposite effect

Section summary

We reviewed evidence for the effectiveness of interventions for the treatment and management of APD and BPD. A number of alternative treatments are available for BPD. Most of these treatments are superior to treatment as usual, but it is difficult to say that one treatment is better than the alternatives because there is so little research on the topic. Despite their differences, all treatments target similar cognitive processes such as emotion regulation and mentalising, so they may all work via a similar mechanism. The search for an effective treatment for APD and psychopathy has not yielded any success stories, and existing psychological therapies may do more harm than good. For this reason, forensic psychiatrists and psychologists are more concerned with managing patients with APD and psychopathy, to prevent them from committing criminal acts in future, rather than treating the underlying personality disorder.

Essential questions

Some possible exam questions that stem from this chapter are:

- Are personality disorders distinct from 'healthy' personalities and 'classic' mental disorders such as schizophrenia, depression, etc.?
- Critically evaluate the influences of genetics, early attachment, and childhood trauma in the development of borderline personality disorder.
- Is antisocial personality disorder a heritable brain disease?
- Can personality disorders be successfully treated?

Further reading

Blair, R. J. R. (2013). The neurobiology of psychopathic traits in youths. *Nature Reviews Neuroscience*, 14(11): 786–799. (A readable overview of the latest research on psychopathy, which attempts to unify the diverse research into a neurobiological model.)

Gask, L., Evans, M., & Kessler, D. (2013). Personality disorder. *BMJ (Online):* 347(7924). (Excellent overview of everything, although it attracted some online criticism for its neglect of the role of attachment and the dismissive coverage of therapeutic communities. For a balanced view, you should read the comments from other researchers at www. bmj.com/content/347/bmj.f5276?tab=responses)

Sempértegui, G. A., Karreman, A., Arntz, A., & Bekker, M. H. J. (2013). Schema therapy for borderline personality disorder: A comprehensive review of its empirical foundations, effectiveness and implementation possibilities. *Clinical Psychology Review*, 33(3): 426–447. (Comprehensive and engaging overview of borderline personality disorder, with an emphasis on schema therapy.)

Tyrer, P. (2013). The classification of personality disorders in ICD-11: Implications for forensic psychiatry. *Criminal Behaviour and Mental Health*, 23(1): 1–5. (Brief, scathing and witty commentary on the categorisation of personality disorders in DSM and ICD.)

References

Abela, J. R. Z. (2001). The hopelessness theory of depression: A test of the diathesis-stress and causal mediation components in third and seventh grade children. *Journal of Abnormal Child Psychology*, 29(3): 241–254.

Abramowitz, A. J., O'Leary, S. G., & Futtersak, M. W. (1988). The relative impact of long and short reprimands on children's off-task behavior in the classroom. *Behavior Therapy*, 19(2): 243–247.

Abramson, L. Y., Seligman, M. E. P., & Teasdale, J. D. (1978). Learned helplessness in humans: Critique and reformulation. *Journal of Abnormal Psychology*, 87(1): 49–74.

Acker, M. M., & O'Leary, S. G. (1988). Effects of consistent and inconsistent feedback on inappropriate child behavior. *Behavior Therapy*, 19(4): 619–624.

Agrawal, A., Balasubramanian, S., Smith, E. K., Madden, P. A. F., Bucholz, K. K., Heath, A. C., & Lynskey, M. T. (2010). Peer substance involvement modifies genetic influences on regular substance involvement in young women. *Addiction*, 105(10): 1844–1853.

Agrawal, A., & Lynskey, M. T. (2008). Are there genetic influences on addiction? Evidence from family, adoption and twin studies. *Addiction*, 103(7): 1069–1081.

Aitken, R. C. B., Lister, J. A., & Main, C. J. (1981). Identification of features associated with flying phobias in aircrew. *British Journal of Psychiatry*, 139: 38–42.

Aleman, A., & Larøi, F. (2011). Insights into hallucinations in schizophrenia: Novel treatment approaches. *Expert Review of Neurotherapeutics*, 11(7): 1007–1015.

Allen, J. P., Mattson, M. E., Miller, W. R., Tonigan, J. S., Connors, G. J., Rychtarik, R. G., et al. (1997). Matching alcoholism treatments to client heterogeneity: Project MATCH posttreatment drinking outcomes. *Journal of Studies on Alcohol*, 58(1): 7–29.

Alloy, L. B., Abramson, L. Y., Whitehouse, W. G., Hogan, M. E., Panzarella, C., & Rose, D. T. (2006). Prospective incidence of first onsets and recurrences of depression in individuals at high and low cognitive risk for depression. *Journal of Abnormal Psychology*, 115(1): 145–156.

Alloy, L. B., Abramson, L. Y., Whitehouse, W. G., Hogan, M. E., Tashman, N. A., L. Steinberg, D., et al. (1999). Depressogenic cognitive styles: Predictive validity, information processing and personality characteristics, and developmental origins. *Behaviour Research and Therapy*, 37(6): 503–531.

Amad, A., Ramoz, N., Thomas, P., Jardri, R., & Gorwood, P. (2014). Genetics of borderline personality disorder: Systematic review and proposal of an integrative model. *Neuroscience and Biobehavioral Reviews*, 40: 6–19.

American Psychiatric Association (2013a). *Diagnostic and Statistical Manual of Mental Disorders* (5th edition). Washington, DC: APA.

American Psychiatric Association (2013b). *Personality Disorders*. Retrieved from http://www.dsm5.org/Documents/Personality Disorders Fact Sheet.pdf

Andersen, S. L., & Teicher, M. H. (2009). Desperately driven and no brakes: Developmental stress exposure and subsequent risk for substance abuse. *Neuroscience and Biobehavioral Reviews*, 33(4): 516–524.

Anderson, I. M., Ferrier, I. N., Baldwin, R. C., Cowen, P. J., Howard, L., Lewis, G., et al. (2008). Evidence-based guidelines for treating depressive disorders with antidepressants: A revision of the 2000 British Association for Psychopharmacology guidelines. *Journal of Psychopharmacology*, 22(4): 343–396.

Anglin, D. M., Cohen, P. R., & Chen, H. (2008). Duration of early maternal separation and prediction of schizotypal symptoms from early adolescence to midlife. *Schizophrenia Research*, 103(1–3): 143–150.

Arcelus, J., Mitchell, A. J., Wales, J., & Nielsen, S. (2011). Mortality rates in patients with anorexia nervosa and other eating disorders: A meta-analysis of 36 studies. *Archives of General Psychiatry*, 68(7): 724–731.

Arntz, A., & van Genderen, H. (2009). *Schema Therapy for Borderline Personality Disorder*. Chichester: Wiley.

Attia, E. (2010). Anorexia nervosa: Current status and future directions. *Annual Review of Medicine*, 61, 425–435.

Auerbach, R. P., Ho, M. H. R., & Kim, J. C. (2014). Identifying cognitive and interpersonal predictors of adolescent depression. *Journal of Abnormal Child Psychology*, 42(6): 913–924.

Ball, J. S., & Links, P. S. (2009). Borderline personality disorder and childhood trauma: Evidence for a causal relationship. *Current Psychiatry Reports*, 11(1): 63–68.

Barch, D. M., Carter, C. S., Arnsten, A., Buchanan, R. W., Cohen, J. D., Geyer, M., et al. (2009). Selecting paradigms from cognitive neuroscience for translation into use in clinical trials: Proceedings of the Third CNTRICS meeting. *Schizophrenia Bulletin*, 35(1): 109–114.

Barkus, E., & Murray, R. M. (2010) Substance use in adolescence and psychosis: Clarifying the relationship. *Annual Review of Clinical Psychology*, 6: 365–389.

Barr, W., Kirkcaldy, A., Horne, A., Hodge, S., Hellin, K., & Gpfert, M. (2010). Quantitative findings from a mixed methods evaluation of once-weekly therapeutic community day services for people with personality disorder. *Journal of Mental Health*, 19(5): 412–421.

Bateman, A., & Fonagy, P. (2008). 8-year follow-up of patients treated for borderline personality disorder: Mentalization-based treatment versus treatment as usual. *American Journal of Psychiatry*, 165(5): 631–638.

Bateman, A. W. (2012). Treating borderline personality disorder in clinical practice. *American Journal of Psychiatry*, 169(6): 560–563.

Bateson, G., Jackson, D., Haley, J., & Weakland, J. (1956). Toward a theory of schizophrenia. *Behavioural Science*, 1: 251–264.

Bauer, D. H. (1976). An exploratory study of developmental changes in children's fears. *Journal of Child Psychology and Psychiatry*, 17: 69–74.

Beard, C., Sawyer, A. T., & Hofmann, S. G. (2012). Efficacy of attention bias modification using threat and appetitive stimuli: A meta-analytic review. *Behavior Therapy*, 43(4): 724–740.

Beatty, M. J., Heisel, A. D., Hall, A. E., Levine, T. R., & La France, B. H. (2002). What can we learn from the study of twins about genetic and environmental influences on interpersonal affiliation, aggressiveness, and social anxiety? A meta-analytic study. *Communication Monographs*, 69(1): 1–18.

Bebbington, P., & Kuipers, L. (1994). The clinical utility of expressed emotion in schizophrenia. *Acta Psychiatrica Scandinavica*, 89 (382)(Supplement): 46–53.

Bebbington, P. E., Bhugra, D., Brugha, T., Singleton, N., Farrell, M., Jenkins, R., et al. (2004). Psychosis, victimisation and childhood disadvantage: Evidence from the second British National Survey of Psychiatric Morbidity. *British Journal of Psychiatry*, 185: 220–226.

Beck, A. T. (1967). *Depression: Clinical, Experimental and Theoretical Aspects*. New York: Harper & Row.

Beck, A. T. (1976). *Cognitive Therapy and the Emotional Disorders*. New York: International Universities Press.

Beck, A. T. (2008). The evolution of the cognitive model of depression and its neurobiological correlates. *American Journal of Psychiatry*, 165(8): 969–977.

Beck, A. T., & Rector, N. A. (2003). A cognitive model of hallucinations. *Cognitive Therapy and Research*, 27(1): 19–52.

Beck, A. T., & Rector, N. A. (2005). Cognitive approaches to schizophrenia. *Theory and Therapy*, 1: 577–606.

Beck, A. T., Steer, R. A., & Carbin, M. G. (1988). Psychometric properties of the Beck Depression Inventory: Twenty-five years of evaluation. *Clinical Psychology Review*, 8(1): 77–100.

Behar, E., DiMarco, I. D., Hekler, E. B., Mohlman, J., & Staples, A. M. (2009). Current theoretical models of generalized anxiety disorder (GAD): Conceptual review and treatment implications. *Journal of Anxiety Disorders*, 23(8): 1011–1023.

Bellack, A. S. (2004). Skills training for people with severe mental illness. *Psychiatric Rehabilitation Journal*, 27(4): 375–391.

Belsky, J., & Beaver, K. M. (2011). Cumulative-genetic plasticity, parenting and adolescent self-regulation. *Journal of Child Psychology and Psychiatry, and Allied Disciplines*, 52(5): 619–626.

Bender, R. E., & Alloy, L. B. (2011). Life stress and kindling in bipolar disorder: Review of the evidence and integration with emerging biopsychosocial theories. *Clinical Psychology Review*, 31(3): 383–398.

Bennett, P. (2005). *Abnormal and Clinical Psychology: An Introductory Textbook*. Maidenhead: Open University Press.

Bennett-Levy, J., Richards, D., Farrand, P., Christensen, H., Griffiths, K., Kavanagh, D., et al. (2010). *Oxford Guide to Low Intensity CBT Interventions*. Oxford: Oxford University Press.

Bentall, R. P. (2003). *Madness Explained: Psychosis and Human Nature*. London: Penguin.

Bentall, R. P., Wickham, S., Shevlin, M., & Varese, F. (2012). Do specific early-life adversities lead to specific symptoms of psychosis? A study from the 2007 Adult Psychiatric Morbidity Survey. *Schizophrenia Bulletin*, 38(4): 734–740.

Bergeron, L., Valla, J., & Breton, J. (1992). Pilot study for the Quebec Child Mental Health Survey: Part 1. Measurement of prevalence estimates among six to 14 year olds. *Canadian Journal of Psychiatry*, 37: 374–380.

Bergström, J., Andersson, G., Ljótsson, B., Rück, C., Andréewitch, S., Karlsson, A., et al. (2010). Internet-versus group-administered cognitive behaviour therapy for panic disorder in a psychiatric setting: A randomised trial. *BMC Psychiatry*, 10(1): art. 54.

Bienvenu, O. J., Davydow, D. S., & Kendler, K. S. (2011). Psychiatric diseases versus behavioral disorders and degree of genetic influence. *Psychological Medicine*, 41(1): 33–40.

Blair, R. J. R. (2001). Neurocognitive models of aggression, the antisocial personality disorders, and psychopathy. *Journal of Neurology, Neurosurgery and Psychiatry*, 71(6): 727–731.

Blair, R. J. R. (2013). The neurobiology of psychopathic traits in youths. *Nature Reviews Neuroscience*, 14(11): 786–799.

Blair, R. J. R., Peschardt, K. S., Budhani, S., Mitchell, D. G. V., & Pine, D. S. (2006). The development of psychopathy. *Journal of Child Psychology and Psychiatry and Allied Disciplines*, 47(3–4): 262–275.

Boileau, I., Dagher, A., Leyton, M., Gunn, R. N., Baker, G. B., Diksic, M., & Benkelfat, C. (2006). Modeling sensitization to stimulants in humans: An [11C] raclopride/positron emission tomography study in healthy men. *Archives of General Psychiatry*, 63(12): 1386–1395.

Bolton, D., Eley, T. C., O'Connor, T. G., Perrin, S., Rabe-Hesketh, S., Rijsdijk, F., & Smith, P. (2006). Prevalence and genetic and environmental influences on anxiety disorders in 6-year-old twins. *Psychological Medicine*, 36(3): 335–344.

Bonin, E.-M., Stevens, M., Beecham, J., Byford, S., & Parsonage, M. (2011). *BMC Public Health*, 11(1): art. 803.

Borkovec, T. D. (1994). The nature, functions, and origins of worry. In G. Davey and F. Tallis (eds), *Worrying: Perspectives on Theory, Assessment and Treatment*. Chichester: Wiley, pp. 5–33.

Borkovec, T. D., Alcaine, O. M., & Behar, E. (2004). Avoidance theory of worry and generalized anxiety disorder. In R. Heimberg, C. Turk and D. Mennin (eds), *Generalized Anxiety Disorder: Advances in Research and Practice*. New York: Guilford, pp. 77–108.

Borkovec, T. D., Robinson, E., Pruzinsky, T., & DePree, J. A. (1983). Preliminary exploration of worry: Some characteristics and processes. *Behaviour Research and Therapy*, 21(1): 9–16.

Bornovalova, M. A., Huibregtse, B. M., Hicks, B. M., Keyes, M., McGue, M., & Iacono, W. (2013). Tests of a direct effect of childhood abuse on adult borderline personality disorder traits: A longitudinal discordant twin design. *Journal of Abnormal Psychology*, 122(1): 180–194.

Bowlby, J. (1969). *Attachment and Loss, Volume 1: Attachment*. London: Pimlico.

Bowlby, J. (1973). *Attachment and Loss, Volume 2: Separation, Anxiety and Anger*. London: Pimlico.

Boysen, G. A., & Vanbergen, A. (2013). A review of published research on adult dissociative identity disorder: 2000–2010. *Journal of Nervous and Mental Disease*, 201(1): 5–11.

Brady, K. T., Back, S. E., & Coffey, S. F. (2004). Substance abuse and posttraumatic stress disorder. *Current Directions in Psychological Science*, 13(5): 206–209.

Brambilla, P., Soloff, P. H., Sala, M., Nicoletti, M. A., Keshavan, M. S., & Soares, J. C. (2004). Anatomical MRI study of borderline personality disorder patients. *Psychiatry Research: Neuroimaging*, 131(2): 125–133.

Briggs-Gowan, M., Horwitz, S., Schwab-Stone, M. E., Leventhal, J., & Leaf, P. (2000). Mental health in pediatric settings: Distribution of disorders and factors related to service use. *Journal of the American Academy of Child & Adolescent Psychiatry*, 39(7): 841–849.

British Psychological Society (2009). *Code of Ethics and Conduct*. London: BPS.

Broeren, S., Lester, K. J., Muris, P., & Field, A. P. (2011). 'They are afraid of the animal, so therefore I am too': Influence of peer modeling on fear beliefs and approach-avoidance behaviors towards animals in typically developing children. *Behaviour Research and Therapy*, 49(1): 50–57.

Brown, G. P., Hammen, C. L., Craske, M. G., & Wickens, T. D. (1995). Dimensions of dysfunctional attitudes as vulnerabilities to depressive symptoms. *Journal of Abnormal Psychology*, 104(3): 431–435.

Brown, T. A., Di Nardo, P. A., Lehman, C. L., & Campbell, L. A. (2001). Reliability of DSM-IV anxiety and mood disorders: Implications for the classification of emotional disorders. *Journal of Abnormal Psychology*, 110(1): 49–58.

Bruce, S. E., Yonkers, K. A., Otto, M. W., Eisen, J. L., Weisberg, R. B., Pagano, M., et al. (2005). Influence of psychiatric comorbidity on recovery and recurrence in generalized anxiety disorder, social phobia, and panic disorder: A 12–year prospective study. *The American Journal of Psychiatry*, 162(6): 1179–1187.

Budge, S. L., Moore, J. T., Del Re, A. C., Wampold, B. E., Baardseth, T. P., & Nienhuis, J. B. (2013). The effectiveness of evidence-based treatments for personality disorders when comparing treatment-as-usual and bona fide treatments. *Clinical Psychology Review*, 33(8): 1057–1066.

Bulik, C. M., Prescott, C. A., & Kendler, K. S. (2001). Features of childhood sexual abuse and the development of psychiatric and substance use disorders. *British Journal of Psychiatry*, 179: 444–449.

Burns, A. M. N., Erickson, D. H., & Brenner, C. A. (2014). Cognitive-behavioral therapy for medication-resistant psychosis: A meta-analytic review. *Psychiatric Services*, 65(7): 874–880.

Butler, A. C., Chapman, J. E., Forman, E. M., & Beck, A. T. (2006). The empirical status of cognitive-behavioral therapy: A review of meta-analyses. *Clinical Psychology Review*, 26(1): 17–31.

Butler, G., Fennell, M., Robson, P., & Gelder, M. (1991). Comparison of behavior therapy and cognitive behavior therapy in the treatment of generalized anxiety disorder. *Journal of Consulting and Clinical Psychology*, 59(1): 167–175.

Button, K. S., Ioannidis, J. P. A., Mokrysz, C., Nosek, B. A., Flint, J., Robinson, E. S. J., & Munafò, M. R. (2013). Power failure: Why small sample size undermines the reliability of neuroscience. *Nature Reviews Neuroscience*, 14(5): 365–376.

Butzlaff, R. L., & Hooley, J. M. (1998). Expressed emotion and psychiatric relapse: A meta-analysis. *Archives of General Psychiatry*, 55(6): 547–552.

Calati, R., Gressier, F., Balestri, M., & Serretti, A. (2013). Genetic modulation of borderline personality disorder: Systematic review and meta-analysis. *Journal of Psychiatric Research*, 47(10): 1275–1287.

Campbell, I. C., Mill, J., Uher, R., & Schmidt, U. (2011). Eating disorders, gene–environment interactions and epigenetics. *Neuroscience and Biobehavioral Reviews*, 35(3): 784–793.

Campbell, S. B. (1986). Developmental issues in childhood anxiety. In R. Gittelman (ed.), *Anxiety Disorders of Childhood*. New York: Guilford, pp. 24–57.

Canino, G., Polanczyk, G., Bauermeister, J. J., Rohde, L. A., & Frick, P. J. (2010). Does the prevalence of CD and ODD vary across cultures? *Social Psychiatry and Psychiatric Epidemiology*, 45(7): 695–704.

Cantor-Graae, E. (2007). The contribution of social factors to the development of schizophrenia: A review of recent findings. *Canadian Journal of Psychiatry*, 52(5): 277–286.

Carter, B. L., & Tiffany, S. T. (1999). Meta-analysis of cue-reactivity in addiction research. *Addiction*, 94(3): 327–340.

Cartwright-Hatton, S., McNicol, K., & Doubleday, E. (2006). Anxiety in a neglected population: Prevalence of anxiety disorders in pre-adolescent children. *Clinical Psychology Review*, 26(7): 817–833.

Caspi, A., Moffitt, T. E., Morgan, J., Rutter, M., Taylor, A., Arseneault, L., et al. (2004). Maternal expressed emotion predicts children's antisocial behavior problems: Using monozygotic-twin differences to identify environmental effects on behavioral development. *Developmental Psychology*, 40(2): 149–161.

Caspi, A., Sugden, K., Moffitt, T. E., Taylor, A., Craig, I. W., Harrington, H., et al. (2003). Influence of life stress on depression: Moderation by a polymorphism in the 5-HTT gene. *Science*, 301(5631): 386–389.

Cha, D. S., & McIntyre, R. S. (2012). Treatment-emergent adverse events associated with atypical antipsychotics. *Expert Opinion on Pharmacotherapy*, 13(11): 1587–1598.

Choi-Kain, L. W., & Gunderson, J. G. (2008). Mentalization: Ontogeny, assessment, and application in the treatment of borderline personality disorder. *American Journal of Psychiatry*, 165(9): 1127–1135.

Choy, Y., Fyer, A. J., & Lipsitz, J. D. (2007). Treatment of specific phobia in adults. *Clinical Psychology Review*, 27: 266–286.

Cisler, J. M., & Koster, E. H. W. (2010). Mechanisms of attentional biases towards threat in anxiety disorders: An integrative review. *Clinical Psychology Review*, 30(2): 203–216.

Clark, D. M. (1986). A cognitive approach to panic. *Behaviour Research and Therapy*, 24(4): 461–470.

Clark, D. M., Ehlers, A., McManus, F., Hackmann, A., Fennell, M., Campbell, H., et al. (2003). Cognitive therapy versus fluoxetine in generalized social phobia: A randomized placebo-controlled trial. *Journal of Consulting and Clinical Psychology*, 71(6): 1058–1067.

Clark, D. M., & Fairburn, C. G. (1997). *Science and Practice of Cognitive Behaviour Therapy*. Oxford: Oxford University Press.

Clark, D. M., Salkovskis, P. M., Hackmann, A., Middleton, H., Anastasiades, P., & Gelder, M. (1994). A comparison of cognitive therapy, applied relaxation and imipramine in the treatment of panic disorder. *The British Journal of Psychiatry*, 164(6): 759–769.

Clark, D. M., Salkovskis, P. M., Hackmann, A., Wells, A., Ludgate, J., & Gelder, M. (1999). Brief cognitive therapy for panic disorder: A randomized controlled trial. *Journal of Consulting and Clinical Psychology*, 67(4): 583–589.

Clark, D. M., & Wells, A. (1995). A cognitive model of social phobia. In R. G. Heimberg and M. R. Liebowitz (eds), *Social Phobia: Diagnosis, Assessment, and Treatment*. New York: Guilford.

Clarke, P. J. F., Notebaert, L., & MacLeod, C. (2014). Absence of evidence or evidence of absence: Reflecting on therapeutic implementations of attentional bias modification. *BMC Psychiatry*, 14, art. 8.

Cody, M. W., & Teachman, B. A. (2010). Post-event processing and memory bias for performance feedback in social anxiety. *Journal of Anxiety Disorders*, 24(5): 468–479.

Colman, I., Murray, J., Abbott, R. A., Maughan, B., Kuh, D., Croudace, T. J., & Jones, P. B. (2009). Outcomes of conduct problems in adolescence: 40 year follow-up of national cohort. *BMJ*, 338, a2981.

Conklin, C. A., & Tiffany, S. T. (2002). Applying extinction research and theory to cue-exposure addiction treatments. *Addiction*, 97(2): 155–167.

Costa Jr, P. T., & McCrae, R. R. (1992). The five-factor model of personality and its relevance to personality disorders. *Journal of Personality Disorders*, 6(4): 343–359.

Couturier, J., Kimber, M., & Szatmari, P. (2013). Efficacy of family-based treatment for adolescents with eating disorders: A systematic review and meta-analysis. *International Journal of Eating Disorders*, 46(1): 3–11.

Cox, G. R., Callahan, P., Churchill, R., Hunot, V., Merry, S. N., Parker, A. G., & Hetrick, S. E. (2012). Psychological therapies versus antidepressant medication, alone and in combination for depression in children and adolescents. *Cochrane Database of Systematic Reviews* (Online), 11, art. CD008324.

Craddock, N., O'Donovan, M. C., & Owen, M. J. (2005). The genetics of schizophrenia and bipolar disorder: Dissecting psychosis. *Journal of Medical Genetics*, 42(3): 193–204.

Craske, M. G., Rapee, R. M., Jackel, L., & Barlow, D. H. (1989). Qualitative dimensions of worry in DSM-III-R generalized anxiety disorder subjects and nonanxious controls. *Behaviour Research and Therapy*, 27(4): 397–402.

Crow, T. J. (1980). Molecular pathology of schizophrenia: More than one disease process? *British Medical Journal*, 280(6207): 66–68.

Cutting, J., & Dunne, F. (1989). Subjective experience of schizophrenia. *Schizophrenia Bulletin*, 15(2): 217–231.

Dagnan, D., Chadwick, P., & Proudlove, J. (2000). Toward an assessment of suitability of people with mental retardation for cognitive therapy. *Cognitive Therapy and Research*, 24(6): 627–636.

Daniels, D., & Plomin, R. (1984). Origins of individual differences in infant shyness. *Developmental Psychology*, 21(1): 118–121.

Davey, G. C. L. (1997). A conditioning model of phobias. In G. C. L. Davey (ed.), *Phobias: A Handbook of Theory, Research and Treatment.* Chichester: Wiley, pp. 301–322.

Davey, G. C. L., de Jong, P. J., & Tallis, F. (1993). UCS inflation in the aetiology of a variety of anxiety disorders: Some case histories. *Behaviour Research and Therapy*, 31: 495–498.

Davidson, J. R. T., Ballenger, J. C., Lecrubier, Y., Rickels, K., Borkovec, T. D., Stein, D. J., & Nutt, D. J. (2001). Pharmacotherapy of generalized anxiety disorder. *Journal of Clinical Psychiatry*, 62(supplement 11): 46–52.

Davies, J. B. (1992). *The Myth of Addiction*. Amsterdam: Harwood.

Davis, R. L., Rubanowice, D., McPhillips, H., Raebel, M. A., Andrade, S. E., Smith, D., et al. (2007). Risks of congenital malformations and perinatal events among infants exposed to antidepressant medications during pregnancy. *Pharmacoepidemiology and Drug Safety*, 16(10): 1086–1094.

Degenhardt, L., & Hall, W. (2012). Extent of illicit drug use and dependence, and their contribution to the global burden of disease. *The Lancet*, 379(9810): 55–70.

Demily, C., & Franck, N. (2008). Cognitive remediation: A promising tool for the treatment of schizophrenia. *Expert Review of Neurotherapeutics*, 8(7): 1029–1036.

Di Forti, M., Morgan, C., Dazzan, P., Pariante, C., Mondelli, V., Marques, T. R., et al. (2009). High-potency cannabis and the risk of psychosis. *British Journal of Psychiatry*, 195(6): 488–491.

Dienes, Z. (2011). Bayesian versus orthodox statistics: Which side are you on? *Perspectives on Psychological Science*, 6(3): 274–290.

Dishion, T. J., Patterson, G. R., & Kavanagh, K. A. (1992). An experimental test of the coercion model: Linking theory, measurement, and intervention. In J. McCord and R. E. Tremblay (eds), *Preventing Antisocial Behavior: Interventions from Birth through Adolescence*. New York: Guilford, pp. 253–282.

Dobbs, D. (2012). Orchid children: How bad-news genes came good. *New Scientist*, 2849: 42–45.

Dollinger, S. J., O'Donnell, J. P., & Staley, A. A. (1984). Lightning-strike disaster: Effects on children's fears and worries. *Journal of Consulting and Clinical Psychology*, 52(6): 1028–1038.

Donovan, C. L., & Penny, R. (2014). In control of weight: The relationship between facets of control and weight restriction. *Eating Behaviors*, 15(1): 144–150.

Dretzke, J., Davenport, C., Frew, E., Barlow, J., Stewart-Brown, S., Bayliss, S., et al. (2009). The clinical effectiveness of different parenting programmes for children with conduct problems: A systematic review of randomised controlled trials. *Child and Adolescent Psychiatry and Mental Health*, 3(1): art. 7.

Drevets, W. C., Price, J. L., & Furey, M. L. (2008). Brain structural and functional abnormalities in mood disorders: Implications for neurocircuitry models of depression. *Brain Structure and Function*, 213(1–2): 93–118.

Drury, V., Birchwood, M., & Cochrane, R. (2000). Cognitive therapy and recovery from acute psychosis: A controlled trial. 3. Five-year follow-up. *British Journal of Psychiatry*, 177: 8–14.

Duggan, C. (2011). Dangerous and severe personality disorder. *British Journal of Psychiatry*, 198(6): 431–433.

Dumas, J. E., La Freniere, P. J., & Serketich, W. J. (1995). 'Balance of power': A transactional analysis of control in mother–child dyads involving socially competent, aggressive and anxious children. *Journal of Abnormal Psychology*, 104(1): 104–113.

Durham, R. C. (2007). Treatment of generalized anxiety disorder. *Psychiatry*, 6(5): 183–187.

Durham, R. C., Murphy, T., Allan, T., Richard, K., Treliving, L. R., & Fenton, G. W. (1994). Cognitive therapy, analytic psychotherapy and anxiety management training for generalised anxiety disorder. *British Journal of Psychiatry*, 165(September): 315–323.

Eberl, C., Wiers, R. W., Pawelczack, S., Rinck, M., Becker, E. S., & Lindenmeyer, J. (2013). Approach bias modification in alcohol dependence: Do clinical effects replicate and for whom does it work best? *Developmental Cognitive Neuroscience*, 4: 38–51.

Edenberg, H. J. (2011). Genes contributing to the development of alcoholism: An overview. *Alcohol Research and Health*, 34(3): 336–338.

Edwards, S. L., Rapee, R. M., & Kennedy, S. (2010). Prediction of anxiety symptoms in pre-school-aged children: Examination of maternal and paternal perspectives. *Journal of Child Psychology and Psychiatry, and Allied Disciplines*, 51(3): 313–321.

Ehlers, A. (1993). Interoception and panic disorder. *Advances in Behaviour Research and Therapy*, 15(1): 3–21.

Eley, T. C., Bolton, D., O'Connor, T. G., Perrin, S., Smith, P., & Plomin, R. (2003). A twin study of anxiety-related behaviours in pre-school children. *Journal of Child Psychology and Psychiatry*, 44(7): 945–960.

Eley, T. C., Gregory, A. M., Lau, J. Y. F., McGuffin, P., Napolitano, M., Rijsdijk, F. V, & Clark, D. M. (2008). In the face of uncertainty: A twin study of ambiguous information, anxiety and depression in children. *Journal of Abnormal Child Psychology*, 36(1): 55–65.

Emmelkamp, P. M. G. (2012). Attention bias modification: The Emperor's new suit? *BMC Medicine*, 10: art. 63.

Emmelkamp, P. M. G., & Vedel, E. (2010). Commentary: Psychological treatments for anti-social personality disorder: Where is the evidence that group treatment and therapeutic community should be recommended? *Personality and Mental Health*, 4(1): 30–33.

Engel, S. G., Wonderlich, S. A., Crosby, R. D., Wright, T. L., Mitchell, J. E., Crow, S. J., & Venegoni, E. E. (2005). A study of patients with anorexia nervosa using ecologic momentary assessment. *International Journal of Eating Disorders*, 38(4): 335–339.

Enock, P. M., Hofmann, S. G., & McNally, R. J. (2014). Attention bias modification training via smartphone to reduce social anxiety: A randomized, controlled multi-session experiment. *Cognitive Therapy and Research*, 38(2): 200–216.

Ersche, K. D., Jones, P. S., Williams, G. B., Turton, A. J., Robbins, T. W., & Bullmore, E. T. (2012). Abnormal brain structure implicated in stimulant drug addiction. *Science*, 335(6068): 601–604.

Eyers, K., & Parker, G. (2008). *Mastering bipolar disorder: An insider's guide to mastering mood swings and finding balance.* Allen & Unwin.

Eysenck, H. J. (1985). *Decline and Fall of the Freudian Empire.* London: Penguin.

Eysenck, M. W., Mogg, K., May, J., Richards, A., & Mathews, A. (1991). Bias in interpretation of ambiguous sentences related to threat in anxiety. *Journal of Abnormal Psychology*, 100(2): 144–150.

Fairburn, C. G., & Cooper, Z. (2011). Eating disorders, DSM-5 and clinical reality. *British Journal of Psychiatry*, 198(1): 8–10.

Fairburn, C. G., Cooper, Z., Doll, H. A., O'Connor, M. E., Bohn, K., Hawker, D. M., et al. (2009). Transdiagnostic cognitive-behavioral therapy for patients with eating disorders: A two-site trial with 60-week follow-up. *American Journal of Psychiatry*, 166(3): 311–319.

Fairburn, C. G., Cooper, Z., & Shafran, R. (2003). Cognitive behaviour therapy for eating disorders: A 'transdiagnostic' theory and treatment. *Behaviour Research and Therapy*, 41(5): 509–528.

Fairburn, C. G., Marcus, M. D., & Wilson, G. T. (1993). Cognitive-behavioral therapy for binge eating and bulimia nervosa: A comprehensive treatment manual. In C. G. Fairburn and G. T. Wilson (eds), *Binge Eating: Nature, Assessment and Treatment.* New York: Guilford, pp. 461–404.

Fairburn, C. G., Norman, P. A., Welch, S. L., O'Connor, M. E., Doll, H. A., & Peveler, R. C. (1995). A prospective study of outcome in bulimia nervosa and the long-term effects of three psychological treatments. *Archives of General Psychiatry*, 52(4): 304–312.

Fairburn, C. G., Shafran, R., & Cooper, Z. (1999). A cognitive behavioural theory of anorexia nervosa. *Behaviour Research and Therapy*, 37(1): 1–13.

Fazel, S., Gulati, G., Linsell, L., Geddes, J. R., & Grann, M. (2009). Schizophrenia and violence: Systematic review and meta-analysis. *PLoS Medicine*, 6(8): art. e1000120

Fedoroff, I. C., & Taylor, S. (2001). Psychological and pharmacological treatments of social phobia: A meta-analysis. *Journal of Clinical Psychopharmacology*, 21(3): 311–324.

Fehm, L. & Margraf, J. (2002). Thought suppression: Specificity in agoraphobia versus broad impairment in social phobia? *Behaviour Research and Therapy*, 40: 57–66.

Ferri, M., Amato, L., & Davoli, M. (2006). Alcoholics Anonymous and other 12-step programmes for alcohol dependence. *Cochrane Database of Systematic Reviews* (Online): 19(3): CD005032.

Field, A. (2003). *Clinical Psychology.* Exeter: Learning Matters.

Field, A. P., Argyris, N. G., & Knowles, K. A. (2001). Who's afraid of the big bad wolf? A prospective paradigm to test Rachman's indirect pathways in children. *Behaviour Research and Therapy*, 39: 1259–1276.

Field, A. P. & Davey, G. C. L. (2001). Conditioning models of childhood anxiety. In W. K. Silverman and P. A. Treffers (eds), *Anxiety Disorders in Children and Adolescents: Research, Assessment and Intervention.* Cambridge: Cambridge University Press, pp. 187–211.

Field, A. P., & Lester, K. J. (2010). Is there room for 'development' in developmental models of information processing biases to threat in children and adolescents? *Clinical Child and Family Psychology Review*, 13(4): 315–332.

Field, M., Marhe, R., & Franken, I. H. A. (2014). The clinical relevance of attentional bias in substance use disorders. *CNS Spectrums*, 19(3): 225–230.

Field, M., Mogg, K., & Bradley, B. P. (2006). Automaticity of smoking behaviour: The relationship between dual-task performance, daily cigarette intake and subjective nicotine effects. *Journal of Psychopharmacology*, 20(6): 799–805.

Fisher, C. A., Hetrick, S. E., & Rushford, N. (2010). Family therapy for anorexia nervosa. *Cochrane Database of Systematic Reviews*, 14(4): CD004780.

Foa, E. B., Franklin, M. E., & Moser, J. (2002). Context in the clinic: How well do cognitive-behavioral therapies and medications work in combination? *Biological Psychiatry*, 52(10): 989–997.

Fonagy, P., & Bateman, A. (2008). The development of borderline personality disorder: A mentalizing model. *Journal of Personality Disorders*, 22(1): 4–21.

Fonagy, P., & Luyten, P. (2009). A developmental, mentalization-based approach to the understanding and treatment of borderline personality disorder. *Development and Psychopathology*, 21(4): 1355–1381.

Fontaine, N., & Viding, E. (2008). Genetics of personality disorders. *Psychiatry*, 7(3): 137–141.

Ford, T., Goodman, R., & Meltzer, H. (2003). The British Child and Adolescent Mental Health Survey: The prevalence of DSM-IV disorders. *Journal of the American Academy of Child & Adolescent Psychiatry*, 42(10): 1203–1211.

Forehand, R., Wells, K. C., & Sturgis, E. T. (1978). Predictors of child noncompliant behavior in the home. *Journal of Consulting and Clinical Psychology*, 46(1): 179.

Forgeard, M. J. C., Haigh, E. A. P., Beck, A. T., Davidson, R. J., Henn, F. A., Maier, S. F., et al. (2011). Beyond depression: Toward a process-based approach to research, diagnosis, and treatment. *Clinical Psychology: Science and Practice*, 18(4): 275–299.

Fox, N. A., Nichols, K. E., Henderson, H. A., Rubin, K., Schmidt, L., Hamer, D., et al. (2005). Evidence for a gene–environment interaction in predicting behavioral inhibition in middle childhood. *Psychological Science*, 16(12): 921–926.

Fredrikson, M., Annas, P., Fischer, H., & Wik, G. (1996). Gender and age differences in the prevalence of specific fears and phobias. *Behaviour Research and Therapy*, 34: 33–39.

Freeston, M. H., Rhéaume, J., Letarte, H., Dugas, M. J., & Ladouceur, R. (1994). Why do people worry? *Personality and Individual Differences*, 17(6): 791–802.

Freitas-Ferrari, M. C., Hallak, J. E. C., Trzesniak, C., Filho, A. S., Machado-de-Sousa, J. P., Chagas, M. H. N., et al. (2010). Neuroimaging in social anxiety disorder: A systematic review of the literature. *Progress in Neuro-Psychopharmacology & Biological Psychiatry*, 34(4): 565–580.

Freud, S. (1954). *The Interpretation of Dreams*. London: George Allen & Unwin Ltd.

Friederich, H. C., Wu, M., Simon, J. J., & Herzog, W. (2013). Neurocircuit function in eating disorders. *International Journal of Eating Disorders*, 46(5): 425–432.

Frith, C. D. (1992). *The Cognitive Neurospsychology of Schizophrenia*. Hove: Erlbaum.

Furmark, T., Tillfors, M., Marteinsdottir, I., Fischer, H., Pissiota, A., Långström, B., & Fredrikson, M. (2002). Common changes in cerebral blood flow in patients with social phobia treated with citalopram or cognitive-behavioral therapy. *Archives of General Psychiatry*, 59(5): 425.

Furukawa, T. A., Watanabe, N., & Churchill, R. (2006). Psychotherapy plus antidepressant for panic disorder with or without agoraphobia: Systematic review. *The British Journal of Psychiatry: The Journal of Mental Science*, 188(4): 305–312.

Gallagher, B., & Cartwright-Hatton, S. (2008). The relationship between parenting factors and trait anxiety: Mediating role of cognitive errors and metacognition. *Journal of Anxiety Disorders*, 22(4): 722–733.

Garratt, G., Ingram, R. E., Rand, K. L., & Sawalani, G. (2007). Cognitive processes in cognitive therapy: Evaluation of the mechanisms of change in the treatment of depression. *Clinical Psychology: Science and Practice*, 14(3): 224–239.

Gask, L., Evans, M., & Kessler, D. (2013). Personality disorder. *BMJ*, 347: art. 7924.

Geddes, J. R., Burgess, S., Hawton, K., Jamison, K., & Goodwin, G. M. (2004). Long-term lithium therapy for bipolar disorder: Systematic review and meta-analysis of randomized controlled trials. *American Journal of Psychiatry*, 161(2): 217–222.

Gerull, F. C., & Rapee, R. M. (2002). Mother knows best: Effects of maternal modelling on the acquisition of fear and avoidance behaviour in toddlers. *Behaviour Research and Therapy*, 40(3): 279–287.

Giancola, P. R., & Tarter, R. E. (1999). Executive cognitive functioning and risk for substance abuse. *Psychological Science*, 10(3): 203–205.

Giesen-Bloo, J., Van Dyck, R., Spinhoven, P., Van Tilburg, W., Dirksen, C., Van Asselt, T., et al. (2006). Outpatient psychotherapy for borderline personality disorder: Randomized trial of schema-focused therapy vs transference-focused psychotherapy. *Archives of General Psychiatry*, 63(6): 649–658.

Giovino, G. A., Mirza, S. A., Samet, J. M., Gupta, P. C., Jarvis, M. J., Bhala, N., et al. (2012). Tobacco use in 3 billion individuals from 16 countries: An analysis of nationally representative cross-sectional household surveys. *The Lancet*, 380(9842): 668–679.

Gloster, A. T., Wittchen, H.-U., Einsle, F., Lang, T., Helbig-Lang, S., Fydrich, T., et al. (2011). Psychological treatment for panic disorder with agoraphobia: A randomized controlled trial to examine the role of therapist-guided exposure in situ in CBT. *Journal of Consulting and Clinical Psychology*, 79(3): 406–420.

Goghari, V. M., Sponheim, S. R., & MacDonald, A. W. (2010). The functional neuroanatomy of symptom dimensions in schizophrenia: A qualitative and quantitative review of a persistent question. *Neuroscience and Biobehavioral Reviews*, 34(3): 468–486.

Goldacre, B. (2012). *Bad Pharma: How Drug Companies Mislead Doctors and Harm Patients*. London: Fourth Estate.

Goldapple, K., Segal, Z., Garson, C., Lau, M., Bieling, P., Kennedy, S., & Mayberg, H. (2004). Modulation of cortical-limbic pathways in major depression: Treatment-specific effects of cognitive behavior therapy. *Archives of General Psychiatry*, 61(1): 34–41.

Goodwin, G. M. (2009). Evidence-based guidelines for treating bipolar disorder: Revised second edition – recommendations from the British association for psychopharmacology. *Journal of Psychopharmacology*, 23(4): 346–388.

Gotlib, I. H., & Joormann, J. (2010) Cognition and depression: Current status and future directions. *Annual Review of Clinical Psychology*, 6: 285–312.

Gottesman, I. I. (1991). *Schizophrenia Genesis: The Origins of Madness*. New York: W. H. Freeman.

Gould, R. A., Otto, M. W., Pollack, M. H., & Yap, L. (1997). Cognitive behavioral and pharmacological treatment of generalized anxiety disorder: A preliminary meta-analysis. *Behavior Therapy*, 28(2): 285–305.

Grant, B. F., Hasin, D. S., Blanco, C., Stinson, F. S., Chou, S. P., Goldstein, R. B., et al. (2005). The epidemiology of social anxiety disorder in the United States: Results from the National Epidemiologic Survey on Alcohol and Related Conditions. *Journal of Clinical Psychiatry*, 66(11): 1351–1361.

Grant, B. F., Hasin, D. S., Stinson, F. S., Dawson, D. A., Ruan, W. J., Goldstein, R. B., et al. (2005). Prevalence, correlates, co-morbidity, and comparative disability of DSM-IV generalized anxiety disorder in the USA: Results from the National Epidemiologic Survey on Alcohol and Related Conditions. *Psychological Medicine*, 35(12): 1747–1759.

Grant, B. F., Stinson, F. S., Dawson, D. A., Chou, S. P., Dufour, M. C., Compton, W., et al., (2004). Prevalence and co-occurrence of substance use disorders and independent mood and anxiety disorders: Results from the national epidemiologic survey on alcohol and related conditions. *Archives of General Psychiatry*, 61(8): 807–816.

Green, M. F. (2006). Cognitive impairment and functional outcome in schizophrenia and bipolar disorder. *Journal of Clinical Psychiatry*, 67(supplement 9): 3–8.

Greenbaum, P. E., Cook, E. W., Melamed, B. G., & Abeles, L. A. (1988). Sequential patterns of medical stress: Maternal agitation and child distress. *Child and Family Behavior Therapy*, 10(1): 9–18.

Greenwood, T. A., Braff, D. L., Light, G. A., Cadenhead, I. S., Calkins, M. E., Dobie, D., et al. (2007). Initial heritability analyses of endophenotypic measures for schizophrenia: The Consortium on the Genetics of Schizophrenia. *Archives of General Psychiatry*, 64(11): 1242–1250.

Gregory, A. M., & Eley, T. C. (2007). Genetic influences on anxiety in children: What we've learned and where we're heading. *Clinical Child and Family Psychology Review*, 10(3): 199–212.

Groesz, L. M., Levine, M. P., & Murnen, S. K. (2002). The effect of experimental presentation of thin media images on body satisfaction: A meta-analytic review. *International Journal of Eating Disorders*, 31(1): 1–16.

Gur, R. E., Calkins, M. E., Gur, R. C., Horan, W. P., Nuechterlein, K. H., Seidman, L. J., & Stone, W. S. (2007). The consortium on the genetics of schizophrenia: Neurocognitive endophenotypes. *Schizophrenia Bulletin*, 33(1): 49–68.

Haaga, D. A. F., Dyck, M. J., & Ernst, D. (1991). Empirical status of cognitive theory of depression. *Psychological Bulletin*, 110(2): 215–236.

Hackmann, A., Clark, D. M., & McManus, F. (2000). Recurrent images and early memories in social phobia. *Behaviour Research and Therapy*, 38(6): 601–610.

Hakamata, Y., Lissek, S., Bar-Haim, Y., Britton, J. C., Fox, N. A., Leibenluft, E., et al. (2010). Attention bias modification treatment: A meta-analysis toward the establishment of novel treatment for anxiety. *Biological Psychiatry*, 68(11): 982–990.

Hall, K., Gibbie, T., & Lubman, D. I. (2012). Motivational interviewing techniques: Facilitating behaviour change in the general practice setting. *Australian Family Physician*, 41: 660–667.

Hallion, L. S., & Ruscio, A. M. (2011). A meta-analysis of the effect of cognitive bias modification on anxiety and depression. *Psychological Bulletin*, 137(6): 940–958.

Hammen, C. (2005) Stress and depression. *Annual Review of Clinical Psychology*, 1: 293–319.

Hanrahan, F., Field, A. P., Jones, F. W., & Davey, G. C. L. (2013). A meta-analysis of cognitive therapy for worry in generalized anxiety disorder. *Clinical Psychology Review*, 33(1): 120–132.

Hare, R. D. (2003). *Hare Psychopathy Checklist: Revised* (PCL-R) (2nd edition). Toronto: Multi-Health Systems.

Harmer, C. J., & Cowen, P. J. (2013). 'It's the way that you look at it': A cognitive neuropsychological account of SSRI action in depression. *Philosophical Transactions of the Royal Society B: Biological Sciences*, 368: art. 20140407.

Harmer, C. J., Shelley, N. C., Cowen, P. J., & Goodwin, G. M. (2004). Increased positive versus negative affective perception and memory in healthy volunteers following selective serotonin and norepinephrine reuptake inhibition. *American Journal of Psychiatry*, 161(7): 1256–1263.

Hasin, D. S. (2012). Combining abuse and dependence in DSM-5. *Journal of Studies on Alcohol and Drugs*, 73(4): 702–704.

Hatch, A., Madden, S., Kohn, M., Clarke, S., Touyz, S., & Williams, L. M. (2010). Anorexia nervosa: Towards an integrative neuroscience model. *European Eating Disorders Review*, 18(3): 165–179.

Hay, P. (2013). A systematic review of evidence for psychological treatments in eating disorders: 2005–2012. *International Journal of Eating Disorders*, 46(5): 462–469.

Haynos, A. F., & Fruzzetti, A. E. (2011). Anorexia nervosa as a disorder of emotion dysregulation: Evidence and treatment implications. *Clinical Psychology: Science and Practice*, 18(3): 183–202.

Heidbreder, C. A., & Newman, A. H. (2010) Current perspectives on selective dopamine D3 receptor antagonists as pharmacotherapeutics for addictions and related disorders. *Annals of the New York Academy of Sciences*, 1187: 4–34.

Hemsley, D. R. (1993). A simple (or simplistic?) cognitive model for schizophrenia. *Behaviour Research and Therapy*, 31(7): 633–645.

Heninger, G. R., Delgado, P. L., & Charney, D. S. (1996). The revised monoamine theory of depression: A modulatory role for monoamines, based on new findings from monoamine depletion experiments in humans. *Pharmacopsychiatry*, 29(1): 2–11.

Henningfield, J. E., Fant, R. V., Buchhalter, A. R., & Stitzer, M. L. (2005). Pharmacotherapy for nicotine dependence. *CA: A Cancer Journal for Clinicians*, 55(5): 281–299.

Hettema, J. M. (2001). A review and meta-analysis of the genetic epidemiology of anxiety disorders. *American Journal of Psychiatry*, 158(10): 1568–1578.

Hettema, J. M., Annas, P., Neale, M. C., Kendler, K. S., & Fredrikson, M. (2003). A twin study of the genetics of fear conditioning. *Archives of General Psychiatry*, 60: 702–708.

Hettema, J. M., Prescott, C. A., & Kendler, K. S. (2001). A population-based twin study of generalized anxiety disorder in men and women. *Journal of Nervous and Mental Disease*, 189(7): 413–420.

Heyman, G. M. (1996). Resolving the contradictions of addiction. *Behavioral and Brain Sciences*, 19(4): 561–610.

Hicks, B. M., Krueger, R. F., Iacono, W. G., McGue, M., & Patrick, C. J. (2004). Family transmission and heritability of externalizing disorders: A twin-family study. *Archives of General Psychiatry*, 61(9): 922–928.

Higgins, S. T., Budney, A. J., Bickel, W. K., Foerg, F. E., Donham, R., & Badger, G. J. (1994). Incentives improve outcome in outpatient behavioral treatment of cocaine dependence. *Archives of General Psychiatry*, 51(7): 568–576.

Hiroto, D. S., & Seligman, M. E. (1975). Generality of learned helplessness in man. *Journal of Personality and Social Psychology*, 31(2): 311–327.

Hirsch, C. R., & Mathews, A. (2012). A cognitive model of pathological worry. *Behaviour Research and Therapy*, 50(10): 636–646.

Ho, M. K., Goldman, D., Heinz, A., Kaprio, J., Kreek, M. J., Li, M. D., et al. (2010). Breaking barriers in the genomics and pharmacogenetics of drug addiction. *Clinical Pharmacology and Therapeutics*, 88(6): 779–791.

Hodge, S., Barr, W., Gpfert, M., Hellin, K., Horne, A., & Kirkcaldy, A. (2010). Qualitative findings from a mixed methods evaluation of once-weekly therapeutic community day services for people with personality disorder. *Journal of Mental Health*, 19(1): 43–51.

Hogarth, L., Balleine, B. W., Corbit, L. H., & Killcross, S. (2013) Associative learning mechanisms underpinning the transition from recreational drug use to addiction. *Annals of the New York Academy of Sciences*, 1282: 12–24.

Hollon, S. D., DeRubeis, R. J., Shelton, R. C., Amsterdam, J. D., Salomon, R. M., O'Reardon, J. P., et al. (2005). Prevention of relapse following cognitive therapy vs medications in moderate to severe depression. *Archives of General Psychiatry*, 62(4): 417–422.

Holmes, E. A., & Mathews, A. (2010). Mental imagery in emotion and emotional disorders. *Clinical Psychology Review*, 30(3): 349–362.

Hooley, J. M. (2007) Expressed emotion and relapse of psychopathology. *Annual Review of Clinical Psychology*, 3: 329–352.

Horder, J., Matthews, P., & Waldmann, R. (2011). Placebo, Prozac and PLoS: Significant lessons for psychopharmacology. *Journal of Psychopharmacology*, 25(10): 1277–1288.

Hudson, J. L., & Rapee, R. M. (2006). Parental perceptions of overprotection specific to anxious children or shared between siblings? *Behaviour Change*, 22(3): 185–195.

Huhn, M., Tardy, M., Spineli, L. M., Kissling, W., Förstl, H., Pitschel-Walz, G., et al. (2014). Efficacy of pharmacotherapy and psychotherapy for adult psychiatric disorders: A systematic overview of meta-analyses. *JAMA Psychiatry*, 71(6): 706–715.

Hulshoff Pol, H. E., & Kahn, R. S. (2008). What happens after the first episode? A review of progressive brain changes in chronically ill patients with schizophrenia. *Schizophrenia Bulletin*, 34(2): 354–366.

Hyman, S. E. (2010) The diagnosis of mental disorders: The problem of reification. *Annual Review of Clinical Psychology*, 6: 155–179.

Ioannidis, J. P. A. (2005). Why most published research findings are false. *PLoS Medicine*, 2(8): 0696–0701.

Jacob, G. A., & Arntz, A. (2013). Schema therapy for personality disorders: A review. *International Journal of Cognitive Therapy*, 6(2): 171–185.

Jacobi, C., Hayward, C., De Zwaan, M., Kraemer, H. C., & Agras, W. S. (2004). Coming to terms with risk factors for eating disorders: Application of risk terminology and suggestions for a general taxonomy. *Psychological Bulletin*, 130(1): 19–65.

Jauhar, S., McKenna, P. J., Radua, J., Fung, E., Salvador, R., & Laws, K. R. (2014). Cognitive-behavioural therapy for the symptoms of schizophrenia: Systematic review and meta-analysis with examination of potential bias. *British Journal of Psychiatry*, 204(1): 20–29.

Jenkins, R., Lewis, P., Bebbington, P., Brugha, T., Farrell, M., Gill, B., & Meltzer, H. (1997). The National Psychiatric Morbidity Surveys of Great Britain: Initial findings from the Household Survey. *Psychological Medicine*, 27: 775–789.

Jentsch, J. D., & Taylor, J. R. (1999). Impulsivity resulting from frontostriatal dysfunction in drug abuse: Implications for the control of behavior by reward-related stimuli. *Psychopharmacology*, 146(4): 373–390.

Jester, J. M., Wong, M. M., Cranford, J. A., Buu, A., Fitzgerald, H. E., & Zucker, R. A. (2014). Alcohol expectancies in childhood: Change with the onset of drinking and ability to predict adolescent drunkenness and binge drinking. *Addiction*, in press, doi: 10.1111/add.12704

Johnson, S. L., Edge, M. D., Holmes, M. K., & Carver, C. S. (2012) The behavioral activation system and mania. *Annual Review of Clinical Psychology*, 8: 243–267.

Jonas, D. E., Amick, H. R., Feltner, C., Bobashev, G., Thomas, K., Wines, R., et al. (2014). Pharmacotherapy for adults with alcohol use disorders in outpatient settings: A systematic review and meta-analysis. *Journal of the American Medical Association*, 311(18): 1889–1900.

Jones, B., Corbin, W. R., & Fromme, K. (2001). A review of expectancy theory and alcohol consumption. *Addiction*, 96: 57–72.

Jones, C., Cormac, I., Mota, J., & Campbell, C. (2000). Cognitive behaviour therapy for schizophrenia. *Cochrane Database of Systematic Reviews*, 2: CD000524.

Jones, M. K., & Menzies, R. G. (2000). Danger expectancies, self-efficacy and insight in spider phobia. *Behaviour Research and Therapy*, 38(6): 585–600.

Kanter, J. W., Manos, R. C., Bowe, W. M., Baruch, D. E., Busch, A. M., & Rusch, L. C. (2010). What is behavioral activation? A review of the empirical literature. *Clinical Psychology Review*, 30(6): 608–620.

Kapur, S., & Mamo, D. (2003). Half a century of antipsychotics and still a central role for dopamine D2 receptors. *Progress in Neuro-Psychopharmacology and Biological Psychiatry*, 27(7): 1081–1090.

Kapur, S., Mizrahi, R., & Li, M. (2005). From dopamine to salience to psychosis – Linking biology, pharmacology and phenomenology of psychosis. *Schizophrenia Research*, 79(1): 59–68.

Kapur, S., & Remington, G. (2001). Atypical antipsychotics: New directions and new challenges in the treatment of schizophrenia. *Annual Review of Medicine*, 52: 503–517.

Karwautz, A., Rabe-Hesketh, S., Hu, X., Zhao, J., Sham, P., Collier, D. A., & Treasure, J. L. (2001). Individual-specific risk factors for anorexia nervosa: A pilot study using a discordant sister-pair design. *Psychological Medicine*, 31(2): 317–329.

Karwautz, A., Wagner, G., Waldherr, K., Nader, I. W., Fernandez-Aranda, F., Estivill, X., et al. (2011). Gene–environment interaction in anorexia nervosa: Relevance of non-shared environment and the serotonin transporter gene. *Molecular Psychiatry*, 16(6): 590–592.

Kaufman, J., Yang, B.-Z., Douglas-Palumberi, H., Grasso, D., Lipschitz, D., Houshyar, S., et al. (2006). Brain-derived neurotrophic factor-5-HTTLPR gene interactions and environmental modifiers of depression in children. *Biological Psychiatry*, 59(8): 673–680.

Kaye, W. H., Fudge, J. L., & Paulus, M. (2009). New insights into symptoms and neurocircuit function of anorexia nervosa. *Nature Reviews Neuroscience*, 10(8): 573–584.

Kaye, W. H., Klump, K. L., Frank, G. K. W., & Strober, M. (2000) Anorexia and bulimia nervosa. *Annual Review of Medicine*, 51: 299–313.

Keel, P. K., & Brown, T. A. (2010). Update on course and outcome in eating disorders. *International Journal of Eating Disorders*, 43(3): 195–204.

Keel, P. K., Brown, T. A., Holland, L. A., & Bodell, L. P. (2012) Empirical classification of eating disorders. *Annual Review of Clinical Psychology*, 8: 381–404.

Keel, P. K., Dorer, D. J., Franko, D. L., Jackson, S. C., & Herzog, D. B. (2005). Postremission predictors of relapse in women with eating disorders. *American Journal of Psychiatry*, 162(12): 2263–2268.

Kellett, S., Bennett, D., Ryle, T., & Thake, A. (2013). Cognitive analytic therapy for borderline personality disorder: Therapist competence and therapeutic effectiveness in routine practice. *Clinical Psychology and Psychotherapy*, 20(3): 216–225.

Kertz, S. J., & Woodruff-Borden, J. (2011). The developmental psychopathology of worry. *Clinical Child and Family Psychology Review*, 14(2): 174–197.

Kessler, R. C., Chiu, W. T., Demler, O., & Walters, E. E. (2005). Prevalence, severity, and comorbidity of 12-month DSM-IV disorders in the National Comorbidity Survey Replication. *Archives of General Psychiatry*, 62(6): 617–627.

Kessler, R. C., Chiu, W. T., Jin, R., Ruscio, A. M., Shear, K., & Walters, E. E. (2006). The epidemiology of panic attacks, panic disorder, and agoraphobia in the National Comorbidity Survey Replication. *Archives of General Psychiatry*, 63(4): 415–424.

Kessler, R. C., & Wang, P. S. (2008) The descriptive epidemiology of commonly occurring mental disorders in the United States. *Annual Review of Public Health*, 29: 115–129.

Khandelwal, S. K., Sharan, P., & Saxena, S. (1995). Eating disorders: An Indian perspective. *International Journal of Social Psychiatry*, 41(2): 132–146.

Kiehl, K. A. (2006). A cognitive neuroscience perspective on psychopathy: Evidence for paralimbic system dysfunction. *Psychiatry Research*, 142(2–3): 107–128.

Kim-Cohen, J., Caspi, A., Taylor, A., Williams, B., Newcombe, R., Craig, I. W., & Moffitt, T. E. (2006). MAOA, maltreatment, and gene–environment interaction predicting children's mental health: New evidence and a meta-analysis. *Molecular Psychiatry*, 11(10): 903–913.

Kirsch, I., Deacon, B. J., Huedo-Medina, T. B., Scoboria, A., Moore, T. J., & Johnson, B. T. (2008). Initial severity and antidepressant benefits: A meta-analysis of data submitted to the food and drug administration. *PLoS Medicine*, 5(2): 0260–0268.

Klein, D. F. (1964). Delineation of two drug-responsive anxiety syndromes. *Psychopharmacologia*, 5(6): 397–408.

Klein, D. F. (1993). False suffocation alarms, spontaneous panics, and related conditions: An integrative hypothesis. *Archives of General Psychiatry*, 50(4): 306.

Koenigsberg, H. W., & Handley, R. (1986). Expressed emotion: From predictive index to clinical construct. *American Journal of Psychiatry*, 143(11): 1361–1373.

Koob, G. F., & Le Moal, M. (1997). Drug abuse: Hedonic homeostatic dysregulation. *Science*, 278(5335): 52–58.

Koob, G. F., & Volkow, N. D. (2010). Neurocircuitry of addiction. *Neuropsychopharmacology*, 35(1): 217–238.

Koskina, A., Campbell, I. C., & Schmidt, U. (2013). Exposure therapy in eating disorders revisited. *Neuroscience and Biobehavioral Reviews*, 37(2): 193–208.

Kraepelin, E. (1922). *Manic-depressive insanity and paranoia*. Edinburgh: E & S. Livingstone.

Kurtz, M. M., & Mueser, K. T. (2008). A meta-analysis of controlled research on social skills training for schizophrenia. *Journal of Consulting and Clinical Psychology*, 76(3): 491–504.

Kuther, T. L. (2002). Rational decision perspectives on alcohol consumption by youth: Revising the theory of planned behavior. *Addictive Behaviors*, 27(1): 35–47.

Kwon, S. M., & Oei, T. P. S. (1992). Differential causal roles of dysfunctional attitudes and automatic thoughts in depression. *Cognitive Therapy and Research*, 16(3): 309–328.

Lakdawalla, Z., Hankin, B. L., & Mermelstein, R. (2007). Cognitive theories of depression in children and adolescents: A conceptual and quantitative review. *Clinical Child and Family Psychology Review*, 10(1): 1–24.

Laskey, B., & Cartwright-Hatton, S. (2009). Parental discipline behaviours and beliefs: Associations with parental and child anxiety. *Child: Care, Health & Development*, 35(5): 717–727.

Lataster, T., van Os, J., Drukker, M., Henquet, C., Feron, F., Gunther, N., & Myin-Germeys, I. (2006). Childhood victimisation and developmental expression of non-clinical delusional ideation and hallucinatory experiences. *Social Psychiatry and Psychiatric Epidemiology*, 41(6): 423–428.

Lau, J. Y. F., & Eley, T. C. (2010) The genetics of mood disorders. *Annual Review of Clinical Psychology*, 6: 313–337.

Laulik, S., Chou, S., Browne, K. D., & Allam, J. (2013). The link between personality disorder and parenting behaviors: A systematic review. *Aggression and Violent Behavior*, 18(6): 644–655.

Lautch, H. (1971). Dental phobia. *British Journal of Psychiatry*, 119: 151–158.

Leff, J., & Vaughn, C. (1985). *Expressed Emotions in Families: Its Significance for Mental Illness*. New York: Guilford.

Levy, K. N. (2005). The implications of attachment theory and research for understanding borderline personality disorder. *Development and Psychopathology*, 17(4): 959–986.

Lewinsohn, P. M., Zinbarg, R., Seeley, J. R., Lewinsohn, M., & Sack, W. H. (1997). Lifetime comorbidity among anxiety disorders and between anxiety disorders and other mental disorders in adolescents. *Journal of Anxiety Disorders*, 11(4): 377–394.

Lewis, M. D. (2011). Dopamine and the neural 'now': Essay and review of addiction: A disorder of choice. *Perspectives on Psychological Science*, 6(2): 150–155.

Liddle, P. F. (1987). The symptoms of chronic schizophrenia: A re-examination of the positive-negative dichotomy. *British Journal of Psychiatry*, 151(August): 145–151.

Lieb, R. (2002). Parental major depression and the risk of depression and other mental disorders in offspring: A prospective-longitudinal community study. *Archives of General Psychiatry*, 59(4): 365–374.

Lieb, R., Becker, E., & Altamura, C. (2005). The epidemiology of generalized anxiety disorder in Europe. *European Neuropsychopharmacology*, 15(4): 445–452.

Limandri, B. J. (2012). The plight of personality disorders in the DSM-5. *Issues in Mental Health Nursing*, 33(9): 598–604.

Linehan, M. M. (1993). *Cognitive-Behavioral Treatment of Borderline Personality Disorder*. New York: Guilford.

Links, P. S., & Eynan, R. (2013). The relationship between personality disorders and axis I psychopathology: Deconstructing comorbidity. *Annual Review of Clinical Psychology*, 9: 529–554.

Lock, J., Le Grange, D., Agras, W. S., Moye, A., Bryson, S. W., & Jo, B. (2010). Randomized clinical trial comparing family-based treatment with adolescent-focused individual therapy for adolescents with anorexia nervosa. *Archives of General Psychiatry*, 67(10): 1025–1032.

Lynch, T. R., Trost, W. T., Salsman, N., & Linehan, M. M. (2007). Dialectical behavior therapy for borderline personality disorder. *Annual Review of Clinical Psychology*, 3: 181–205.

Lyon, H. M., Bentall, R. P., & Startup, M. (1999). Social cognition and the manic defense: Attributions, selective attention, and self-schema in bipolar affective disorder. *Journal of Abnormal Psychology*, 108(2): 273–282.

MacLeod, C., & Mathews, A. (2012) Cognitive bias modification approaches to anxiety. *Annual Review of Clinical Psychology*, 8: 189–217.

MacLeod, C., Rutherford, E., Campbell, L., Ebsworthy, G., & Holker, L. (2002). Selective attention and emotional vulnerability: Assessing the causal basis of their association through the experimental manipulation of attentional bias. *Journal of Abnormal Psychology*, 111(1): 107–123.

Maier, S. F., & Seligman, M. E. (1976). Learned helplessness: Theory and evidence. *Journal of Experimental Psychology: General*, 105(1): 3–46.

Malik, V. S., Willett, W. C., & Hu, F. B. (2013). Global obesity: Trends, risk factors and policy implications. *Nature Reviews Endocrinology*, 9(1): 13–27.

Manning, N. (2010). Therapeutic communities: A problem or a solution for psychiatry? A sociological view. *British Journal of Psychotherapy*, 26(4): 434–443.

Marco, E. M., MacRì, S., & Laviola, G. (2011). Critical age windows for neurodevelopmental psychiatric disorders: Evidence from animal models. *Neurotoxicity Research*, 19(2): 286–307.

Marjoram, D., Tansley, H., Miller, P., MacIntyre, D., Owens, D. G. C., Johnstone, E. C., & Lawrie, S. (2005). A Theory of Mind investigation into the appreciation of visual jokes in schizophrenia. *BMC Psychiatry*, 5: art. 12.

Marsh, A. A., & Blair, R. J. R. (2008). Deficits in facial affect recognition among antisocial populations: A meta-analysis. *Neuroscience and Biobehavioral Reviews*, 32(3): 454–465.

Matheson, S. L., Shepherd, A. M., Pinchbeck, R. M., Laurens, K. R., & Carr, V. J. (2013). Childhood adversity in schizophrenia: A systematic meta-analysis. *Psychological Medicine*, 43(2): 225–238.

Mathews, A., & MacLeod, C. (1994). Cognitive approaches to emotion and emotional disorders. *Annual Review of Psychology*, 45(1): 25–50.

Mathews, A., Mogg, K., Kentish, J., & Eysenck, M. (1995). Effect of psychological treatment on cognitive bias in generalized anxiety disorder. *Behaviour Research and Therapy*, 33(3): 293–303.

McCall, W. V. (2001). Electroconvulsive therapy in the era of modern psychopharmacology. *International Journal of Neuropsychopharmacology*, 4(3): 315–324.

McGee, R., Feehan, M., Williams, S., & Anderson, J. (1992). DSM-III disorders from age 11 to age 15 years. *Journal of the American Academy of Child & Adolescent Psychiatry*, 31: 50–59.

McGuire, P. K., & Frith, C. D. (1996). Disordered functional connectivity in schizophrenia. *Psychological Medicine*, 26(4): 663–667.

McGuire, P. K., Silbersweig, D. A., Wright, I., Murray, R. M., David, A. S., Frackowiak, R. S. J., & Frith, C. D. (1995). Abnormal monitoring of inner speech: A physiological basis for auditory hallucinations. *The Lancet*, 346(8975): 596–600.

McGurk, S. R., Twamley, E. W., Sitzer, D. I., McHugo, G. J., & Mueser, K. T. (2007). A meta-analysis of cognitive remediation in schizophrenia. *American Journal of Psychiatry*, 164(12): 1791–1802.

McIntosh, V. V. W., Carter, F. A., Bulik, C. M., Frampton, C. M. A., & Joyce, P. R. (2011). Five-year outcome of cognitive behavioral therapy and exposure with response prevention for bulimia nervosa. *Psychological Medicine*, 41(5): 1061–1071.

McLean, C. P., & Anderson, E. R. (2009). Brave men and timid women? A review of the gender differences in fear and anxiety. *Clinical Psychology Review*, 29(6): 496–505.

McLeod, B. D., Weisz, J. R., & Wood, J. J. (2007). Examining the association between parenting and childhood depression: A meta-analysis. *Clinical Psychology Review*, 27(8): 986–1003.

McNally, R. J. (1990). Psychological approaches to panic disorder: A review. *Psychological Bulletin*, 108(3): 403–419.

McVey, G. L., Lieberman, M., Voorberg, N., Wardrope, D., & Blackmore, E. (2003). School-based peer support groups: A new approach to the prevention of disordered eating. *Eating Disorders*, 11(3): 169–185.

Mellor, C. S. (1970). First rank symptoms of schizophrenia. I. The frequency in schizophrenics on admission to hospital. II. Differences between individual first rank symptoms. *British Journal of Psychiatry*, 117(536): 15–23.

Menzies, R. G., & Clarke, J. C. (1993a). The etiology of fear of heights and its relationship to severity and individual response patterns. *Behaviour Research and Therapy*, 31: 355–366.

Menzies, R. G., & Clarke, J. C. (1993b). The etiology of childhood water phobia. *Behaviour Research and Therapy*, 31: 499–501.

Merikangas, K. R., & Pato, M. (2009). Recent developments in the epidemiology of bipolar disorder in adults and children: Magnitude, correlates, and future directions. *Clinical Psychology: Science and Practice*, 16(2): 121–133.

Mesholam-Gately, R. I., Giuliano, A. J., Goff, K. P., Faraone, S. V., & Seidman, L. J. (2009). Neurocognition in first-episode schizophrenia: A meta-analytic review. *Neuropsychology*, 23(3): 315–336.

Metalsky, G. I., Joiner Jr, T. E., Hardin, T. S., & Abramson, L. Y. (1993). Depressive reactions to failure in a naturalistic setting: A test of the hopelessness and self-esteem theories of depression. *Journal of Abnormal Psychology*, 102(1): 101–109.

Meyer, U., & Feldon, J. (2010). Epidemiology-driven neurodevelopmental animal models of schizophrenia. *Progress in Neurobiology*, 90(3): 285–326.

Meyer-Lindenberg, A., & Tost, H. (2012). Neural mechanisms of social risk for psychiatric disorders. *Nature Neuroscience*, 15(5): 663–668.

Michael, T., Zetsche, U., & Margraf, J. (2007). Epidemiology of anxiety disorders. *Psychiatry*, 6(4): 136–142.

Miklowitz, D. J., & Goldstein, M. J. (1993). Mapping the intrafamilial environment of the schizophrenic patient. In R. L. Cromwell and C. R. C. R. Snyder (eds), *Schizophrenia: Origins, Processes, Treatments and Outcome.* New York: Oxford University Press.

Miller, W. R. (1996). Motivational interviewing: Research, practice, and puzzles. *Addictive Behaviors*, 21(6): 835–842.

Millon, T. (2012) On the history and future study of personality and its disorders. *Annual Review of Clinical Psychology*, 8: 1–19.

Mineka, S., Davidson, M., Cook, M., & Weir, R. (1984). Observational conditioning of snake fears in rhesus monkeys. *Journal of Abnormal Psychology*, 93: 355–372.

Miranda, J., Gross, J. J., Persons, J. B., & Hahn, J. (1998). Mood matters: Negative mood induction activates dysfunctional attitudes in women vulnerable to depression. *Cognitive Therapy and Research*, 22(4): 363–376.

Mitchell, J. E., Roerig, J., & Steffen, K. (2013). Biological therapies for eating disorders. *International Journal of Eating Disorders*, 46(5): 470–477.

Mochcovitch, M. D., & Nardi, A. E. (2010). Selective serotonin-reuptake inhibitors in the treatment of panic disorder: A systematic review of placebo-controlled studies. *Expert Review of Neurotherapeutics*, 10(8): 1285–93. doi:10.1586/ern.10.110

Mogg, K., Baldwin, D. S., Brodrick, P., & Bradley, B. P. (2004). Effect of short-term SSRI treatment on cognitive bias in generalised anxiety disorder. *Psychopharmacology*, 176(3–4): 466–470.

Mogg, K., Bradley, B. P., Field, M., & De Houwer, J. (2003). Eye movements to smoking-related pictures in smokers: Relationship between attentional biases and implicit and explicit measures of stimulus valence. *Addiction*, 98(6): 825–836.

Mogg, K., Bradley, B. P., Williams, R., & Mathews, A. (1993). Subliminal processing of emotional information in anxiety and depression. *Journal of Abnormal Psychology*, 102(2): 304–311.

Mogoaşe, C., David, D., & Koster, E. H. W. (2014). Clinical efficacy of attentional bias modification procedures: An updated meta-analysis. *Journal of Clinical Psychology*, in press, doi: 10.1002/jclp.22081.

Monroe, S. M., & Harkness, K. L. (2005). Life stress, the 'kindling' hypothesis, and the recurrence of depression: Considerations from a life stress perspective. *Psychological Review*, 112(2): 417–445.

Moore, T. H., Zammit, S., Lingford-Hughes, A., Barnes, T. R., Jones, P. B., Burke, M., & Lewis, G. (2007). Cannabis use and risk of psychotic or affective mental health outcomes: A systematic review. *The Lancet*, 370(9584): 319–328.

Morey, L. C., & Hopwood, C. J. (2013) Stability and change in personality disorders. *Annual Review of Clinical Psychology*, 9: 499–528.

Morgenstern, J., & Longabaugh, R. (2000). Cognitive-behavioral treatment for alcohol dependence: A review of evidence for its hypothesized mechanisms of action. *Addiction*, 95(10): 1475–1490.

Morissette, S. B., Tull, M. T., Gulliver, S. B., Kamholz, B. W., & Zimering, R. T. (2007). Anxiety, anxiety disorders, tobacco use, and nicotine: A critical review of interrelationships. *Psychological Bulletin*, 133(2): 245–272.

Morrison, A. P., Turkington, D., Pyle, M., Spencer, H., et al. (2014). Cognitive therapy for people with schizophrenia spectrum disorders not taking antipsychotic drugs: A single-blind randomised controlled trial. *The Lancet*, 383(9926): 1395–1403.

Mowrer, O. H. (1960). *Learning Theory and Behaviour*. New York: Wiley.

Mulder, R., & Chanen, A. M. (2013). Effectiveness of cognitive analytic therapy for personality disorders. *British Journal of Psychiatry*, 202(2): 89–90.

Munafò, M. R., Durrant, C., Lewis, G., & Flint, J. (2009). Gene × environment interactions at the serotonin transporter locus. *Biological Psychiatry*, 65(3): 211–219.

Muris, P., Merckelbach, H., & Collaris, R. (1997). Common childhood fears and their origins. *Behaviour Research and Therapy*, 35 (10): 929–937.

Muris, P., Merckelbach, H., Meesters, C., & Van Lier, P. (1997). What do children fear most often? *Journal of Behaviour Therapy and Experimental Psychiatry*, 28: 263–267.

Murphy, A., Taylor, E., & Elliott, R. (2012). The detrimental effects of emotional process dysregulation on decision making in substance dependence. *Frontiers in Integrative Neuroscience*, 6: art. 101.

Murray, C. J. L., & Lopez, A. D. (1996). *The Global Burden of Disease*. Geneva: World Health Organisation, Harvard School of Public Health, World Bank.

National Institute for Health and Care Excellence (NICE) (2005*). Depression in Children and Young People: Identification and Management in Primary, Secondary and Community Care*. Retrieved 18 September 2014 from www.nice.org.uk/guidance/cg28

National Institute for Health and Care Excellence (NICE) (2011). *CG113 Generalised Anxiety Disorder and Panic Disorder (with or without agoraphobia) in Adults*. Retrieved 18 September 2014 from www.nice.org.uk/guidance/cg113

National Institute for Health and Care Excellence (NICE) (2013a). *CG159 Social Anxiety Disorder: Recognition, Assessment and Treatment*. Retrieved 18 September 2014 from www.nice.org.uk/guidance/cg159

National Institute for Health and Care Excellence (NICE) (2013b). *CG158 Antisocial Behaviour and Conduct Disorders in Children and Young People: Recognition, Intervention and Management*. Retrieved 18 September 2014 from www.nice.org.uk/guidance/cg158

National Institute of Mental Health (2014). *Anxiety Disorders*. Retrieved 12 August 2014 from www.nimh.nih.gov/HEALTH/PUBLICATIONS/ANXIETY-DISORDERS/INDEX. SHTML#pub7

National Prescribing Centre (2010). *Case Study 1: A Young Man with First Episode Psychosis*. Retrieved 30 July 2014 from http://www.npc.nhs.uk/therapeutics/cns/schizophrenia/case1_schizophrenia.php

Neumark-Sztainer, D. R., Wall, M. M., Haines, J. I., Story, M. T., Sherwood, N. E., & van den Berg, P. A. (2007). Shared risk and protective factors for overweight and disordered eating in adolescents. *American Journal of Preventive Medicine*, 33(5): 359–369.e353.

Newman, M. G., & Llera, S. J. (2011). A novel theory of experiential avoidance in generalized anxiety disorder: A review and synthesis of research supporting a contrast avoidance model of worry. *Clinical Psychology Review*, 31(3): 371–382.

Newman, M. G., Llera, S. J., Erickson, T. M., Przeworski, A., & Castonguay, L. G. (2013). Worry and generalized anxiety disorder: A review and theoretical synthesis of evidence on nature, etiology, mechanisms, and treatment. *Annual Review of Clinical Psychology*, 9: 275–297.

Newton, E., Landau, S., Smith, P., Monks, P., Shergill, S., & Wykes, T. (2005). Early psychological intervention for auditory hallucinations: An exploratory study of young people's voices groups. *Journal of Nervous and Mental Disease*, 193(1): 58–61.

Nilsson, J., Östling, S., Waern, M., Karlsson, B., Sigström, R., Guo, X., & Skoog, I. (2012). The 1-month prevalence of generalized anxiety disorder according to DSM-iv, DSM-v, and ICD-10 among nondemented 75-year-olds in Gothenburg, Sweden. *American Journal of Geriatric Psychiatry*, 20(11): 963–972.

Nisbett, R. E., & Wilson, T. D. (1977). Telling more than we can know: Verbal reports on mental processes. *Psychological Review*, 84(3): 231–259.

O'Connor, T., Heron, J., Golding, J., Glover, V., & Team, T. A. S. (2003). Maternal antenatal anxiety and behavioural/emotional problems in children: A test of a programming hypothesis. *Journal of Child Psychology and Psychiatry*, 44(7): 1025–1036.

O'Donovan, M. C., Craddock, N., Norton, N., Williams, H., Peirce, T., Moskvina, V., et al. 2008). Identification of loci associated with schizophrenia by genome-wide association and follow-up. *Nature Genetics*, 40(9): 1053–1055.

Öhman, A., Flykt, A., & Esteves, F. (2001). Emotion drives attention: Detecting the snake in the grass. *Journal of Experimental Psychology: General*, 130: 466–478.

Ollendick, T. H. & King, N. J. (1991). Origins of childhood fears: An evaluation of Rachman's theory of fear acquisition. *Behaviour Research and Therapy*, 29: 117–123.

O'Neill, A., & Frodl, T. (2012). Brain structure and function in borderline personality disorder. *Brain Structure and Function*, 217(4): 767–782.

Ost, L.-G. (1987). Age of onset in different phobias. *Journal of Abnormal Psychology*, 96: 223–229.

Palmer, R. L. (1993). Weight concern should not be a necessary criterion for the eating disorders: A polemic. *International Journal of Eating Disorders*, 14(4): 459–465.

Parry-Jones, W. L., & Parry-Jones, B. (1994). Implications of historical evidence for the classification of eating disorders. *British Journal of Psychiatry*, 165(September): 287–292.

Patterson, G. R. (1982). *Coercive Family Process: A Social Learning Approach* (Vol. 3). Eugene: Castalia.

Patterson, G. R., & Stouthamer-Loeber, M. (1984). The correlation of family management practices and delinquency. *Child Development*, 55(4): 1299–1307.

Petry, N. M., & Bickel, W. K. (1998). Polydrug abuse in heroin addicts: A behavioral economic analysis. *Addiction*, 93(3): 321–335.

Pharoah, F., Mari, J., Rathbone, J., & Wong, W. (2010). Family intervention for schizophrenia. *Cochrane Database of Systematic Reviews*, 12: CD000088.

Piet, J., & Hougaard, E. (2011). The effect of mindfulness-based cognitive therapy for prevention of relapse in recurrent major depressive disorder: A systematic review and meta-analysis. *Clinical Psychology Review*, 31(6): 1032–1040.

Pitschel-Walz, G., Leucht, S., Bäuml, J., Kissling, W., & Engel, R. R. (2001). The effect of family interventions on relapse and rehospitalization in schizophrenia: A meta-analysis. *Schizophrenia Bulletin*, 27(1): 73–92.

Post, R. M. (1992). Transduction of psychosocial stress into the neurobiology of recurrent affective disorder. *American Journal of Psychiatry*, 149(8): 999–1010.

Power, T. G., & Chapieski, M. L. (1986). Childrearing and impulse control in toddlers: A naturalistic investigation. *Developmental Psychology*, 22(2): 271–275.

Powers, M. B., Sigmarsson, S. R., & Emmelkamp, P. M. G. (2008). A meta-analytic review of psychological treatments for social anxiety disorder. *International Journal of Cognitive Therapy*, 1(2): 94–113.

Prochaska, J. O., DiClemente, C. C., & Norcross, J. C. (1992). In search of how people change: Applications to addictive behaviors. *American Psychologist*, 47(9): 1102–1114.

Quiggle, N. L., Garber, J., Panak, W. F., & Dodge, K. A. (1992). Social information processing in aggressive and depressed children. *Child Development*, 63(6): 1305–1320.

Rachman, S. (1977). The conditioning theory of fear acquisition: A critical examination. *Behaviour Research and Therapy*, 15: 375–387.

Rachman, S. (1991). Neoconditioning and the classical theory of fear acquisition. *Clinical Psychology Review*, 17: 47–67.

Rachman, S., Gruter-Andrew, J., & Shafran, R. (2000). Post-event processing in social anxiety. *Behaviour Research and Therapy*, 38(6): 611–617.

Radtke, K. M., Ruf, M., Gunter, H. M., Dohrmann, K., Schauer, M., Meyer, A., & Elbert, T. (2011). Transgenerational impact of intimate partner violence on methylation in the promoter of the glucocorticoid receptor. *Translational Psychiatry*, 1: e21.

Rapee, R., Mattick, R., & Murrell, E. (1986). Cognitive mediation in the affective component of spontaneous panic attacks. *Journal of Behavior Therapy and Experimental Psychiatry*, 17(4): 245–253.

Rapee, R. M., Brown, T. A., Antony, M. M., & Barlow, D. H. (1992). Response to hyperventilation and inhalation of 5.5% carbon dioxide-enriched air across the DSM-III—R anxiety disorders. *Journal of Abnormal Psychology*, 101(3): 538–552.

Rapee, R. M., & Heimberg, R. G. (1997). A cognitive-behavioral model of anxiety in social phobia. *Behaviour Research and Therapy*, 35(8): 741–756.

Rapee, R. M., Kennedy, S., Ingram, M., Edwards, S., & Sweeney, L. (2005). Prevention and early intervention of anxiety disorders in inhibited preschool children. *Journal of Consulting & Clinical Psychology*, 73(3): 488–497.

Rapee, R. M., MacLeod, C., Carpenter, L., Gaston, J. E., Frei, J., Peters, L., & Baillie, A. J. (2013). Integrating cognitive bias modification into a standard cognitive behavioural treatment package for social phobia: A randomized controlled trial. *Behaviour Research and Therapy*, 51(4–5): 207–215.

Rapoport, J. L., Giedd, J. N., & Gogtay, N. (2012). Neurodevelopmental model of schizophrenia: Update 2012. *Molecular Psychiatry*, 17(12): 1228–1238.

Read, J., Van Os, J., Morrison, A. P., & Ross, C. A. (2005). Childhood trauma, psychosis and schizophrenia: A literature review with theoretical and clinical implications. *Acta Psychiatrica Scandinavica*, 112(5): 330–350.

Rector, N. A., Beck, A. T., & Stolar, N. (2005). The negative symptoms of schizophrenia: A cognitive perspective. *Canadian Journal of Psychiatry*, 50(5): 247–257.

Regier, D. A., Narrow, W. E., Clarke, D. E., Kraemer, H. C., Kuramoto, S. J., Kuhl, E. A., & Kupfer, D. J. (2013). DSM-5 field trials in the United States and Canada, part II: Test-retest reliability of selected categorical diagnoses. *American Journal of Psychiatry*, 170(1): 59–70.

Reichborn-Kjennerud, T., Ystrom, E., Neale, M. C., Aggen, S. H., Mazzeo, S. E., Knudsen, G. P., et al. (2013). Structure of genetic and environmental risk factors for symptoms of DSM-IV borderline personality disorder. *JAMA Psychiatry*, 70(11): 1206–1214.

Reid, W. H., & Gacono, C. (2000). Treatment of antisocial personality, psychopathy, and other characterologic antisocial syndromes. *Behavioral Sciences and the Law*, 18(5): 647–662.

Reiman, E. M., Raichle, M. E., Robins, E., Butler, F. K., Herscovitch, P., Fox, P., & Perlmutter, J. (1986). The application of positron emission tomography to the study of panic disorder. *American Journal of Psychiatry*, 143(4): 469–477.

Reynolds, S., Wilson, C., Austin, J., & Hooper, L. (2012). Effects of psychotherapy for anxiety in children and adolescents: A meta-analytic review. *Clinical Psychology Review*, 32(4): 251–262.

Rice, F. (2010). Genetics of childhood and adolescent depression: Insights into etiological heterogeneity and challenges for future genomic research. *Genome Medicine*, 2(9): 68.

Richards, D. (2011). Prevalence and clinical course of depression: A review. *Clinical Psychology Review*, 31(7): 1117–1125.

Ripke, S., Neale, B. M., Corvin, A., Walters, J. T. R., Farh, K. H., Holmans, P. A., et al. (2014). Biological insights from 108 schizophrenia-associated genetic loci. *Nature*, 511(7510): 421–427.

Roberts, M. W., McMahon, R. J., Forehand, R., & Humphreys, L. (1978). The effect of parental instruction-giving on child compliance. *Behavior Therapy*, 9(5): 793–798.

Robinson, R., & Cartwright-Hatton, S. (2008). Maternal disciplinary style with preschool children: Associations with children's and mothers' trait anxiety. *Behavioural and Cognitive Psychotherapy*, 36(1): 49–59.

Robinson, T. E., & Berridge, K. C. (1993). The neural basis of drug craving: An incentive-sensitization theory of addiction. *Brain Research Reviews*, 18(3): 247–291.

Rocca, P., Fonzo, V., Scotta, M., Zanalda, E., & Ravizza, L. (1997). Paroxetine efficacy in the treatment of generalized anxiety disorder. *Acta Psychiatrica Scandinavica*, 95(5): 444–450.

Roth, D., Antony, M. M., & Swinson, R. P. (2001). Interpretations for anxiety symptoms in social phobia. *Behaviour Research and Therapy*, 39(2): 129–138.

Rothbaum, F., & Weisz, J. R. (1994). Parental caregiving and child externalizing behavior in nonclinical samples: A meta-analysis. *Psychological Bulletin*, 116(1): 55–74.

Roy-Byrne, P. P., Craske, M. G., & Stein, M. B. (2006). Panic disorder. *The Lancet*, 368(9540): 1023–1032.

Ruscio, A. M., & Borkovec, T. D. (2004). Experience and appraisal of worry among high worriers with and without generalized anxiety disorder. *Behaviour Research and Therapy*, 42(12): 1469–1482.

Ruscio, A. M., Chiu, W. T., Roy-Byrne, P., Stang, P. E., Stein, D. J., Wittchen, H. U., & Kessler, R. C. (2007). Broadening the definition of generalized anxiety disorder: Effects on prevalence and associations with other disorders in the National Comorbidity Survey Replication. *Journal of Anxiety Disorders*, 21(5): 662–676.

Saha, S., Chant, D., Welham, J., & McGrath, J. (2005). A systematic review of the prevalence of schizophrenia. *PLoS Medicine*, 2(5): 0413–0433.

Salkovskis, P. M., Clark, D. M., & Gelder, M. G. (1996). Cognition–behaviour links in the persistence of panic. *Behaviour Research and Therapy*, 34(5–6): 453–458.

Salkovskis, P. M., Clark, D. M., Hackmann, A., Wells, A., & Gelder, M. G. (1999). An experimental investigation of the role of safety-seeking behaviours in the maintenance of panic disorder with agoraphobia. *Behaviour Research and Therapy*, 37: 559–574.

Sanders, A. R., Duan, J., Levinson, D. F., Shi, J., He, D., Hou, C., et al. (2008). No significant association of 14 candidate genes with schizophrenia in a large European ancestry sample: Implications for psychiatric genetics. *American Journal of Psychiatry*, 165(4): 497–506.

Sanders, M. R. (2012). Development, evaluation, and multinational dissemination of the Triple P-Positive Parenting Program. *Annual Review of Clinical Psychology*, 8(1): 345–379.

Saulsman, L. M., & Page, A. C. (2004). The five-factor model and personality disorder empirical literature: A meta-analytic review. *Clinical Psychology Review*, 23(8): 1055–1085.

Scher, C. D., Ingram, R. E., & Segal, Z. V. (2005). Cognitive reactivity and vulnerability: Empirical evaluation of construct activation and cognitive diatheses in unipolar depression. *Clinical Psychology Review*, 25(4): 487–510.

Schienle, A., Hettema, J. M., Cáceda, R., & Nemeroff, C. B. (2011). Neurobiology and genetics of generalized anxiety disorder. *Psychiatric Annals*, 41(2): 111–123.

Schneider, K. (1923). *Die Psychopathischen Persönlichkeiten*. Berlin: Springer.

Schultz, W. (2013). Updating dopamine reward signals. *Current Opinion in Neurobiology*, 23(2): 229–238.

Schwartz, M. W., Woods, S. C., Porte Jr, D., Seeley, R. J., & Baskin, D. G. (2000). Central nervous system control of food intake. *Nature*, 404(6778): 661–671.

Scott, J., Stanton, B., Garland, A., & Ferrier, I. N. (2000). Cognitive vulnerability in patients with bipolar disorder. *Psychological Medicine*, 30(2): 467–472.

See, J., MacLeod, C., & Bridle, R. (2009). The reduction of anxiety vulnerability through the modification of attentional bias: A real-world study using a home-based cognitive bias modification procedure. *Journal of Abnormal Psychology*, 118(1): 65–75.

Segal, Z. V., Gemar, M., & Williams, S. (1999). Differential cognitive response to a mood challenge following successful cognitive therapy or pharmacotherapy for unipolar depression. *Journal of Abnormal Psychology*, 108(1): 3–10.

Seligman, M. E. (1971). Phobias and preparedness. *Behavior Therapy*, 2: 307–320.

Seligman, M. E. (1975). *Helplessness*. New York: Freeman.

Seligman, M. E., Maier, S. F., & Geer, J. H. (1968). Alleviation of learned helplessness in the dog. *Journal of Abnormal Psychology*, 73: 256–262.

Selten, J. P., & Cantor-Graae, E. (2005). Social defeat: Risk factor for schizophrenia? *British Journal of Psychiatry*, 187(August): 101–102.

Sempértegui, G. A., Karreman, A., Arntz, A., & Bekker, M. H. J. (2013). Schema therapy for borderline personality disorder: A comprehensive review of its empirical foundations, effectiveness and implementation possibilities. *Clinical Psychology Review*, 33(3): 426–447.

Seto, M. C., & Barbaree, H. E. (1999). Psychopathy, treatment behavior, and sex offender recidivism. *Journal of Interpersonal Violence*, 14(12): 1235–1248.

Shafran, R., Lee, M., Payne, E., & Fairburn, C. G. (2007). An experimental analysis of body checking. *Behaviour Research and Therapy*, 45(1): 113–121.

Shenton, M. E., Dickey, C. C., Frumin, M., & McCarley, R. W. (2001). A review of MRI findings in schizophrenia. *Schizophrenia Research*, 49(1–2): 1–52.

Silverman, W. K., & Nelles, W. B. (1989). An examination of the stability of mothers' ratings of child fearfulness. *Journal of Anxiety Disorders*, 3: 1–5.

Simmons, J. P., Nelson, L. D., & Simonsohn, U. (2011). False-positive psychology: Undisclosed flexibility in data collection and analysis allows presenting anything as significant. *Psychological Science*, 22(11): 1359–1366.

Simon, N. W., Mendez, I. A., & Setlow, B. (2007). Cocaine exposure causes long-term increases in impulsive choice. *Behavioral Neuroscience*, 121(3): 543–549.

Skapinakis, P., Lewis, G., Davies, S., Brugha, T., Prince, M., & Singleton, N. (2011). Panic disorder and subthreshold panic in the UK general population: Epidemiology, comorbidity and functional limitation. *European Psychiatry: The Journal of the Association of European Psychiatrists*, 26(6): 354–362.

Skodol, A. E. (2012) Personality disorders in DSM-5. *Annual Review of Clinical Psychology*, 8: 317–344.

Skog, O. J., & Melberg, H. O. (2006). Becker's rational addiction theory: An empirical test with price elasticities for distilled spirits in Denmark 1911–31. *Addiction*, 101(10): 1444–1450.

Slutske, W. S., Heath, A. C., Dinwiddie, S. H., & Madden, P. A. F. (1997). Modeling genetic and environmental influences in the etiology of conduct disorder: A study of 2,682 adult twin pairs. *Journal of Abnormal Psychology*, 106(2): 266–279.

Smedslund, G., Berg, R. C., Hammerstrøm, K. T., Steiro, A., Leiknes, K. A., Dahl, H. M., & Karlsen, K. (2011). Motivational interviewing for substance abuse. *Cochrane Database of Systematic Reviews*, 5: CD008063.

Smith, M. L., Glass, G. V., & Miller, T. I. (1980). *The Benefits of Psychotherapy*. Baltimore: John Hopkins University Press.

Staal, W. G., Hulshoff, H. E., Schnack, H. G., Hoogendoorn, M. L. C., Jellema, K., & Kahn, R. S. (2000). Structural brain abnormalities in patients with schizophrenia and their healthy siblings. *American Journal of Psychiatry*, 157(3): 416–421.

Stacy, A. W., & Wiers, R. W. (2010). Implicit cognition and addiction: A tool for explaining paradoxical behavior. *Annual Review of Clinical Psychology*, 6: 551–575.

Stahl, S. M., & Buckley, P. F. (2007). Negative symptoms of schizophrenia: A problem that will not go away. *Acta Psychiatrica Scandinavica*, 115(1): 4–11.

Stanley, B., & Siever, L. J. (2010). The interpersonal dimension of borderline personality disorder: Toward a neuropeptide model. *American Journal of Psychiatry*, 167(1): 24–39.

Stead, L. F., Perera, R., Bullen, C., Mant, D., Hartmann-Boyce, J., Cahill, K., & Lancaster, T. (2012). Nicotine replacement therapy for smoking cessation. *Cochrane Database of Systematic Reviews*, 11: CD000146.

Steele, H., & Siever, L. (2010). An attachment perspective on borderline personality disorder: Advances in gene–environment considerations. *Current Psychiatry Reports*, 12(1): 61–67.

Stephan, K. E., Friston, K. J., & Frith, C. D. (2009). Dysconnection in schizophrenia: From abnormal synaptic plasticity to failures of self-monitoring. *Schizophrenia Bulletin*, 35(3): 509–527.

Stewart, J., de Wit, H., & Eikelboom, R. (1984). Role of unconditioned and conditioned drug effects in the self-administration of opiates and stimulants. *Psychological Review*, 91(2): 251–268.

Stice, E., Shaw, H., & Marti, C. N. (2007) A meta-analytic review of eating disorder prevention programs: Encouraging findings. *Annual Review of Clinical Psychology*, 3: 207–231.

Stirling, J. D., Hellewell, J. S. E., & Ndlovu, D. (2001). Self-monitoring dysfunction and the positive symptoms of schizophrenia. *Psychopathology*, 34(4): 198–202.

Stoffers, J. M., Völlm, B. A., Rücker, G., Timmer, A., Huband, N., & Lieb, K. (2012). Psychological therapies for people with borderline personality disorder. *Cochrane Database of Systematic Reviews*, 8: CD005652.

Striegel-Moore, R. H., & Franko, D. L. (2008) Should binge eating disorder be included in the DSM-V? A critical review of the state of the evidence. *Annual Review of Clinical Psychology*, 4: 305–324.

Szentagotai, A., & David, D. (2010). The efficacy of cognitive-behavioral therapy in bipolar disorder: A quantitative meta-analysis. *Journal of Clinical Psychiatry*, 71(1): 66–72.

Taylor, M., Cavanagh, J., Hodgson, R., & Tiihonen, J. (2012). Examining the effectiveness of antipsychotic medication in first-episode psychosis. *Journal of Psychopharmacology*, 26(supplement 5): 27–32.

Teachman, B. A., & Woody, S. R. (2003). Automatic processing in spider phobia: Implicit fear associations over the course of treatment. *Journal of Abnormal Psychology*, 112(1): 100–109.

The NHS Information Centre, Lifestyle Statistics (2013). *Statistics on Alcohol: England, 2013*. London: The Health and Social Care Information Centre.

Tiffany, S. T. (1990). A cognitive model of drug urges and drug-use behavior: Role of automatic and nonautomatic processes. *Psychological Review*, 97(2): 147–168.

Tolin, D. F. (2010). Is cognitive-behavioral therapy more effective than other therapies? A meta-analytic review. *Clinical Psychology Review*, 30(6): 710–720.

Touyz, S., Le Grange, D., Lacey, H., Hay, P., Smith, R., Maguire, S., et al. (2013). Treating severe and enduring anorexia nervosa: A randomized controlled trial. *Psychological Medicine*, 43(12): 2501–2511.

Trace, S. E., Baker, J. H., Peñas-Lledó, E., & Bulik, C. M. (2013) The genetics of eating disorders. *Annual Review of Clinical Psychology*, 9: 589–620.

Treasure, J., Claudino, A. M., & Zucker, N. (2010). Eating disorders. *The Lancet*, 375(9714): 583–593.

Trull, T. J., & Durrett, C. A. (2005) Categorical and dimensional models of personality disorder. *Annual Review of Clinical Psychology*, 1: 355–380.

Turkington, D., Sensky, T., Scott, J., Barnes, T. R., Nur, U., Siddle, R., et al. (2008). A randomized controlled trial of cognitive-behavior therapy for persistent symptoms in schizophrenia: A five-year follow-up. *Schizophrenia Research*, 98(1–3): 1–7.

Turner, S. M., Beidel, D. C., & Costello, A. (1987). Psychopathology in the offspring of anxiety disorders patients. *Journal of Consulting and Clinical Psychology*, 55(2): 229–235.

Tyrer, P. (2013). The classification of personality disorders in ICD-11: Implications for forensic psychiatry. *Criminal Behaviour and Mental Health*, 23(1): 1–5.

Tyrer, P., & Mackay, A. (1986). Schizophrenia: No longer a functional psychosis. *Trends in Neurosciences*, 9(11–12): 537–538.

Van Ameringen, M., Mancini, C., & Oakman, J. M. (1998). The relationship of behavioral inhibition and shyness to anxiety disorder. *Journal of Nervous and Mental Disease*, 186(7): 425–431.

Van der Bruggen, C. O., Stams, G. J. J. M., & Bögels, S. M. (2008). Research review: The relation between child and parent anxiety and parental control: A meta-analytic review. *Journal of Child Psychology and Psychiatry, and Allied Disciplines*, 49(12): 1257–1269.

Van Houtem, C. M. H. H., Laine, M. L., Boomsma, D. I., Ligthart, L., van Wijk, A. J., & De Jongh, A. (2013). A review and meta-analysis of the heritability of specific phobia subtypes and corresponding fears. *Journal of Anxiety Disorders*, 27(4): 379–388.

Van Os, J., & Kapur, S. (2009). Schizophrenia. *The Lancet*, 374(9690): 635–645.

Varese, F., Barkus, E., & Bentall, R. P. (2012). Dissociation mediates the relationship between childhood trauma and hallucination-proneness. *Psychological Medicine*, 42(5): 1025–1036.

Varese, F., Smeets, F., Drukker, M., Lieverse, R., Lataster, T., Viechtbauer, W., et al. (2012). Childhood adversities increase the risk of psychosis: A meta-analysis of patient-control, prospective- and cross-sectional cohort studies. *Schizophrenia Bulletin*, 38(4): 661–671.

Varese, F., Udachina, A., Myin-Germeys, I., Oorschot, M., & Bentall, R. P. (2011). The relationship between dissociation and auditory verbal hallucinations in the flow of daily life of patients with psychosis. *Psychosis: Psychological, Social and Integrative Approaches*, 3(1): 14–28.

Viding, E., Blair, R. J. R., Moffitt, T. E., & Plomin, R. (2005). Evidence for substantial genetic risk for psychopathy in 7-year-olds. *Journal of Child Psychology and Psychiatry, and Allied Disciplines*, 46(6): 592–597.

Vocks, S., Tuschen-Caffier, B., Pietrowsky, R., Rustenbach, S. J., Kersting, A., & Herpertz, S. (2010). Meta-analysis of the effectiveness of psychological and pharmacological treatments for binge eating disorder. *International Journal of Eating Disorders*, 43(3): 205–217.

Volkow, N. D., Fowler, J. S., Wang, G. J., & Swanson, J. M. (2004). Dopamine in drug abuse and addiction: Results from imaging studies and treatment implications. *Molecular Psychiatry*, 9(6): 557–569.

Wakefield, J. C., & First, M. B. (2012). Validity of the bereavement exclusion to major depression: Does the empirical evidence support the proposal to eliminate the exclusion in DSM-5? *World Psychiatry*, 11(1): 3–10.

Walkup, J. T., Albano, A. M., Piacentini, J., Birmaher, B., Compton, S. N., Sherrill, J. T., et al. (2008). Cognitive behavioral therapy, sertraline, or a combination in childhood anxiety. *New England Journal of Medicine*, 359(26): 2753–2766.

Warren, S. L., Huston, L., Egeland, B., & Sroufe, L. A. (1997). Child and adolescent anxiety disorders and early attachment. *Journal of the American Academy of Child and Adolescent Psychiatry*, 36(5): 637–644.

Watson, B., & Lingford-Hughes, A. (2007). Pharmacological treatment of addiction. *Psychiatry*, 6(7): 309–312.

Watson, J.B., & Rayner, R. (1920). Conditioned emotional reactions. *Journal of Experimental Psychology*, 3: 1–14.

Webster-Stratton, C. (1985). Mother perceptions and mother–child interactions: Comparison of a clinic-referred and a nonclinic group. *Journal of Clinical Child Psychology*, 14(4): 334–339.

Webster-Stratton, C., Hollinsworth, T., & Kolpacoff, M. (1989). The long term effectiveness and clinical significance of three cost-effective training programs for families with conduct-problem children. *Journal of Clinical Child Psychology*, 57(4): 550–553.

Weinberger, D. R., Torrey, E. F., Neophytides, A. N., & Wyatt, R. J. (1979). Lateral cerebral ventricular enlargement in chronic schizophrenia. *Archives of General Psychiatry*, 36(7): 735–739.

Weiner, I., & Arad, M. (2009). Using the pharmacology of latent inhibition to model domains of pathology in schizophrenia and their treatment. *Behavioural Brain Research*, 204(2): 369–386.

Wells, A. (1995). Meta-cognition and worry: A cognitive model of generalized anxiety disorder. *Behavioural and Cognitive Psychotherapy*, 23(3): 301–320.

Wells, A., Clark, D. M., Salkovskis, P., Ludgate, J., Hackmann, A., & Gelder, M. (1995). Social phobia: The role of in-situation safety behaviors in maintaining anxiety and negative beliefs. *Behavior Therapy*, 26(1): 153–161.

Wells, A., & King, P. (2006). Metacognitive therapy for generalized anxiety disorder: An open trial. *Journal of Behavior Therapy and Experimental Psychiatry*, 37(3): 206–212.

Wells, A., & Papageorgiou, C. (2001). Brief cognitive therapy for social phobia: A case series. *Behaviour Research and Therapy*, 39(6): 713–720.

Wermter, A.-K., Laucht, M., Schimmelmann, B., Banaschweski, T., Sonuga-Barke, E., Rietschel, M., & Becker, K. (2010). From nature versus nurture, via nature and nurture, to gene × environment interaction in mental disorders. *European Child & Adolescent Psychiatry*, 19(3): 199–210.

Wertheim, E. H., Koerner, J., & Paxton, S. J. (2001). Longitudinal predictors of restrictive eating and bulimic tendencies in three different age groups of adolescent girls. *Journal of Youth and Adolescence*, 30(1): 69–81.

Wicks, S., Hjern, A., Gunnell, D., Lewis, G., & Dalman, C. (2005). Social adversity in childhood and the risk of developing psychosis: A national cohort study. *American Journal of Psychiatry*, 162(9): 1652–1657.

Wiers, R. W., Ames, S. L., Hofmann, W., Krank, M., & Stacy, A. W. (2010). Impulsivity, impulsive and reflective processes and the development of alcohol use and misuse in adolescents and young adults. *Frontiers in Psychology*, 1: art. 144.

Wiers, R. W., Eberl, C., Rinck, M., Becker, E. S., & Lindenmeyer, J. (2011). Retraining automatic action tendencies changes alcoholic patients' approach bias for alcohol and improves treatment outcome. *Psychological Science*, 22(4): 490–497.

Wikler, A. (1948). Recent progress in research on the neurophysiologic basis of morphine addiction. *American Journal of Psychiatry*, 105(5): 329–338.

Williams, J. M. G., Mathews, A., & MacLeod, C. (1996). The emotional stroop task and psychopathology. *Psychological Bulletin*, 120: 3–24.

Williamson, S., Harpur, T. J., & Hare, R. D. (1991). Abnormal processing of affective words by psychopaths. *Psychophysiology*, 28(3): 260–273.

Wilson, E. J., MacLeod, C., Mathews, A., & Rutherford, E. M. (2006). The causal role of interpretive bias in anxiety reactivity. *Journal of Abnormal Psychology*, 115(1): 103–111.

Wilson, P., Rush, R., Hussey, S., Puckering, C., Sim, F., Allely, C., et al. (2012). How evidence-based is an 'evidence-based parenting program'? A PRISMA systematic review and meta-analysis of Triple P. *BMC Medicine*, 10(1): 130.

Winters, K. C., & Neale, J. M. (1985). Mania and low self-esteem. *Journal of Abnormal Psychology*, 94(3): 282–290.

Wolpe, J., & Lang, P. J. (1974, reprinted 2008). A fear survey schedule for use in behavior therapy. In E. J. Thomas (ed.), *Behavior Modification Procedure: A Sourcebook*. New Brunswick, NJ, pp. 228–232.

Wood, J., McLeod, B. D., Sigman, M., Hwang, W.-C., & Chu, B. C. (2003). Parenting and childhood anxiety: Theory, empirical findings and future directions. *Journal of Child Psychology & Psychiatry & Allied Disciplines*, 44(1): 134–151.

World Health Organisation (1992). *The ICD-10 Classification of Mental and Behavioural Disorders: Diagnostic Criteria for Research*. Geneva: World Health Organisation.

Wykes, T., Hayward, P., Thomas, N., Green, N., Surguladze, S., Fannon, D., & Landau, S. (2005). What are the effects of group cognitive behaviour therapy for voices? A randomised control trial. *Schizophrenia Research*, 77(2–3): 201–210.

Wykes, T., Huddy, V., Cellard, C., McGurk, S. R., & Czobor, P. (2011). A meta-analysis of cognitive remediation for schizophrenia: Methodology and effect sizes. *American Journal of Psychiatry*, 168(5): 472–485.

Wykes, T., Steel, C., Everitt, B., & Tarrier, N. (2008). Cognitive behavior therapy for schizophrenia: Effect sizes, clinical models, and methodological rigor. *Schizophrenia Bulletin*, 34(3): 523–537.

Yang, Y., & Raine, A. (2009). Prefrontal structural and functional brain imaging findings in antisocial, violent, and psychopathic individuals: A meta-analysis. *Psychiatry Research: Neuroimaging*, 174(2): 81–88.

Young, J., Klosko, S., & Weishaar, M. (2003). *Schema Therapy: A Practitioner's Guide*. New York: Guilford.

Yu, R., Geddes, J. R., & Fazel, S. (2012). Personality disorders, violence, and antisocial behavior: A systematic review and meta-regression analysis. *Journal of Personality Disorders*, 26(5): 775–792.

Yule, W., Udwin, O., & Murdoch, K. (1990). The 'Jupiter' sinking: Effects in children's fears, depression and anxiety. *Journal of Child Psychology and Psychiatry*, 31(7): 1051–1061.

Ziauddeen, H., Farooqi, I. S., & Fletcher, P. C. (2012). Obesity and the brain: How convincing is the addiction model? *Nature Reviews Neuroscience*, 13(4): 279–286.

Zimmermann, G., Favrod, J., Trieu, V. H., & Pomini, V. (2005). The effect of cognitive behavioral treatment on the positive symptoms of schizophrenia spectrum disorders: A meta-analysis. *Schizophrenia Research*, 77(1): 1–9.

Zipfel, S., Wild, B., Grob, G., Friederich, H. C., Teufel, M., Schellberg, D., et al., (2014). Focal psychodynamic therapy, cognitive behaviour therapy, and optimised treatment as usual in outpatients with anorexia nervosa (ANTOP study): Randomised controlled trial. *The Lancet*, 383(9912): 127–137.

Zoccola, P. M., Dickerson, S. S., & Yim, I. S. (2011). Trait and state perseverative cognition and the cortisol awakening response. *Psychoneuroendocrinology*, 36(4): 592–595.

Index